STAYING ALIVE

··

STAYING ALIVE

Critical Perspectives on Health, Illness, and Health Care

··

Edited by
Dennis Raphael, Toba Bryant,
and Marcia Rioux

Foreword by
Gary Teeple

Canadian Scholars' Press Inc
Toronto

Staying Alive: Critical Perspectives on Health, Illness, and Health Care
Edited by Dennis Raphael, Toba Bryant, and Marcia Rioux

First published in 2006 by
Canadian Scholars' Press Inc.
180 Bloor Street West, Suite 801
Toronto, Ontario
M5S 2V6

www.cspi.org

Canadian Scholars' Press gratefully acknowledges financial support for our publishing activities from the Government of Canada through the Book Publishing Industry Development Program (BPIDP).

Library and Archives Canada Cataloguing in Publication

Staying alive : critical perspectives on health, illness and health care / edited by Dennis Raphael, Toba Bryant, and Marcia Rioux ; foreword by Gary Teeple.

Includes bibliographical references and index.

ISBN 978-1-55130-296-6

1. Social medicine--Canada. 2. Medical care--Canada. I. Raphael, Dennis II. Bryant, Toba III. Rioux, Marcia H.

RA418.3.C3S68 2006   302.1'042'0971   C2006-900054-9

Cover design by George Kirkpatrick
Cover photo: "Looking from the Inside" from http://www.sxc.hu. Copyright © Christopher Bruno, 2005. Reprinted by permission of Stock.Xchng/Christopher Bruno.
Page design and layout by Brad Horning

09 10   5 4 3

Printed and bound in Canada by Marquis Book Printing Inc.

Canadä

TABLE OF CONTENTS

COPYRIGHT ACKNOWLEDGEMENTS

Part I opener: "Old and Young" from http://www.sxc.hu. Copyright © David Peter Hansen, 2005. Reprinted by permission of stock.xchng/David Peter Hansen.

Part II opener: "MARA" from http://www.sxc.hu. Copyright © Aldo Peralta, 2005. Reprinted by permission of stock.xchng/Aldo Peralta.

Part III opener: "Pediatrics" from http://www.sxc.hu. Copyright © Tomasz Kobosz, 2005. Reprinted by permission of stock.xchng/ Tomasz Kobosz.

Part IV opener: "Depressed" from http://www.sxc.hu. Copyright © David Peter Hansen, 2005. Reprinted by permission of stock.xchng/David Peter Hansen.

Fig. 1.4: "Income Distribution and Life Expectancy" from *British Medical Journal* 304(6820). Copyright © *British Medical Journal*, 1992. Reprinted by permission of *British Medical Journal*.

Fig. 1.5: "Working-Aged Male Mortality by Proportion of Income Belonging to the Less Well-Off Half of Households, US States (1990) and Canadian Provinces (1991)" from "Working-Aged Male (25-64) Mortality by Median Share US States and Canadian Provinces" in *British Medical Journal* 320 (7239). Copyright © *British Medical Journal*, 2000. Reprinted by permission of *British Medical Journal*.

Fig. 1.6: "Mortality, Income, Distribution, US Cities" from "Income Inequality and Mortality in Metropolitan Areas of the United States" in *American Journal of Public Health* 88: 1074–1080. Copyright ©, 1998. Reprinted by permission of *American Journal of Public Health*.

Fig. 2.1: "Navarro's Depiction of the Health Effects of the Labour Process in Capitalism" from *Crisis, Health, and Medicine: A Social Critique*. Copyright © Tavistock Publications, 1986. Reprinted by permission of Tavistock Publications.

Table 3.1: Gottschalk and Smeeding, "Ratio of the Top Ten 10 Percent of Income Earners to the Bottom 10 Percent and the Gini Index of Inequality," adapted from "Empirical Evidence of Income Inequality in Industrialized Countries" in *The Handbook of Income Distribution*, vol. 1. Copyright © Elsevier, 2000. Reprinted by permission of Elsevier.

Table 4.1: "The Recognition of the Right to Health Internationally," adapted from "The International Human Right to Health: What Does This Mean for Our Nation and World?" from *Indiana Law Review*, vol. 34. Copyright © Indiana Law Review, 2001. Reprinted by permission of *Indiana Law Review*.

Fig. 4.1: "Linkages Between Health and Human Rights" from Health and Human Rights Publication Series, no. 1. Copyright © World Health Organization, July 2002. Reprinted by permission of World Health Organization.

Box 4.3: "Health Good Practice ® Right to Health Good Practice," from "Human Rights Situations and Reports of Special Rapporteurs and Representatives, 58th Session, 10 October" from *UN Special Rapporteur's Report to the United Nations General Assembly*.

Table 5.1: "The Union Wage Advantage in 2002" from *In Solidarity: The Union Advantage*. Copyright © Canadian Labour Congress; Statistics Canada, Labour Force Survey, 2003. Reprinted by permission of Canadian Labour Congress/Statistics Canada.

Table 5.2: Andrew Jackson, "25 Key Indicators of Social Development" from *Canada Beats USA—But Loses Gold to Sweden*. Copyright © Canadian Council on Social Development, 2002. Reprinted by permission of Canadian Council on Social Development.

Fig. 5.1: "Social Determinants of Health in Broader Perspective" from *Policies and Strategies To Promote Social Equity in Health*. Copyright © Insititute for Futures Studies, 1991. Reprinted by permission of Insititute for Futures Studies.

Fig. 5.2: "Child Poverty in Rich Nations" from *A League Table of Child Poverty in Rich Nations*. Copyright © Innocenti Research Centre, 2000. Reprinted by permission of Innocenti Research Centre.

Table 7.1: "Age-Adjusted Prevalence Conditions by Immigrant Status, Canadian-born and Immigrant, Canada, 1994-1995" from *National Population Survey*, Cat. No. 82F0001XCB. Copyright © Statistics Canada, 1994-95. Reprinted by permission of Statistics Canada.

Fig. 7.1: "Sexual Assaults and Thefts of Personal Property More Likely to Be Perpetrated against Women" from *Women in Canada, Canadian Centre for Justice Statistics Profile Series, Statistics Canada*, Cat. No. 85F0033MIE. Copyright © Statistics Canada, 2001. Reprinted by permission of Statistics Canada.

Box 7.1: "Canadian Women, Poverty, and the Minimum Wage." Copyright © The UN Platform for Action Committee, 2004. Reprinted by permission of The UN Platform for Action Committee.

Box 7.2: Geoff McMaster "Poverty Hurts Women Most—Activist" from *Express News*. April 26, 2002. Copyright © Geoff McMaster/*Express News*, 2002. Reprinted by permission of *Express News*.

Box 7.3: "Degree of Women's Homelessness Underestimated, Study Finds," from *The Canadian Women's Health Network Magazine*, vol. 6, no. 2/3; adapted from *Common Occurrence: The Impact of Homelessness on Women's Health (Sistering 2002)*. Copyright © The Canadian Women's Health Network <www.cwhn.ca>, 2003. Reprinted by permission of The Canadian Women's Health Network/*Sistering*.

Box 7.4: "Health Canada and Gender Analysis" from *Healthy Living: Factsheets* <http://www. hc-sc.gc.ca/english/women/facts_issues/facts_gender.htm>. Copyright © Health Canada—Bureau of Women's Health and Gender Analysis, 2004. Reprinted by permission of Health Canada—Bureau of Women's Health and Gender Analysis.

Box 7.5: Carmelina Prete, "Encouraging Signs for Aboriginal People Living off Reserves" from *The Hamilton Spectator*, September 25, 2003. Copyright © *The Hamilton Spectator*, 2003. Reprinted by permission of *The Hamilton Spectator*.

Table 8.1: "Social Spending as a Percentage of Gross Domestic Product, 1998" from *Society at a Glance: OECD Social Indicators*, vol. I 2003, no. 76 22. Copyright © Organisation for Economic Co-operation and Development, 2003. Reprinted by permission of Organisation for Economic Co-operation and Development.

Table 8.2: Mark Robert Rank, "Rates of Poverty Using Relative and Absolute Rates for Various Groups in Canada, the U.S., the U.K., and Sweden during the 1990s" from *One Nation,*

FOREWORD

The study of health and health care has a long history in the physical and social sciences. The last few decades, however, have brought dramatic changes to health-related issues that have culminated in a new context for old questions, a context that demands fresh insights and new awareness. The very meaning of health, for instance, can no longer be defined as simply "the absence of disease," given what we now know about the complexity of social relations and the human being. How health is defined in practice and how illness is treated, moreover, can now be seen as issues decided by numerous self-seeking social and economic interests. And public health policy can now be understood as the outcome of conflict between parties whose concerns about health are secondary to other matters.

These are a few of the important issues addressed in this book, *Staying Alive: Critical Perspectives on Health, Illness, and Health Care*. By using broad methodological approaches, such as social epidemiology, critical sociology, and, more particularly, political economy and a human rights analysis, the authors in this volume achieve incisive and novel insights in the study of health and health care, especially in Canada. They are insights, the editors argue, that are intended to assist in bringing about change to the health system.

Given the scientific and technological revolutions in medical research and health practice in the past half century, a political economy approach lends itself very well to grasping the multidimensional nature of the current health system or, perhaps better, the health industry. The investment of capital, public and private, now plays a central role in all aspects of medicine. Whether it is the state or the corporate sector that finances hospitals, medical and nursing schools, health-related salaries and wages, insurance, pharmaceutical drugs, or medical research and equipment, it is clear that there are many powerful interests involved. And this is not to mention the professional associations and unions that represent many of the categories of people employed in the health system. In short, there are numerous and complex conflicting forces that are very difficult to grasp as a dynamic but contradictory whole without the use of an approach such as political economy.

Only by examining these competing constituents of a system concerned with health, illness, and its remedies can we fathom how they are defined, how and what treatment is authorized, and who decides these matters, among other questions. Why and how change takes place in the health industry, furthermore, can be fully

1

understood only by studying the interests involved; the conflicting demands for higher profits, wages and salaries, and state expenditures; for continued monopolies and patents over knowledge, technology, and procedures; and for the mere preservation of the status quo. These are all factors whose interaction sets the boundaries of the health system. At the same time, these conflicts obscure the real sources of illness and overshadow the interests of the patient.

In more general terms, a political economy approach allows us to comprehend the present structure of the health industry as both a product and bulwark of contemporary capitalism. Because the health system possesses all the fundamental ideological relations of mainstream society, it facilitates the reproduction of the status quo. Sexism, racism, class and religious notions, commodified solutions, and other biases are all deeply embedded in the definition of health and illness and their associated practices. It also reproduces key forms of societal power relations, namely, interactions that are hierarchical, authoritarian, patriarchal, unequal, unidirectional, and professionally and bureaucratically indifferent—relations that assume certain monopolies over knowledge, treatment, and technology. In a word, the prevailing ideas and forms of social linkages are reproduced in the health sector; they confront citizens in their most vulnerable moments, reaffirming the systemic inequalities of the system as a whole.

To understand how the definitions of health, illness, and medical care are related to a specific mode of production in a specific era, and to be able to challenge accepted paradigms about these issues, requires research methods that go beyond those of the mainstream that confine research and understanding within the boundaries of the system. One of the great strengths of this book is that it takes the reader/student outside these boundaries.

Another of its strengths is the examination of health care as a human right in a social justice context. From this perspective, it would be a mistake to assume that the medical system is merely part of systemic reproduction. In most industrial countries, citizens' right to medical care within a state-sponsored health system is not only a consequence of the need to reproduce and legitimize the system as a whole, but also the outcome of class struggle and the market's inability to address health-related issues adequately or, in some respects, at all.

There are today numerous international agreements that define universal rights to health. And in the industrial countries there is a substantial commitment of national resources by the state to medicine that goes far to decommodify the practice of health care, that is, to keep it relatively free of market principles and practice. In fact, it is commonly argued on the political left that "socialized medicine" represents a gain for the working classes at the expense of the powers that be. Arguably, it is accurate to say that all social legislation that benefits working people is a class victory of sorts and speaks in part of an implicit or explicit class struggle as its inspiration. But it must be remembered that so-called socialized medicine is state sponsored rather than genuinely socialized; the latter implies medical care as defined, organized, run, and critically assessed by the whole of society without contradictory and self-serving interests at the heart of it.

Whatever the health rights won by working people, state-sponsored medical care is always paradoxical. First, although it benefits the working classes by providing them with various degrees and forms of decommodified medical assistance, it remains subordinate to state direction, and so it is ultimately dependent on the vibrancy of the class struggle and the conditions of capital accumulation. Changes in this struggle and/or in these conditions provide opportunities for alterations in the degree and form of state-sponsored medical care. Second, despite the benefits to the working classes and the partial political (rather than merely market) basis to state sponsorship, the entire health industry remains defined by the political and economic system that gave rise to it. It follows that in capitalist countries the concepts of health, illness, and care are delimited by the boundaries of the capitalist mode of production. That is to say, the human is defined largely as labour power; the concept of health is rooted in notions of the ability to work and to maintain commodity consumption; illness is broadly viewed as a physical condition that prevents work; and medical care emphasizes the physical reproduction of humans as labour power and the consumption of "therapeutic" commodities.

Paradoxical victories, however, cannot be an argument for not engaging in struggle for change. The long and many-sided fights for state-sponsored medical care, and more and better care, are important because these medical services do benefit working people; they are efficacious within limits; they prevent personal and family bankruptcies in the face of serious accidents, illness, or disease; and treatment is to a degree decommodified. Nevertheless, the paradox extends to all the efforts to defend the existing system in the face of seemingly unrelenting criticism and budgetary and/or service cutbacks. If they are not fought, the gains are gradually diminished or even lost, but at the same time the fight to maintain the status quo conceals the problematic structure of health care in its present form as a product of contending interests in a marketplace society. These defensive actions also obscure the social and economic bases of health and illness because, by defending the current structure of health, the focus remains on care and cures for acute conditions; preventative medicine and the extensive critique of capitalism that it would entail have little space on the agenda. Kept within a human rights discourse, moreover, the struggle itself is restricted to legal and structural boundaries set by the established powers; lawyers, officials, and experts prevail while the critical consciousness and participation of the classes concerned are undermined and depoliticized.

This book, through its critical perspectives, examines many of the questions raised here, among others; in general, it is concerned with the numerous contradictions of health, illness, and care in a capitalist society, and how to understand them. As a concluding note, some of these broad incongruities are worth summarizing. First, an economic system whose principles and practices themselves lie at the heart of most medical problems is unlikely to be able to address them adequately or successfully;

if the definitions of health, illness, and care are constructed as part of systemic social reproduction, they are likely to contain all the built-in assumptions, biases, and limitations of the system itself. For a critical understanding, it is necessary to step outside the confines of the system. A related inconsistency is the pursuit of cures for conditions that are chronically caused by the system itself. The only real "cure" in this situation is prevention, but this cannot be admitted in a marketplace society without calling the whole system into question. Third, because health and illness are quintessentially social phenomena, it is incongruous to define health or sickness and its treatment as pertaining to one individual, one class or stratum, or any one category of people, and not all. That there are different levels of health care across strata, classes, and nations is simply testimony to the inequalities of capitalist economies; in principle, human health implies the health of everyone, not just some. Fourth, a health care system that is the product of several contending self-interested forces can hardly be expected to have an impartial appreciation of human health or those suffering illness. In a capitalist medical system, the patient becomes client, a means to an end, or even the object of competition in the encounters between the conflicting forces that define the system.

It could be argued that the health industry is not about human health any more than the automobile industry is about transportation. While the need for transport underlies auto manufacturing and highway construction, how the need is addressed is arguably the least efficient and most costly of all forms of transport, not to mention a common risk to life and a major contributor to ecological destruction. The need for health services similarly underlies the health industry, but how the need is addressed is more individual than social, more costly than necessary (given corporate involvement), more interest-based than health-centred, more "curative" than preventative, and in many ways hazardous to one's health. There is, for example, little demonstrable relation between expenditures for medical care and lower rates of morbidity and mortality; most major chronic illnesses stubbornly persist in the face of modern medical intervention; and thousands die each year of hospital errors and thousands more from adverse pharmaceutical drug reactions. It is difficult to see health as the first concern of the health system.

This book, above all, provides us with critical methods to understand the health system, particularly in Canada, at this historical juncture. Hopefully, it will also lead to changes.

Gary Teeple
Professor of Sociology
Simon Fraser University
Vancouver, August 2005

PREFACE

Concerns about health and the health care system have reached a fever pitch in Canada in recent years. The public is subjected to a daily onslaught of media stories about the causes and treatment of disease and the threats to the sustainability of the Canadian health care system. Traditionally, the study of health has been informed by a variety of perspectives that for too long have been isolated from each other and from an explicit concern with having findings applied to solving the health problems identified by research.

Much of the isolation can be attributed to the nature of the disciplines that have evolved to ask and answer questions about health, illness, and the health care system. Epidemiology has been the primary tool wielded by the medical profession in quest of the causes of disease and illness. Its application, however, has been narrow, with little appreciation of the complex of political, economic, and social factors that set the stage for the onset of disease and illness. The emerging field of social epidemiology is a favourable counterweight to this tradition.

Sociology has made major contributions to understanding the causes of illness and different groups' experience of disease and illness by casting a wider net for the factors that explain health, illness, and the organization of health services. It has, however, been less concerned with identifying the forces that drive these different experiences of health and illness. Like epidemiology, there has been relatively little penetration of concepts and understanding into the sociology of health from the study of public policy and its implications for solving the problems that epidemiologists and sociologists identify.

More recently, however, two new perspectives have emerged that offer solutions to some of these problems. The political economy of health is explicitly concerned with the political and economic structures that shape citizens' experience of health and illness. It is specifically focused on understanding how the creation and distribution of resources influence the health and well-being of populations in general and specific groups in particular. The perspective has a strong commitment to identifying how these structures can be changed to promote health and well-being. The human rights perspective shares a concern with these broader issues, but places these issues within legal and ethical frameworks. The introduction of an explicit values and social justice dimension in discussion of health and health care issues constitutes a strong imperative for action.

5

This volume was conceived with a view to bringing together these important yet usually isolated perspectives with the purpose of (a) identifying key issues in health, illness, and health care; (b) relating these to current policy environments; (c) identifying the complex origins of the problems identified; and (d) contributing in a meaningful way to their solution. Thus, we aim to put into action Marx's well-quoted dictum: "The philosophers have attempted to understand the world in different ways, the point, however, is to change it."

The contributors are established authorities in their field who have demonstrated a commitment to translate theory and empirical findings into action. Most contributors are sociologists, but all have been heavily influenced by sociological perspectives and insights. All of the contributors are concerned with public policy and its role in determining the degree of health and illness in society; the organization and distribution of political, economic, and social resources within society; and the organization, quality, accessibility, and delivery of health care services.

The focus of this book is on the Canadian scene with relevant comparisons to the U.S. and other countries. It is organized into four parts. Part I provides an overview and critical review of four major health paradigms: the epidemiological, sociological, political economy, and human rights perspectives. The basic assumptions of each paradigm are provided as are overviews of recent activity and findings of those working within the area. Part II explores the emerging field of the social determinants of health. There is a focus on social class, gender, and race as indicators of differential access to the economic and social resources available within a society. A unique contribution is the analysis of the role played by political ideology and public policy in shaping the distribution of these economic and social resources.

Part III focuses on the health care system. It provides a comparative history of the Canadian health care system, an overview of current attempts at reform, and a detailed analysis of the effects upon the system and its participants of recent trends toward privatization. Part IV considers critical issues in health and health care that illustrate some of the key themes of the volume: gender and its interaction with health and health care; the construction of illness and disability; health policy through the lens of pharmaceuticals and the health care system; and the promotion of population health.

This volume was envisioned as being appropriate for courses on the sociology of health and illness, but its content is clearly relevant for both undergraduate and graduate courses in the health sciences, nursing, medicine, and other allied health professions. Its concern with policy makes it appropriate for undergraduate and graduate studies in public policy. We welcome feedback concerning its usefulness in educating students and professionals engaged in promoting health, preventing illness, and planning and delivering health care services in Canada and elsewhere.

We are grateful to Megan Mueller, Editorial Director, Social Sciences and History at Canadian Scholars' Press, for her ongoing support of our efforts to raise the profile of the critical health issues facing Canadians. We also acknowledge the ongoing contributions to Canadians' health made by social welfare and health service providers, advocates, researchers, and policy analysts whose ongoing efforts to promote the health and well-being of Canadians remain steadfast even in these difficult times.

Dennis Raphael
Toba Bryant
Marcia Rioux
Toronto, August 2005

Note from the Publisher

Thank you for selecting *Staying Alive: Critical Perspectives on Health, Illness, and Health Care*, a contributed volume edited by Dennis Raphael, Toba Bryant, and Marcia Rioux.

The editors and publisher have devoted considerable time and careful development (including meticulous peer reviews) to this book. We appreciate your recognition of this effort and accomplishment.

Teaching Features

This original contributed volume distinguishes itself on the market in many ways. One key feature is the book's well-written and comprehensive part openers, which make the chapters all the more accessible to undergraduate students. The part openers truly add cohesion to each section and to the whole book. The themes of the book are very clearly presented in these section openers.

The art program of this book is quite sophisticated. Each part opener features an opening photograph and all of the chapters contain a wide array of boxed inserts, figures, charts, graphs, logs, timelines, tables, and even maps.

This book is equally rich in pedagogy for the undergraduate student. Each chapter includes insightful learning objectives, an introduction, conclusions, references, critical thinking questions, annotated further readings, annotated relevant Web sites, an extensive glossary, as well as endnotes (where applicable). Contributor biographies are at the end of the book, as is the index.

PERSPECTIVES ON HEALTH, ILLNESS, AND HEALTH CARE

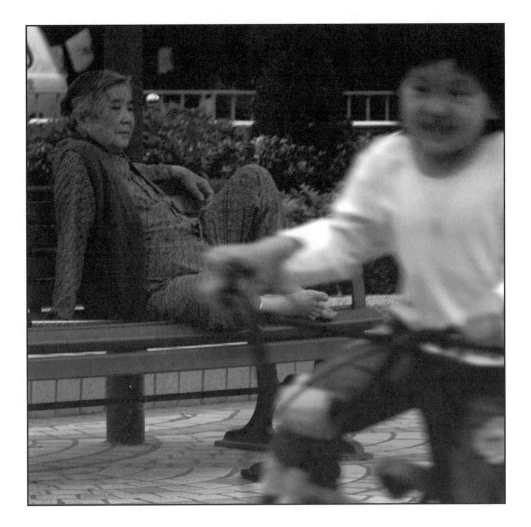

The study of health, illness, and health care is carried out within various conceptual frameworks. These perspectives or paradigms shape our understandings of health issues by identifying the broad dimensions or contexts within which these issues exist. These perspectives identify particular areas of concern, direct the research approaches we take to investigate these issues, and specify the appropriate means of addressing the problems that are identified. Each perspective has value for the study of health, illness, and health care in Canada. Together they provide a means of looking at health in a comprehensive way. Such an approach can lead to the development of innovative theory and enlightened practice.

The study of health issues has traditionally been dominated by two perspectives: the epidemiological and the sociological. Epidemiology is a branch of medicine that studies the causes, distribution, and control of disease in populations. Much of epidemiology is concerned with identifying individual risk factors that are precursors to disease and illness. In contrast, the sociological perspective has its roots in the social sciences and deals with a much wider range of health issues than the causes and distribution of disease. Society, how its organization affects health, and how individuals understand both society and health are the concerns of sociology.

The political economy and human rights perspectives are also presented. The political economy point of view examines the powerful political, economic, and social forces that shape our understanding of the world in general and health issues in particular. In Canada, the economic system and the beliefs associated with capitalism are prime determinants of both health and our understanding of health. The human rights perspective places issues of health and health care within ethical and legal frameworks that guide our expectations of what society considers fair and is obligated to offer its citizens. This view directs our attention to how society meets its commitments to a number of international agreements and commonly accepted ethical principles.

In Chapter 1, Stephen Bezruchka outlines the scope and methods of epidemiology. He provides a brief historical overview of the roots of epidemiology and describes how it is practised today. Epidemiology has its origins in medicine and is primarily concerned with the origins of illness and disease. Bezruchka makes the distinction between studying health and illness at the cellular, organ, individual, and population level. While most of epidemiology is focused at the organ level—identifying the origins of illnesses that affect our bodily systems—there is increasing interest in how the organization of societies affects human health and well-being. He argues that the gap between rich and poor in a society may very well turn out to be the key factor in producing health.

In Chapter 2, Ivy Bourgeault provides an overview of sociological approaches to studying health, illness, and health care. Sociological approaches are concerned with human society and its structures and institutions as well as social relations and experiences of its members. The major trends in sociological thinking about health—functionalism, conflict theory, and materialism, as well as symbolic interactionist and social constructionist approaches—are presented as are the concerns of each approach. Bourgeault also recognizes the contributions of feminist, post-colonial, and post-structualist perspectives. Sociological perspectives go well beyond the causes of disease and address the organization of society and how it affects the distribution of health among the population, the experience of illness, how people understand health and disease, and the organization of health care systems.

In Chapter 3, David Coburn provides the key concepts that constitute a critical materialist approach to understanding how politics and economics shape health and health care systems in societies. By understanding the structure of society and how this structure determines the distribution of resources, differences in health among individuals within a society, as well as differences in health among societies, can be understood. He uses the example of neo-liberalism—the belief that the marketplace should determine the organization of society—to show how political ideology and policies shape health patterns in a society and the organization of health care systems. He demonstrates how a political economy approach can help us to understand why some nations are healthier than others and why Canada has a universal national health care system while the U.S. does not.

In Chapter 4, Marcia Rioux outlines the basis of an ethical and legal approach to health and health care. The dimensions of a human rights approach to health are presented and it is shown how these principles have been institutionalized in various international human rights agreements that define a right to health. These principles guarantee both the determinants of health—such as housing, income, employment, and security—as well as the right to receive health care when it is needed. She shows the implications of this approach for addressing current health issues of the day such as HIV/AIDS, reproductive health, mental health and disability, and access to health care. All of these and other issues have clear ethical and legal components.

· ·

CHAPTER ONE

EPIDEMIOLOGICAL APPROACHES

Stephen Bezruchka

· ·

Learning Objectives

At the conclusion of this chapter, the reader will be able to
- describe the differences in considering health at the level of a cell or organ versus an individual or population
- list critical factors that produce health in populations
- discuss limitations of modern methods of epidemiology in understanding health from a population perspective

Introduction

Epidemiology is the study of health and its determinants in specified populations with the often unstated goal of improving health. The root word, "epidemic," derives its origin from a study of the causes of diseases. The word has been so used for the last 125 years, and epidemiology as a discipline is mainly concerned with illness or disease rather than health and well-being. This chapter traces the historical roots of epidemiology's evolution, its main concepts, and discusses how the way it is practised limits its potential to improve the health of populations. This chapter considers what health means at various biological and social levels, and the sources of health in populations. It is argued that the gap between rich and poor in a society is the key factor in producing health. Discussion of various natural experiments will help the reader grasp this concept.

Early Epidemiology

The origins of epidemiology and a classic example of its approach comes from John Snow, who studied people who succumbed to cholera in London 150 years ago (Gordis 1996). By plotting the incidence of death on maps he discovered an association between deaths in various districts and the sources of drinking water. He went door to door, counting deaths and asking about those homes' water sources. He hypothesized that the scourge was spread by contaminated water from evacuations of infected people. Once these sources were identified, Snow removed the offending pumps' handles even though he did not understand that it was bacteria that spread the disease. Subsequently, deaths declined.

As Snow demonstrated, if we wish to produce health we can do so without understanding all the links between the causes and outcomes of disease. When Snow's study is discussed in standard textbooks, the action he undertook to control the epidemic is rarely mentioned. This lack of concern with improving health once the causes of disease are identified is all too common in the practice of epidemiology today.

Epidemiologists today mostly conduct studies and report results. Action is not usually considered part of the discipline's domain. This reality can be equated with going to the doctor to find out what is wrong with you and then having to find a non-physician to provide treatment. We need a more positive and action-oriented approach to producing health.

Another health official in London at that time, William Farr, the registrar-general in London, recognized that poverty was an important associate of poor health (Farr 2000). Others, before and since, have remarked on this, usually considering that the responsible agents are behaviours and environmental exposures associated with poverty. In this chapter, we scientifically develop the concept that there is something intrinsic about poverty and material deprivation that is unhealthy. This approach is also missing from many standard texts. If studies demonstrate this but there is no action by the field of epidemiology, we may wonder why.

Health as a Concept Differs on the Level Being Considered

The next section considers health from a cellular level, then at an individual human level, and finally at the population level to give a perspective on how health can be produced within a society. Consider a human being and ask of what an individual consists. In biology classes we looked at cells under a microscope and saw small structures with nuclei and chromosomes in which DNA resided. There were also cell walls that contained proteins and energy sources. Cells come in many varieties: heart muscle cells, brain cells, stomach lining cells, blood cells, and so on. As a medical student, I spent considerable time learning the different features of those cells, and how to identify them.

In one sense, you and I are nothing more than a community of different kinds of cells stuck together in various organ systems. These organs include our nervous system, which makes our limbs move when and how we want them to; our digestive system, which extracts and stores nutrients from food; our cardiovascular system, which moves oxygen and energy to various parts of our body, and scavenges waste; our musculoskeletal system, which allows us to maintain our shape and move, and so on. We consist of cells arranged in these various communities, along with water and some other biochemical material.

Suppose we isolate one of these cells, such as a heart muscle cell, and ask what that cell needs to be healthy? Cell biologists would say a cell needs nutrients and oxygen. Glucose is the key nutrient or energy substance in our blood that powers cells. Oxygen is necessary as well as a few trace elements. The same is true for other cells. If your heart cells do not get enough oxygen or glucose because of a faulty nutrient-delivery system, these cells die and you will have a heart attack. The same is true for any cell in the body. If it is not nourished properly, the cell will not work as it should. Such cells will not be healthy and premature death may occur.

The argument could be made that since human beings are but an assembly of cells that need oxygen and glucose plus some trace elements, then humans need just what their cells need to be healthy. If cells benefit from oxygen and glucose, the more we get, the better. We should consume as much food as possible to get as much glucose as we can, and breathe as much oxygen as we can. Then since each one of our cells will be healthy, so should we.

But stuffing ourselves full of food is folly, as our increasing obesity rates demonstrate. Healthy adults breathing high concentrations of oxygen over long periods get lung disease. And babies given pure oxygen go blind. The logic of doing what is best for our component parts—our cells—and generalizing this prescription to the community of cells that comprise a human being may not be the best advice for us as humans to be healthy.

At the individual level—the community of cells that comprise us—our individual health is improved by following all the do's and don'ts such as eating right, exercising, not smoking, wearing a seat belt, using a condom, and getting a good night's sleep. That is good health advice for an individual human. None of those recommendations make any sense to one of your cells. You cannot ask cells to exercise or to not smoke or to wear a seat belt or to get a good night's sleep and so on. That isn't what cells can choose to do. There are no cellular-relevant versions of individual health advice.

If you follow health advice for individuals, your cells should be healthy as a by-product. If you exercise, eat right, and don't smoke, then your heart muscle cell should be healthier than if you didn't follow those behaviours. If you do what is best for an individual human to produce health, your cells will be healthier than if you don't. Individual health advice is for individual humans, and cellular health advice is for cells and we should keep them separate because humans are a community of cells and the organization of the cells must be considered.

What about others levels of organization—communities, states/provinces, or nations? These locations contain populations of humans. Are we making a logical fallacy by assuming that what is the best advice for the constituents of that population, namely you and I, would be the best health advice for the population? Our health advisers tell us that we should exercise, eat right, not smoke, wear seat belts, use condoms, and our population will be healthy. Are they making the same oversight that I prophesied in going from the health advice for a cell to that of an individual human? Looking at Japan as an example of a population suggests there may be considerable cause for rethinking our health advice to populations of all rich countries. They smoke the most, yet by almost any definition of health, they lead the world (Marmot 2004). We have all learned how bad smoking is for our health. Smoking is not good for your health, but compared to other factors that affect populations, its effect may be secondary.

There are factors that exist at a population level that produce health that have no individual counterparts, just as the individual health advice had no cellular counterparts. If the population factors are gotten right, then what individuals in that population do or don't do for their own health may not matter as much. They are healthy as a by-product of the way the jurisdiction is organized, just as our cells are healthy if we do what's right for us as individuals. If this is the case, then we can produce the population factors in a particular society and obtain health, or we may decide to organize society in such as way that the population will not be healthy. Citizens in Canada and elsewhere may be unaware of how population level factors impact their health. The task then is to make them aware.

Associations of cells as organs and the factors that produce disease in these organs are the primary concern of most epidemiologists. They study the incidence and prevalence of diseases such as heart disease, lung cancer, and Alzheimer's and attempt to identify the precipitating exposures that lead to these afflictions. This focus leads the discipline to consider risk factors in an individual that produce unhealthy organs. A *risk factor* is a behaviour or other characteristic that is associated with the condition studied. Such a focus may not be more effective than looking at the health of a cell. Certainly when we come to action, removing the pump handle as John Snow did affected a population. These environmental actions may be preferable to trying to get individuals in London to modify their risk factors that affect intestinal (organ) health (cholera), such as boiling their water, or walking to another pump. It is increasingly apparent that we need to look for the pump handle in modern society.

The Cause of the Cause

There is an Indian story—Clifford Geertz, the famous anthropologist, recounts hearing it as a story from India—about an Englishman who, having been told that the world rested on a platform on the back of an elephant, which rested in turn on the back of a turtle, asked what the turtle rested on. Another turtle. And that turtle? "Ah Sahib, after that it is turtles all the way down."

In any discussion of disease and the causes of disease, we can look at the cause of the cause of the cause—that is, we need to go back to the source of the problem. This can be difficult since discussion of disease and its causes is often limited by various societal norms and understandings as to the appropriate way to identify and deal with a problem. There are three questions to ponder. What are the facts? What is the interpretation of the facts? And what are the presuppositions that frame a discussion? What questions are you not supposed to ask? In looking at the health of populations, what are the basic foundations of health? What is the turtle at the bottom of the pile of turtles?

Population Health Epidemiology

John Snow went door to door in what is called "shoe leather epidemiology" to collect information on water sources and deaths. Such observational data form the backbone of epidemiologic investigations. For a disease-focused approach, one needs to know whether or not someone has the disease, and then obtain a variety of supplemental information to discern what is going on. Suppose one studied lung cancer in a population where everyone smoked. It would be very difficult to discover smoking as a cause of lung cancer if you studied the disease in a population where everyone smoked since you could not compare the incidence of disease between smokers and non-smokers. Smoking as a risk factor for lung cancer would not be apparent. The kinds of questions asked to study health in a population depend on the characteristics of that population and the questions themselves. If you ask the wrong question, or study the wrong population, you get led astray as suggested by our smoking example.

One could ask why "turtles all the way down" are not the focus in epidemiology today. Epidemiologists have graduate training (usually in public health schools) and work in public health departments at various levels. Their employers tend to have a narrow focus, and their projects are short-term and focused on behavioural interventions. These foci may not be the most effective in producing health. Much research is done by private businesses or federal agencies with close ties to private business. The theme is often to create a product, a drug, or an instrument for a procedure, or a communications campaign. The focus is likely to be on individuals or their organs. The outcome is usually something an individual should do. Ask a doctor about a drug. Eat this food. Use this exercise appliance. There are severe limitations with this illness or disease focus (Schwartz et al. 1999).

Another explanation for the kind of work done by epidemiologists relates to the development of powerful computers. This allows analysis of complicated studies of individual diseases. The focus on the individual and the ability to process vast amounts of data keep many researchers stuck in the individual risk factory. At the same time studies demonstrate how difficult it is to change individual behaviours, especially by telling people what they should do. We should not neglect basic treatments of populations comparable to removing the pump handle.

A common approach in modern epidemiology limits the validity of discoveries. A similar problem to studying lung cancer in a society where everyone smokes exists in most contemporary studies of diseases. Unless you look at people who are similar in important respects, you won't find what you are looking for. They must have similar incomes, or education, or wealth, or status in society. In the jargon of epidemiology, you have to control for socio-economic status in a study, or you won't find an effect. Controlling means that you factor out the importance of that variable in the analysis. Then you cannot ask questions about the variable. Hence socio-economic status must be very important in producing health. If it wasn't, then one wouldn't need to control for socio-economic status in studying other factors. How you frame the question profoundly impacts what answer you get.

Defining what a disease is can be very political (Illich 1976). Homosexuality used to be labelled a disease in medical textbooks in the U.S., and it still is in some countries. On the other hand, in Canada formal unions among gays are sanctioned, and it is no longer considered a disease here. Fibromyalgia and chronic fatigue syndrome are conditions that haven't yet appeared on the universally recognized disease stage. A disease focus may provide much useful information, but this schema may not produce health in populations.

Figure 1.1: Time-line

>10,000 years ago	2,500 years ago	1848	1855	Present
Pre-history Gatherer/hunter era	Plato said for a democracy to function, gap between richest and poorest should be no more than 1 in 4	Rudolph Virchow (Prussia) recognized politics was just medicine practiced on a larger scale	John Snow published his book on the pump handle	Pre-eminence of risk factor disease with population perspective beginning

Learning from Health Data on Populations

To understand what produces health in a population we need a definition of health. The World Health Organization states that "health is a state of complete physical, mental and social well-being and not merely the absence of disease or infirmity" (WHO 1986: 1). A more measurable definition might be asking individuals how healthy they consider themselves. For a population, consider the average length of life (life expectancy), or the infant mortality rate. Out of 1,000 infants born, how many die in their first year of life? These can give us numbers, allowing us to ask what may maximize health.

To determine the life expectancy of a population, one needs to know the death rates for the people and their ages in a given year. One then constructs a table in which a hypothetical population would die at those rates and determine the average length of life. The number of person years lived by the population gives you this number. Life expectancies are computed for all countries recording vital events, births, and deaths. The United Nations' annual *Human Development Report* is a convenient data source (UNDP 2004). The top 30 countries are shown in Figure 1.2. For the data reported in 2004, estimating life expectancy for 2002, the range is from 81.5 years for Japan to 32.7 for Zambia, the least healthy in our list of 177 countries.

The U.S. is undoubtedly the world's richest and most powerful country with half of all billionaires and vast military might, yet it is far from being the healthiest.

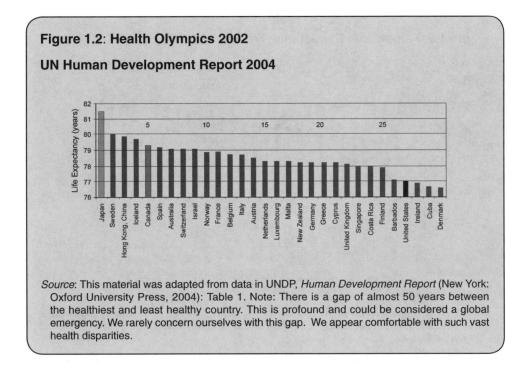

Figure 1.2: Health Olympics 2002

UN Human Development Report 2004

Source: This material was adapted from data in UNDP, *Human Development Report* (New York: Oxford University Press, 2004): Table 1. Note: There is a gap of almost 50 years between the healthiest and least healthy country. This is profound and could be considered a global emergency. We rarely concern ourselves with this gap. We appear comfortable with such vast health disparities.

Canada is right up there, but Japan's lead is considerable. But if the U.S. is only 4.5 years behind Japan, that could appear insignificant. Another perspective is that if the U.S. eliminated heart disease as a cause of death, its number one killer, it still wouldn't be the healthiest country. The health gap is huge! No U.S. doctor could envisage curing heart disease. Fifty-five years ago, best estimates would put the U.S. in the top five, and Japan would be considerably below the 27th ranking enjoyed by the U.S. in 2002, so there has been a profound deterioration in health in the U.S. compared to other countries. Figure 1.3 presents female life expectancy trends for five countries from 1960 to 1990, demonstrating how Japan's health improved faster in comparison to other rich countries, and how the U.S. became last in that cohort.

Imagine how excited John Snow must have been to draw his revealing maps. Our graphs of the "Health Olympics" provide similar insight. The U.S. and Japan have more than changed places. Why? Epidemiologists can collect other data such as measures of health care, air pollution, smoking rates, economic growth, dietary habits, education, etc., to see if there is some association between those data and our measure of health. This is termed looking for confounders or other explanations.

Consider health care. An easy measure is the per-capita expenditure. The U.S. spends half of the world's health care budget, almost U.S. $6,300 per person, in total as much as every other country combined. The U.S. is not buying health with its

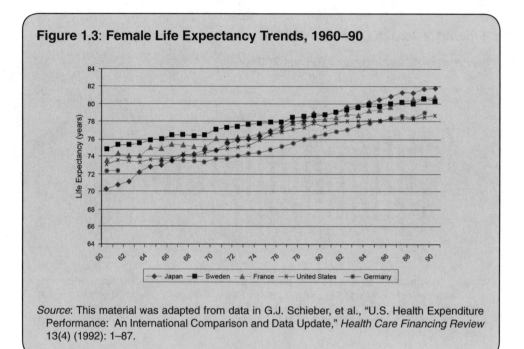

Figure 1.3: Female Life Expectancy Trends, 1960–90

Source: This material was adapted from data in G.J. Schieber, et al., "U.S. Health Expenditure Performance: An International Comparison and Data Update," *Health Care Financing Review* 13(4) (1992): 1–87.

health care money. We naturally assume that health and health care are synonymous, but they are not.

Similar analyses demonstrate that none of the usual factors explain why the U.S. is so unhealthy. We discovered that men in Japan smoke the most of all the countries in Figure 1.2! You could conclude that smoking is what makes Japan so healthy. Another interpretation is that although smoking is not good for your health, other factors are worse and they supercede the bad effects of smoking.

Richard Wilkinson is an economic historian and epidemiologist who has been studying the health of countries for decades, trying to determine the factors related to their health. He demonstrated that the usual factors did not offer satisfactory explanations. By 1986 he had found that the gap between the rich and poor in a country appeared to be correlated with the population's health. This was not something commonly considered, but by 1992, his findings were published in the *British Medical Journal*. Figure 1.4 has life expectancy data for 1981 for 11 countries. You can see how well a country's health lines up with how much income the bottom 70 percent of households earn. This paper helped spawn the study of population health today.

Association does not apply causation. How do we interpret the studies that epidemiologists produce? Guidelines have existed for at least 50 years, and were

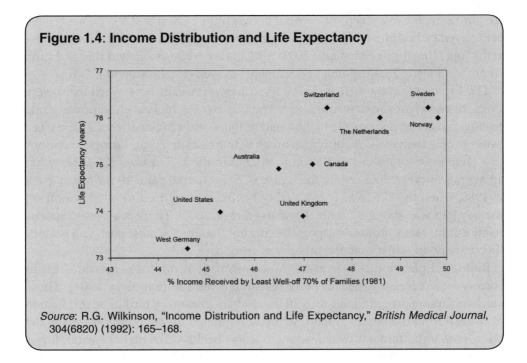

Figure 1.4: Income Distribution and Life Expectancy

Source: R.G. Wilkinson, "Income Distribution and Life Expectancy," *British Medical Journal*, 304(6820) (1992): 165–168.

summarized in the U.S. surgeon general's report of 1964 linking smoking and bad health. To consider a finding to be causative, there would have to be many studies on different populations, by different investigators, on different time periods that demonstrated the association. There must be a *dose-response relationship*—that is, more of one should produce more of the other. The chicken-and-egg dilemma needs to be determined. Which direction did the cause go? And finally, there had to be some pathologic mechanism through which the effect could occur.

The ensuing decade and a half has found researchers investigating the health hierarchy hypothesis. At this point, the conclusions are tentative, but extremely suggestive. Most of the research demonstrates many important findings that could lead us to the equivalent of removing the handle on the pump if our goal is to produce health without knowing everything about disease and its causes.

To summarize the findings, relative poverty is bad for your health. That is, for almost any condition, being lower in the socio-economic ladder is bad for you. In other words, poorer people have different body chemistry and physiology than those of greater means. Poverty has an effect that is not just related to personal behaviours engaged in by poorer or richer people. The Institute of Medicine in the U.S., a branch of the National Academy of Sciences that operates under a congressional charter to advise the federal government, issued a report stating: "more egalitarian societies (i.e., those with a less steep differential between the richest and the poorest) have better average health, because a dollar at the bottom 'buys' more health than a dollar at the top." (Institute of Medicine 2003: 59). This is a well-established rule of thumb common in many Health Canada documents as well (Health Canada 1998).

The gap between the rich and poor in society represents how much the society cares for and shares with its members. The U.S. has the highest child poverty rate among rich countries, despite having half of the world's billionaires. Canada has a better profile than the U.S., but fares much worse than do many European nations (see chapters 5 and 8 in this volume). A CEO in the U.S. makes 531 times what an average worker does, while the figure is 20 for Canada and 10 for Japan. Back in 1980, when the U.S. was considerably healthier compared to other countries, the pay gap was about 40 to one (Anderson et al. 2000). There is a dose-response relationship. Many studies support the concept that for the most part, you get sick if you are poor, rather than the other way around.

Biological plausibility is present. Mechanisms that produce chronic stress in society have received considerable research attention (Sapolsky 2004). These mechanisms are programmed early in life, and are present by birth. The production of cortisol from the adrenal gland, which is regulated by the hippocampus in the brain, is an important pathway leading to worse health when higher cortisol levels are sustained. We have many individual studies as well as population data that demonstrate this (Kristenson et al. 1998).

In developed nations such as Canada, medical care is not as important in producing health in a population as are these other factors (Jamrozik and Hobbs 2002). For the non-specialist and specialist alike, this is the most difficult concept to grasp. The conclusion of the chapter on medical care and health from the *Oxford Textbook of Public Health* is "The impact of personal medical services on the health and survival of individuals seems readily apparent. With modern investigations and treatments, patients are now regularly saved and make very good recoveries from infections, injuries, and a variety of other conditions that were almost uniformly fatal even a few years ago. Surprisingly it is more difficult to demonstrate conclusively the impact of these medical advances on the health of whole communities" (Jamrozik and Hobbs 2002: 238). A major reason for this difficulty is in part because whenever medical care has been studied, it has been found to be a leading cause of death (Davis 2004). Whereas health care definitely helps some, it harms others, and for populations, whenever it has been studied, there appears to be little or no net benefit. Recognizing this is very difficult for most people. I write this as a practising emergency physician. (See "An Overview of Medical Harm" at the end of this chapter.)

Whenever it has been studied (hospital chart reviews or doctors' strikes), medical care is a leading cause of death, so even Bunker's health gains are suspect (see Box 1.1).

Box 1.1: **Evaluating the Impact of Health Care on Health**

Bunker's (2001) study looked at curative and preventive care in the U.S. during the last century and the effects on life expectancy gain:

- approximately five years, with 1.5 from preventive care and 3.5 from curative care
- used gain based on results of idealized care from clinical trials of treatments
- did not consider the difference between efficacy (idealized situation of best practice) and effectiveness (as care is delivered in community)

Inequality in Society Is Bad for Your Health

The most commonly used measure of inequality is that of income differences. This is so since these data appear regularly in the census and other sources. Income is a flawed measure—especially among countries—because there are a variety of behind-the-scenes redistribution mechanisms in different countries. Through taxes, transfers, and other payments, Sweden reduces its poverty rate based on income over 80 percent in comparison to about 40 percent for Canada and less than 20 percent for the U.S. Some countries provide health care, education, and other benefits that people in countries like the U.S. and Canada have to purchase directly. There may be a threshold of disparity for income inequality to have an effect. Canada has less income inequality than the U.S. because of various social and economic policies. The relationship between income distribution and health among Canadian provinces is less pronounced than the situation among U.S. states (see Figure 1.5.) On the other hand, in Chile, which has a large gap between the rich and poor, there is a relationship between health and income inequality.

The geographic level at which income distribution is measured affects the health outcome. In a small neighbourhood, most people are similar economically. It would be unlikely that a small income gap in a small area would be related to health. In the U.S. we see the relationship at the city and state level throughout the country, but not at the county level, within a state, for example (Brodish et al. 2000). For the U.S., looking at cities and their health related to income gaps yields striking findings. Figure 1.6 divides the cities into income brackets by quarters or quartiles. Each grouping of cities is then divided into quartiles by income inequality from the highest inequality to the most equal. For poor or rich quartiles, the cities with a small gap between rich and poor have almost the same mortality. The same is true for poor or rich cities with a big gap between rich and poor. The finding hints at the idea that the rich may be at least as affected by the gap between the rich and the poor as the poor are. Epidemiologists speak of the ecological fallacy for population

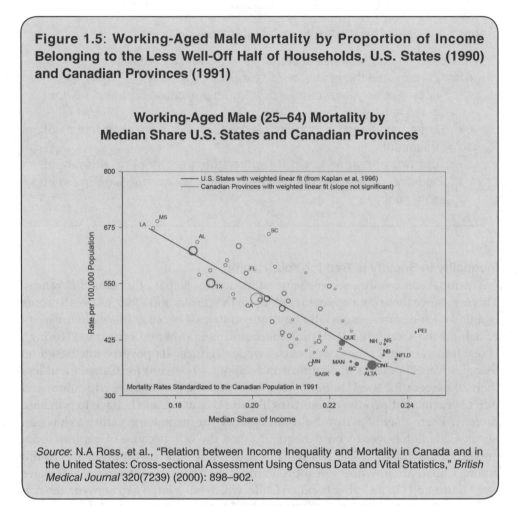

Figure 1.5: **Working-Aged Male Mortality by Proportion of Income Belonging to the Less Well-Off Half of Households, U.S. States (1990) and Canadian Provinces (1991)**

Working-Aged Male (25–64) Mortality by
Median Share U.S. States and Canadian Provinces

Source: N.A Ross, et al., "Relation between Income Inequality and Mortality in Canada and in the United States: Cross-sectional Assessment Using Census Data and Vital Statistics," *British Medical Journal* 320(7239) (2000): 898–902.

findings that may mislead what happens with individuals. For example, the finding that populations with more poverty have worse health than populations with less poverty implies that poorer people will have poorer health, but this must be demonstrated; it could be the opposite, namely that rich individuals have worse health and where there are more poor, there are also more rich. We have one study on individuals that goes beyond the fallacy limitation that suggests that the rich may be more affected by inequality than the poor. This is the first such study, so we should be cautious in saying it is generally true. If it were verified by other research, it would be a powerful selling point for changing the structure of society so everyone is better off.

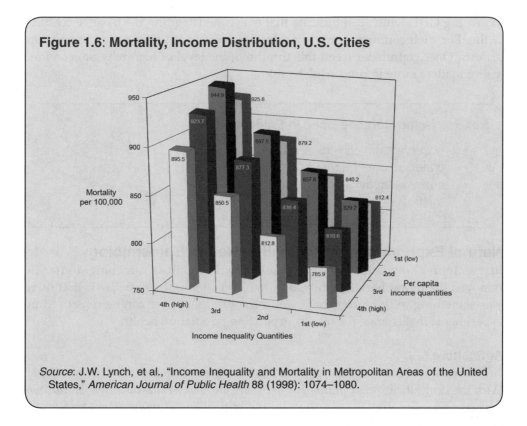

Figure 1.6: Mortality, Income Distribution, U.S. Cities

Source: J.W. Lynch, et al., "Income Inequality and Mortality in Metropolitan Areas of the United States," *American Journal of Public Health* 88 (1998): 1074–1080.

Basic Needs

The nature of caring and sharing in a society determines its health. Can we generalize from what we discovered in rich countries? Are egalitarian societies always healthier than those with a big gap between the rich and poor? Let's look at Nepal where I have spent 10 of the last 35 years, much of it in providing and teaching about health care. The health-hierarchy relationship is difficult to study in such a primarily rural agrarian society that does not record births and deaths. Life expectancies are crude estimates. Determining how many infants die in the first year of life is a little easier. How to measure hierarchy is also problematic for such a population, since few people fill out survey forms, and shoe-leather epidemiology will wear out many pairs of shoes in this mostly roadless nation. Nevertheless, in Nepal the highest infant mortality rate is found in districts with the most egalitarian structure. These districts have significant food deficits and everyone is uniformly poor and starving. Having enough food and clean water and shelter takes precedence over economic justice. One finds that for countries with a low gross domestic product (GDP) (a few hundred dollars up to a couple of thousand dollars per person per year), life expectancy estimates increase with increasing GDP, which can indicate that everyone is getting the basic necessities of life. For such countries, providing food, water, and shelter for everyone take priority. Once countries exceed this threshold, the level of hierarchy or economic justice matters more in producing health.

Box 1.2: Some Methods Used in Epidemiology

- observational ecological studies (e.g., Figure 1.2)
- cohort studies (Figure 1.3)
- cross-sectional study (Figures 1.4, 1.5, 1.6)
- multi-level modelling

Natural Experiments in Population Health Epidemiology

Just as John Snow could observe the decline in deaths from cholera after he removed the pump handle, which boosted his belief in the hypothesis that there was something in the water that caused the disease, so we can be reassured by experiments that change the factors producing population health.

Agriculture

Before the advent of agriculture our health was remarkably good (Cohen 1991). With the domestication of plants and animals, human health declined. In hunter-gatherer societies vigilant sharing was the critical social value. They had few if any possessions and the key resource that was shared with everyone, whether they were related or not, was meat from an occasional big game kill. Given food, shelter, and safety sufficient to sustain health, if everyone is poor, then no one is poorer than anyone else. But with the development of agriculture a food surplus could be produced, and some individuals would proclaim themselves lord or master and coerce others to produce food for the lord, as well as build a castle and protect him. Caring and sharing declined. Poverty appeared. Diets changed and food variety declined (Larsen 1995). Famines began. Living in close proximity to domestic animals resulted in many infectious organisms changing hosts to produce human disease. The nature of human relationships changed as exploitation began. Throughout recorded history until the last century, the health of human populations has been less than that of primitive societies. The recent improvements in health depend on forms of societal redistribution that favoured poorer people along with technological changes that had an impact.

Japan at the End of the Second World War

Japan became the healthiest country in the world because of economic policies resulting from the U.S. occupation of that defeated country after the end of the Second World War (Bezruchka 2003). The "medicine" administered by perhaps the world's greatest population health doctor, General Douglas MacArthur, had three ingredients. The first was demilitarization. Japan was forbidden to have an army and had to resolve disputes peacefully as written into the constitution that MacArthur wrote. The second ingredient was democratization. Everyone got the vote, and labour unions obtained the right to organize and bargain collectively. A public health clause in the constitution required the government to do all it could to improve health. MacArthur legislated a maximum wage of 65,000 yen per year. The final ingredient was decentralization. The concentration of wealth and power that existed in pre-war Japan was broken up. The 11 large family corporations or *zaibatsu* that controlled most aspects of economic life were dismantled. The most successful land-reform program in history was carried out. Before the war, the land in this rice-farming economy was owned by 37,000 landlords and farmed by millions of tenants. MacArthur purchased the land at a fixed price per hectare and sold it to the tenants at that price, while giving them a 30-year interest-free loan to pay for it. With the dismantling of Japan's hierarchy, the resulting improvement in health was "unequaled in any country in the world in medical history in a comparable period of time" (Willoughby and Chamberlain 1954: 345).

The Former Soviet Union

Japan demonstrates what can happen when hierarchies are dismantled. Countries of the former Soviet Union demonstrate what can happen when huge hierarchies are created overnight (Wilkinson 2005). Russia was a very hierarchical society during the Tsarist period, and lagged about 25 life expectancy years behind the U.S. in 1900. The command economy in Russia dismantled the wealth gap so that by 1960, the two countries had comparable health indicators. Health gains in Russia faltered in the 1970s and 1980s as its people felt deprived of the apparent wealth in the West depicted by outside media. With the dismantling of the former Soviet Union, fabulous wealth was created so that Russia now has the third largest number of billionaires in the world while 10 years ago it had none.

As the gap between rich and poor grew astronomically, health in Russia declined, something that has been unprecedented in the modern world (Marmot 2004). The only other example where health has declined substantially in the last century also occurred in the last decade, in high AIDS-prevalent countries of sub-Saharan Africa. Life expectancy in Russia has dropped about seven years for men and somewhat less for women. The decline has still not abated. The carnage has resulted in between 10 million and 20 million deaths that would not have occurred if health had remained at pre-dissolution levels. The gap between rich and poor in Russia today is greater than Tsarist levels. People in Russia are about as unaware of their health declines as people in the U.S. are unaware of their poor health standing. The health decline in Russia has been absolute, meaning there are more deaths than before. The U.S. has seen a relative health decline, meaning health has not improved as much as in other rich countries.

> **Box 1.3: What Produces Health in a Population**
>
> - Basic needs (food, water, shelter, and security) are met.
> - Once those are satisfied, then the nature of caring and sharing in that society, typically measured by distribution of wealth, resources, income, education, political power, status of women, and health care is what is most important.
> - More egalitarian societies have better average health.

Conclusions

A positive and action-oriented approach to producing health would be to popularize what is known regarding the poor health status of countries such as the U.S., which have large gaps between the rich and poor relative to other rich countries. These gaps result from lack of an egalitarian policy frame as the cause. If Canadians have no interest in producing health, they can continue to pursue policies that will increase the gap between our rich and poor that move Canada toward the U.S. model. This will further the already growing hierarchy in Canada. Or if they want to live as a healthier population, they can take policy steps that are diametrically opposite to the current ones. In a democracy there is this choice. It should be an informed one.

References

Anderson, S., J. Cavanagh, C. Collins, C. Hartman, and F. Yeskel. (2000). *Executive Excess 2000: Seventh Annual CEO Compensation Survey.* Washington and Boston: Institute for Policy Studies and United for a Fair Economy.

Bennett, N.G., D.E. Bloom, and S.F. Ivanov. (1998). "Demographic Implications of the Russian Mortality Crisis." *World Development* 26(11): 1921–1937.

Bezruchka, S. (1999). "Social Ordering in Developing Countries: Does Hierarchy Have the Same Effect as in Post-industrial Nations? A Look at Nepal." *Annals of the New York Academy of Sciences* 896: 490–492.

_____. (2001). "Societal Hierarchy and the Health Olympics." *Canadian Medical Association Journal* 164(12): 1701–1703.

_____. (2003). "Inequality and Population Health: The Case of Post-war Japan." San Francisco, Annual Meeting APHA.

Brodish, P.H., M. Massing, and H.A. Tyroler. (2000). "Income Inequality and All-Cause Mortality in the 100 Counties of North Carolina." *Southern Medical Journal* 93(4): 386–391.

Cohen, M.N. (1991). *Health and the Rise of Civilization.* New Haven: Yale University Press.

Davis, P. (2004). "Health Care as a Risk Factor." *Canadian Medical Association Journal* 170(11): 1688-1689.

Farr, W. (2000). "Vital Statistics: Memorial Volume of Selections from the Reports and Writings. 1885." *Bulletin of the World Health Organization* 78(1): 88–95.

Gordis, L. (1996). *Epidemiology.* Philadelphia: Saunders.

Hertzman, C. (2000). "The Case for an Early Childhood Development Strategy." *Canadian Journal of Policy Research* 1: 11–18.

Illich, I. (1976). *Medical Nemesis*. New York: Pantheon.

Institute of Medicine. (2003). *The Future of the Public's Health in the 21st Century*. Washington: National Academy Press.

Jamrozik, K., and M.S.T. Hobbs. (2002). "Medical Care and Public Health." In *Oxford Textbook of Public Health*, edited by R. Detels, J. McEwen, R. Beaglehole, and H. Tanaka, 215–242. Oxford: Oxford University Press.

Kristenson, M., K. Orth-Gomér, Z. Kucineskine, B. Bergdohl, and H. Calkauskas. (1998). "Attenuated Cortisol Response to a Standardized Stress Test in Lithuanian versus Swedish Men: The LiVicordia Study." *International Journal of Behavioral Medicine* 5(1): 17–30.

Larsen, C.S. (1995). "Biological Changes in Human Populations with Agriculture." *Annual Review of Anthropology* 24: 185–213.

Lynch, J.W., G. A. Kaplan, E.R. Pamuk, R. Cohen, C. Heck, J. Balfour, and I. Yen. (1998). "Income Inequality and Mortality in Metropolitan Areas of the United States." *American Journal of Public Health* 88: 1074–1080.

Manchester, W. (1978). *American Caesar: Douglas MacArthur 1880–1964*. Boston: Little, Brown.

Marmot, M. (2004). *Status Syndrome: How Our Position on the Social Gradient Affects Longevity and Health*. London: Bloomsbury.

McClain, J.L. (2002). *Japan: A Modern History*. New York: Norton.

McKee, M. (2001). "The Health Consequences of the Collapse of the Soviet Union: Industrialization and Health in Historical Perspective." In *Poverty, Inequality, and Health: An International Perspective*," edited by D.A. Leon and G. Walt, 17–36. Oxford: Oxford University Press.

Morgenson, G. (2004). "Explaining (or Not) Why the Boss Is Paid So Much." *New York Times* (January 25, 2004): B1.

Ross, N.A., M. Wolfson, J. Dunn, J.M. Berthelot, G. Koplan, and J. Lynch. (2000). "Relation between Income Inequality and Mortality in Canada and in the United States: Cross-sectional Assessment Using Census Data and Vital Statistics." *British Medical Journal* 320(7239): 898–902.

Sapolsky, R.M. (2004). *Why Zebras Don't Get Ulcers: The Acclaimed Guide to Stress, Stress-Related Diseases and Coping*. New York: Henry Holt.

Schieber, G.J., J.D. Poullier, and L. Greenwald. (1992). "U.S. Health Expenditure Performance: An International Comparison and Data Update." *Health Care Financing Review* 13(4): 1–87.

Schwartz, S., E. Sosser, and M. Surser. (1999). "A Future for Epidemiology." *Annual Review of Public Health* 20(1): 15–33.

Subramanian, S.V., and I. Kawachi. (2004). "Income Inequality and Health: What Have We Learned So Far?" *Epidemiological Review* 26(1): 78–91.

UNDP. (2004). *Human Development Report 2004: Cultural Liberty in Today's Diverse World*. New York: Oxford University Press.

Walberg, P. M. McKee, V. Shkolnikov, L. Chenet, and D. Leon. (1998). "Economic Change, Crime, and Mortality Crisis in Russia: Regional Analysis." *British Medical Journal* 317(7154): 312–318.

Wilkinson, R.G. (2005). *The Impact of Inequality*: *How to Make Sick Societies Healthier*. New York: New Press.

Wilkinson, R., and M. Marmot, eds. (2003). *Social Determinants of Health*: *The Solid Facts*. Copenhagen: World Health Organization Regional Office for Europe.

Willoughby, C.A., and J. Chamberlain. (1954). *MacArthur 1941-1951*. New York: McGraw-Hill.

World Health Organization (WHO). (1986). Ottawa Charter for Health Promotion. Geneva: WHO.

● ●

Critical Thinking Questions

1. Why is there little interest among epidemiologists and the general population in the broader factors that produce health in a society?
2. What can be done on an individual basis to improve health in a population?
3. Why are the terms "health" and "health care" often considered synonymously?
4. What could be done to improve some of the broader factors that influence health?
5. What public policies in Canada appear to be supporting health and what are those that are threatening health?

Further Readings

Hofrichter, R., ed. (2003). *Health and Social Justice*: *Politics, Ideology, and Inequity in the Distribution of Disease.* San Francisco: Jossey-Bass.
This collection of articles by many authors looks at the political issues behind the health of societies.

Kawachi, I., and B.P. Kennedy. (2002). *The Health of Nations*: *Why Inequality Is Harmful to Your Health.* New York: New Press.
A single-author approach to the consumption cancer in the U.S. that is close to the root of most problems.

Kawachi, I., B.P. Kennedy, and R.G. Wilkinson, eds. (1999). *The Society and Population Health Reader*, vol. I: Income Inequality and Health. New York: New Press.
This collection of articles examines the relationship between hierarchy and health. It provides fundamental fodder for understanding the science in order to communicate with others.

Marmot, M. (2004). *The Status Syndrome: How Our Position on the Social Gradient Affects Longevity and Health.* New York: Times Books.
A perspective from the pioneering social epidemiologist in England communicating the results of many studies.

Wilkinson, R. (1996). *Unhealthy Societies: The Afflictions of Inequality.* London: Routledge.
A compilation by the leading thinker presenting the psychosocial nature of health.

_____. (2001). *Mind the Gap: Hierarchies, Health and Human Evolution.* New Haven: Yale University Press.
A small readable extension of the basic premise that the gap is bad for society.

_____. (2005). *The Impact of Inequality: How to Make Sick Societies Healthier.* New York: New Press.
A readable summary of how a just society is healthier.

Medical Care and Health
Bunker, J.P. (2001). "The Role of Medical Care in Contributing to Health Improvements within Societies." *International Journal of Epidemiology* 30(6): 1260–1268.

Davis, P. (2004). "Health Care as a Risk Factor." *Canadian Medical Association Journal* 170(11): 1688–1689.

An Overview of Medical Harm
Frankel, S. (2001). "Commentary: Medical Care and the Wider Influences upon Population Health: A False Dichotomy." *International Journal of Epidemiology* 30(6): 1267–1268.
Considers factors not addressed by Bunker in health care producing health.

Hart, J.T. (2001). "Commentary: Can Health Outputs of Routine Practice Approach Those of Clinical Trials?" *International Journal of Epidemiology* 30(6): 1263–1267.
Reflects on whether idealized trials are found in the community.

Mendelsohn, R.S. (1990). *Confessions of a Medical Heretic.* New York: McGraw-Hill.
A polemical look at what doctors do and don't do.

The following three papers consider that when doctors don't work, we are at least not worse off, and possibly better.

Roemer, M.I. (1979). "LA Study of Physician Malpractice Slowdown: Comment." *American Journal of Public Health* 69(8): 825–826.

_____. (1981). "More Data on Post-surgical Deaths Related to the 1976 Los Angeles Doctor Slowdown." *Social Science and Medicine* [C] 15(3): 161–163.

Siegel-Itzkovich, J. (2000). "Doctors' Strike in Israel May Be Good for Health." *British Medical Journal* 320(7249): 1561.

Relevant Web Sites

Centre for Social Justice
www.social justice.org
   The Centre for Social Justice is an advocacy organization that seeks to strengthen the struggle for social justice. It is committed to working for change in partnership with various social movements and recognizes that effective change requires the active participation of all sectors of our community. The centre's work may change from year to year, but there is an ongoing interest in working strategically to narrow the gap between rich and poor, challenging the corporate domination of Canadian politics, and pressing for policy changes that promote economic and social justice.

Inequality
www.inequality.org
   Inequality.org's mission is, first of all, to illuminate the causes and multidimensional consequences of the growing inequality of wealth, income, power, and opportunity in America; and, second, to move this critical national problem onto the front burner of American politics and public discourse.

John Snow
www.ph.ucla.edu/epi/snow.html
   A look at the profound influence this man has had on the subject of epidemiology.

Population Health Forum
http://depts.washington.edu/eqhlth/
   The Population Health Forum, an organization of health activists originally launched at the University of Washington, raises awareness of, promotes dialogue about, and explores how political, economic, and social inequalities interact to reduce the overall health status of our society. It hosts forums, sponsors discussions, develops curriculum, teaches courses, sponsors workshops, and provides speakers to promote knowledge and to advocate for action in service of a healthier society. There is a listserv for updates on population health that you can subscribe to on the site.

UC Atlas of Global Inequality
http://ucatlas.ucsc.edu/
The Atlas explores the interaction between global integration (globalization) and inequality. It has generated maps examining some aspects of material inequality, life and death, global connectedness, and economic globalization. It has expanded coverage of health and gender, and added more interactive capacities, enabling users to make comparisons among countries. It has also portrayed aspects of inequality within countries starting with the health consequences of wealth and poverty.

United for a Fair Economy
www.faireconomy.org/
UFE raises awareness that concentrated wealth and power undermine the economy, corrupt democracy, deepen the racial divide, and tear communities apart. It supports and helps build social movements for greater equality.

Glossary

Cohort: A group of people followed over time; usually they are born in a specified short period.

Confounding: A term used when two or more processes that have not been separated in the analysis have an impact on the outcome studied.

Controlling for a factor: This means statistically adjusting in the analysis for a variable (factor) so that there is no impact of this factor on the outcome one is studying.

Life expectancy: The average number of years lived by a population if the age-specific mortality rates in place when the calculation was done continued until everyone had died.

• •

CHAPTER TWO

SOCIOLOGICAL PERSPECTIVES ON HEALTH AND HEALTH CARE

Ivy Lynn Bourgeault

• •

Learning Objectives

At the conclusion of this chapter, the reader will be able to
- identify the unique features of various sociological approaches to studying health, illness, and health care and how these have evolved historically
- identify the different levels of analysis that can be applied to studies of health, illness, and health care from macro to micro
- understand the key assumptions behind various sociological approaches from conflict to co-operation and from realism to relativism/social constructionism
- understand how contemporary sociological perspectives build upon and react to pre-existing perspectives

---

Introduction

Sociology is the systematic study of human society, including its social structures and institutions, as well as social relations and experiences. Ideally, it also involves studying the interactions between these various elements. Sociology offers a variety of means to understand the incidence and experience of illness and health within societies as well as the social organization of the delivery of health care and differential access to health care resources. The specific application of sociology to the field of health, illness, and health care has been termed "medical sociology."

Medical sociology has its roots in public health and social medicine initiatives during the 19th century, but it grew into a separate field in the late 1940s and early 1950s, drawing mainly from currents within its parent discipline of sociology (Bloom 2002). A key distinction made within this field—between the *sociology in medicine* and the *sociology of medicine*—stems from these early roots. First explicitly articulated by Robert Strauss (1957), sociological studies in medicine are oriented toward applying sociological theory or concepts toward a better understanding of health-related problems or creation of more informed public health policy, whereas sociological studies of medicine are oriented toward a better understanding of society or sociological concepts through the lens of health problems, medical settings, or the organization of health care. Some have argued that there is a trend from the sociology *in* to the sociology *of* medicine and even more broadly to the sociology of health fostered by the increasing institutionalization of sociology within universities (Coburn and Eakin 1998; Cockerham and Ritchey 1997). This reflects a movement away from a medically defined approach to one that is more theoretically oriented, deriving its inspiration—much like the rest of sociology—from the founding traditions of Durkheim, Weber, and Marx and, more recently, from feminist, anti-racism, and postmodernist scholars. While the distinction between sociology *in* and *of* is important to make, it is difficult to tease apart these orientations in practice because many medical sociologists are engaged both in advancing sociology through insights garnered from health and health care and in using their knowledge to create practical change.

In this chapter, I trace the historical evolution of sociological perspectives as applied to health from the grand theories of functionalism, conflict theory, and materialism to symbolic interactionist and social constructionist approaches that focus more specifically on the meaning and experience of health and illness in society. More recent developments in the sociology of health that build upon or react to these founding traditions—namely, feminism, anti-racism, and postmodernism—are also presented. Across all perspectives, I note in particular how each treats the role and experience of patients, or those who seek care, and the providers of that care. In order to provide an overview of this nature it requires a fair degree of simplification of many intricate ideas in each of these literatures. At the end of this chapter, I thus suggest some key works from which the reader could gather more detailed accounts and expanded discussions.

Evolution of Sociological Perspectives on Health and Health Care

Structural Functionalism

Structural functionalism, or simply functionalism, is a theoretical orientation derived in large part from a Durkheimian (1858–1917) tradition that highlights the importance of studying social systems. It focuses on the interrelationships between individuals and groups within society and the way in which it is structured to function in order to maintain the society as a whole (Lachmann 1991). This perspective is associated most closely with the work of A.R. Radcliffe-Brown, a British social anthropologist, who argued in the 1920s that the elements of society—i.e., its social structure—have indispensable functions for one another such that the continued existence of the one element is dependent on that of the others and on society as whole.[1] The focus of inquiries in this field tends toward individual and group *roles* within society and how these are linked to the consensus-based functioning of society.

The application of structural functionalism to the field of medical sociology began with the introduction of *The Social System* (1951) by Talcott Parsons (1902–1979), who devoted considerable space in this text to the function of modern medical practice within society and the complementary roles of physicians and patients. His conceptualization of the sick role in particular became one of the most cited sociological concepts in the field (Matcha 2000). Parsons (1951) described illness as a state of disturbance in the "normal" functioning of the total human individual, including both the state of the organism as a biological system and of his personal and social adjustments (1951: 431). Because of this dual impact—biological and social—the role of a sick person in society is both biologically and socially defined as deviant. Because of this deviant aspect, a new social role—the sick role—had to be defined. Being sick, therefore, constituted a social role with "institutionalised expectations and the corresponding sentiments and sanctions" (1951: 436) in order for equilibrium, wellness, and a functioning society to be maintained. The four elements constituting this sick role include two rights or exemptions and two obligations (see Box 2.1).

Box 2.1: The Sick Role

- The exemption from normal social role responsibilities
- The exemption from responsibility for his or her illness
- The state of being ill is itself undesirable and the person has the obligation to want to "get well" and return to a normal social role
- The sick person also has the obligation to seek technically competent help and comply with treatment regimens

Source: Adapted from Talcott Parsons, *The Social System* (New York: The Free Press, 1951).

To complement this sick role, the provider's role is to legitimate the condition, to treat the condition, and make the person well again. In order to do so, physicians are granted privileged and penetrating access to patients' bodies and their private lives. Balancing these powers are physicians' allegiance to a code of ethics and an altruistic orientation. Neither of these negate the controlling nature of medical practice, but from this perspective it is seen as functional and hence unproblematic.

Being more theoretical than empirical, Parsons's conceptualization came under significant criticism for how it masks the variability in the temporary or legitimate nature of different illnesses, and the diversity in the actual behaviour of sick individuals and of their providers. Twaddle (1969), for example, claimed that there are multiple configurations of the sick role of which Parsons's is but one. Mechanic and Volkart (1960) also noted how Parsons's description was most relevant to acute illnesses, and not the increasingly prevalent chronic illnesses and disabilities that would entail a permanent role status. With respect to the provider's role, Szasz and Hollender (1956) refined Parsons's work by elaborating different doctor-patient models arising from different types of illness. The first matched patient passivity and physician assertiveness—most akin to Parsons's sick role—as the most common reaction to acute illness. The second was characterized by physician guidance and patient co-operation where a less acute illness was involved. The third model was characterized by physicians providing advice on a treatment plan that patients had most of the responsibility to implement; this latter case was most relevant for chronic illnesses and certain forms of disability.[2]

For the most part these early criticisms were still based on the structural functional assumptions of consensus-based society made up of interconnected social roles. What was called for were more possibilities of the various roles there could be. Broader criticisms, however, were levelled at the basic premises of this perspective—specifically, how society was not necessarily consensus-based and that the wielding of power was not always functional but rather is associated with several negative features. This more critical focus is exemplified in two key strands of sociological theory—*interactionism* and *materialism*.

Symbolic Interactionism and Social Constructionism[3]

The school of symbolic interactionist thought is derived from a Weberian (1864–1920) tradition where the focus is not on social institutions but on interacting individuals and the meanings they create. The term was first coined by Herbert Blumer in 1937, drawing upon the work of George Herbert Mead (1863–1931) with whom he studied at the University of Chicago, and Charles Cooley (1864–1929). As he later described in 1969, it involves the following key principles: (1) "human beings act towards things on the basis of the meanings that things have for them"; (2) these meanings "arise out of social interaction"; and (3) social action results from a "fitting together of individual lines of action" (Jary and Jary 1991: 509). Stemming from these key principles, interactionists focus less on objective, macro-structural aspects of social systems than they do on the subjective aspects of social life and people as "pragmatic actors."[4]

One of the key symbolic interactionist theorists who contributed to the field of medical sociology is Canadian-born sociologist Erving Goffman (1922–1982). Because of his interest in how individuals develop their identity through the way in which others view them, he undertook an in-depth observational study of patients' subjective experience in mental institutions. In his book *Asylums* (1961), he described how mental hospitals are "total institutions" in that they contain "a large number of like-situated individuals, cut off from the wider society for an appreciable period of time, [who] together lead an enclosed, formally administered round of life"(1961: xiii). Such institutions thereby controlled large parts of the lives of its inhabitants—including privacy—in a way that damaged their individual self-image, replacing it with an institutionalized one. Patienthood becomes a total way of life for these people and their behaviour is interpreted solely through the lens of their mental illness (Weitz 1996).

In his later work, *Stigma* (1963), Goffman examines what he refers to as the management of a spoiled identity. He describes three main forms of stigma: (1) abominations of the body in the form of physical deformities; (2) blemishes of character in the form of socially deviant behaviour; and (3) groups with minority status in society (Cockerham and Ritchey 1997). A variant of symbolic interactionism following along these studies by Goffman is *labelling theory*, which posits that the impact of labelling a person as ill or deviant means that others will respond to him or her in accordance with that label, which will be very difficult to shed. Labelling theory and Goffman's conceptualization of stigma led to a spate of studies on the stigmatizing features of various illnesses from leprosy to epilepsy (Conrad and Schneider 1980), as well as how stigma can change over time and vary significantly across cultures.

Other examinations from interactionist scholars on the subjective experience of people with illness include Everett Hughes (1971), who proposed the concept of *illness career*. Anselm Strauss and others (1984) similarly conceptualized the illness experience in terms of the work that needed to be accomplished both with respect to their illness and to their everyday life:

> … the various key problems facing the sick persons and their families involve them not only in a variety of different kinds of *work*—crisis work, symptom control work, regimen work—but in a host of other tasks that can for convenience be called comfort work, clinical safety work, the work of preparing for dying, the work of keeping marital relationships, and such. (Strauss et al. 1984: 18)

Other key themes from this literature are the importance of family relations, information awareness and sharing, how illness represents a *biographical disruption* (Bury 1982) and involves the *reconstitution of the self* (Charmaz 1987), and the management of regimens and uncertainty (Conrad 1987).

Just as interactionists have delved into the subjective experience of people suffering from a variety of ailments, they have also examined the experience of health care providers. This began most notably with Becker and colleagues' (1961) treatment of medical socialization in *Boys in White*. In contrast to earlier functionalist perspectives on medical education—best exemplified by Robert Merton and his colleagues (1957) in *The Student Physician* where medical training was oriented toward the mastery of skills and knowledge necessary for practice—Becker argued that medical socialization involved a process of "getting through." Any initial idealism that medical students had toward the practice of medicine quickly shifted to cynicism about their ability to cope with the vast knowledge they were expected to master. Canadian sociologists Jack Haas and William Shaffir (1977) referred to how medical students come to take on a *cloak of competence* as a form of impression management to convince others and themselves that they are competent and confident to face the immense responsibilities of their privileged role.

A related school of thought that emerged out of symbolic interactionism is that of social constructionism. First described by Berger and Luckmann (1967: ii) in the *The Social Construction of Reality*, they argued that "everyday knowledge is creatively produced by individuals and is oriented toward particular practical problems." Thus, social constructionists begin by taking as problematic the very issues that appear to be self-evident. "Facts," they argue, are created by way of social interactions and people's interpretations of these interactions. One of the most popular areas of focus within the social constructionist perspective addressed the social construction of illness, which paralleled a surge in criticisms against biomedicine in the 1970s. The specialty of psychiatry in particular came under intense scrutiny. According to this argument, disease entities do not exist in any objective sense, but are political accomplishments. That is, "disease" is a label that has been successfully applied to particular bodily processes. Thus, all medical "facts" are argued to be socially created products.

Further, medical knowledge is depicted as mediating social relations such that disease categories reinforce existing social structures. Irving Zola (1972) referred to this latter phenomenon as "medicine as an institution of social control." The means by which medicine has come to exert such control is by "'medicalizing' much of daily living and by making medicine and the labels 'healthy' and 'ill' relevant to an ever increasing part of human existence" (Zola 1972: 487).[5] *Medicalization*, accordingly, is defined as the process by which a cluster of symptoms/life events/ deviant behaviour comes to be defined, medically, as a disease (see Box 2.2). Once so defined, responsibility and control lie within the domain of medicine. Conrad and Schneider (1980) describe three levels by which this occurs: (1) at the conceptual level where a medical vocabulary is used to define a problem; (2) at the institutional level where medical personnel supervise treatment organizations or otherwise act as gatekeepers to state benefits; and (3) at the interactional level where physicians actually treat patients' difficulties as medical problems.

Concepts emerging from the symbolic interactionist and social constructionist schools of thought have been very powerful both analytically and in terms of their impact on medical sociology. Many sociology scholars continue to study the illness experience and medicalization process (see discussion in section on feminism below). Conrad and Leiter (2004), for example, still find it a powerful tool to analyze such recent phenomenon as erectile dysfunction and the "wonder drug" Viagra. But as productive as these perspectives have been, they have come under criticism for their tendency to focus on the micro level of analysis and inadequately acknowledge the importance of the macro context (perhaps more applicable for

---

Box 2.2: The Process of Medicalization of Deviance

1. *behaviour is first defined as deviant* before the emergence of a medical definition.
2. *prospecting:* the "discovery" of a medical conception of the disease/deviant behaviour is first announced in a medical journal
3. *claims-making:* both medical and non-medical interests engage in "claims-making" activities to promote the new medical designation
4. *legitimacy:* securing medical turf, which usually involves some type of appeal to the state for recognition of the medical designation
5. *institutionalization* of medical designation in an official medical and/or legal classification system and in the establishment of treatment organizations

Source: Adapted from P. Conrad and J.W. Schneider, *Deviance and Medicalization: From Badness to Sickness* (Philadelphia: Temple University Press, 1992).

---

the social interactionists than the constructionists) and also for its more reflexive stance and elusive treatment of power. Because of these limitations, these theories are considered by some to be more descriptive than explanatory.

Materialism

Sometimes referred to as "conflict theory,"[6] a materialist perspective gives primacy to a macro or structural level of analysis similar to the structural functionalists, but argues that society is based not on consensus but conflict. Social inequality is the primary focus of materialist scholars who derive much of their inspiration from the works of Karl Marx (1818–1883). Marx argued that society is structured into two key social strata: those who own the *means of production* (land, labour, and capital)—*the capitalist class*—and those who do not—the *proletariat*. The capitalist class derives profit (or capital accumulation) from exploiting the labour power of the proletariat—that is, workers are paid less than the value of the product they produce. The pursuit of profit keeps wages low and increases the productivity of workers. Both have clear implications for health.

Vicente Navarro (1976, 1986) is one of the main contemporary theorists who has directly applied Marxist concepts to the study of health and health care. In his focus on the labour process under capitalism, he argues that there is a contradiction between the pursuit of profit and ensuring the safety of workers. That is, the capitalist mode of production actually produces disease (see Figure 2.1), or what some have referred to as the *social production of disease* hypothesis. This could be directly in terms of physical, chemical, or biological pathogens at the workplace or in terms of the stress or risks of accidents as a result of the increasing intensification and fragmentation of work and alienation from the work process. He argues, for example, that "morbidity and mortality are higher among individuals doing routine types of work requiring low levels of skills than among individuals working in jobs that demand a large number of skills and which allow for some type of control over one's own work"(Navarro 1986: 123).

The insights garnered from Navarro's expansion of Marxist concepts have been applied equally to the industrial labour force as well as to certain segments of the

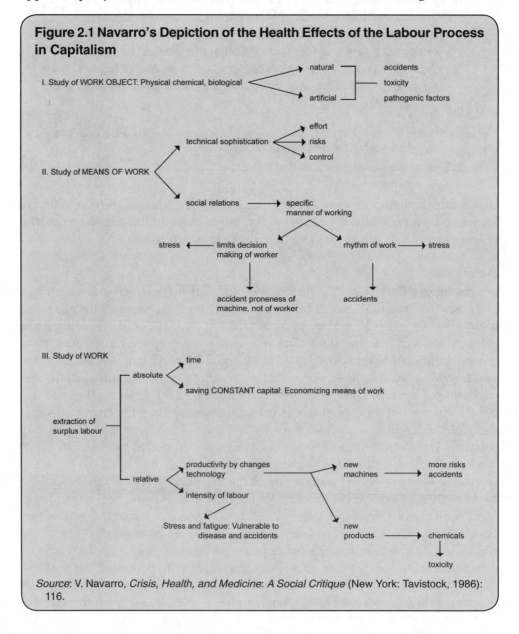

Figure 2.1 Navarro's Depiction of the Health Effects of the Labour Process in Capitalism

Source: V. Navarro, *Crisis, Health, and Medicine: A Social Critique* (New York: Tavistock, 1986): 116.

health labour force. Barbara Ellen Smith (1981), for example, examined the social production of black lung disease, which miners contract in the workplace. She described:

> The instability of the industry frequently resulted in irregular work and a lowering of the piece rate, both of which forced miners to work faster and/or longer hours in an attempt to maintain their standard of living. The impact on health and safety conditions was almost invariably negative, as miners necessarily reduced non-productive, safety-oriented tasks, such as roof timbering, to a minimum. Working longer hours in mines where "towards quitting time [the air] becomes so foul that the miners' lamps will no longer burn" no doubt increased the respiratory disease risk. Moreover, a financially mandated speedup encouraged miners to re-enter their work areas as soon as possible after blasting the coal loose from the face, an operation that generated clouds of dust and powder smoke. (Smith 1981: 345)

Canadian sociologists Novek, Yassi, and Spiegel (1990) make a similar argument in their examination of how the intensification of work in a Canadian meat-packing plant—a direct consequence of the increasing competitiveness in the market—resulted in a dramatic increase in the number and severity of accidents among workers. Workers within the health care system are not immune to these effects. Indeed, the work of Canadian sociologists Pat and Hugh Armstrong (2002) and their colleagues is particularly instructive in this regard. They argue, for example, that the application of management strategies—derived in large part from the private for-profit sector—to the health care system in an effort to control escalating costs resulted in such work intensification that nurses referred to it as a "90-second minute" (Armstrong and Armstrong 2002: 117).[7]

In addition to the negative health impacts of capitalist society on the labour process, the driving down of wages and general economic inequality have also been shown to influence health. Although not explicitly employing a Marxist perspective, many studies of social class differences in health status employ a materialist perspective in the spirit of their arguments. One of the most famous is the 1982 Black Report on inequalities in health (Townsend et al. 1992), which addresses the persistence of class differences in health in Britain despite the supposed "equal access to health services" following the introduction of the National Health Service. In a summary of the Report, Blane (1985) identifies four possible explanations for the differences found (see Box 2.3).

Although the labour process of health care providers is influenced by the logic of capitalism as is any other form of work, materialist scholars note the unique situation that the medical profession holds. For example, although Navarro might agree that the profession of medicine acts as an institution of social control, he argues that it is not the ultimate source of control. His argument in *Medicine under Capitalism* is that "the system of medicine is determined primarily—although not exclusively—by

Box 2.3: Explanation of Social Class Differences in Health Status

1. *Measurement Artifact*:
   - The relationship between social class and health are inherent in the measures (particularly in the measurement of social class).
   - In actuality, this problem may result in an understating of class differences in health rather than an overstatement.
2. *Social Selection*:
   - Also known as the "drift hypothesis," this argues that health affects social mobility and therefore social class, so that those less healthy are less likely to achieve higher levels of social class.
   - Yes, this occurs, but it explains only a minor amount of the differences found and mainly for some diseases in childhood and later life (e.g., schizophrenia).
3. *Cultural/Behavioural*:
   - Gradients in health status are the result of social class differences in behaviours.
   - Yes, but, behaviour cannot be separated from its context; moreover, behaviours are either intervening variables or indicators of structural influences on health.
4. *Materialist*:
   - Class differences in health are the result of social structural differences between the classes (poverty, poor housing, low educational attainment, and the level of business activity) and the competitive character of capitalism.

Source: Adapted from D. Blane, "An Assessment of the Black Report's Explanation of Health Inequalities," *Sociology of Health and Illness* 7(3) (1985): 423-445.

the same forces that determine the overall social formation" (Navarro 1976: vii), that being capitalism. Thus, the power of the medical profession is derivative of the dialectical relationship between capital and medicine specifically in terms of the *congruence* between the ideology of Western biomedicine and the logic of capitalism. The medical ideology of seeing illness in individualistic terms rather than in terms of social and environmental causes is consistent with the ideology of individualism in capitalist society.

The congruence of an individualizing focus on illness arises as a salient issue in Smith's (1981) examination of black lung disease. For example, she describes how it was initially ignored by the medical profession as an *"ordinary* condition that need not cause worry" or in some extreme cases as a form of "malingering," "compensationitis" (Smith 1981: 345). When the cause of black lung came to be identified as respirable coal mine dust, the profession responded with the designation "coal workers' pneumoconiosis," but only for the most severe cases. She argues:

> Medical science's understanding of black lung has not derived from observation unencumbered by a social and economic context, but has been profoundly shaped by that context; as a result, it has performed crucial political and ideological functions. In one era, it served to "normalize" and thereby mask the existence of disease altogether; in the more recent period, it has tended to minimize and individualize the problem. (357)

Overall, studies that apply a materialist perspective have led to new and critical areas of medical sociology inquiry. But some consider Marxism to be a simplistic depiction of society (and it is important to stress that the description herein is a very simplified version of Marxist theory) and others criticize its usefulness in light of the fall of communism (c.f. Turner 1995). Also, because of the macro nature of many of these arguments, they are difficult to test empirically and some argue that data in this case are at best more suggestive than determinative. Many contemporary scholars, however, believe that the basic tenets of his arguments are reaffirmed in the highly stratified class structures in advanced capitalism and in the relations between high- and low-income nations (c.f. Jasso-Aguilar, Waitzkin and Landwehr 2004; Waitzkin 1983). Other theoretical perspectives have grown out of, in response to, or otherwise borrowed from the materialist perspective to examine other social cleavages in society, particularly feminism and anti-racism.

Feminism

Whereas materialism is concerned with social inequity arising from the system of capitalism, feminism is concerned with gender inequalities arising from the system of *patriarchy*. Although "patriarchy" has been used *descriptively* to denote the male-dominated nature of past and present societies, it is also used *analytically* to denote an autonomous system of relations between men and women, comparable to an economic system of production, such as capitalism (Fox 1988). Thus, feminists argue that society is inherently gendered such that men and women have fundamentally different experiences and access to power and that these differences are not natural but socially constructed. By extension, feminists have sought to understand society from the standpoint of women.

Feminists criticize the key theoretical perspectives outlined above—structural functionalism, symbolic interactionism, and conflict theory—for failing to adequately represent or otherwise take into consideration women's perspectives. But at the same time as criticizing these theoretical perspectives, feminists also draw upon and expand upon them with specific reference to the situation and experience of women. For example, some feminist sociologists draw heavily upon symbolic interactionism focusing on women's lived experience. Other feminist theory has conflict elements in it—perhaps best exemplified by radical feminism's assumption that men and women are poised in adversarial positions, that men have power over women, and that society and its various social relationships can be best understood in terms of that situation (Eisenstein 1983).[8] Thus, feminist studies look both at the micro and macro levels of analysis. Canadian feminist sociologist Dorothy Smith's (1993) *institutional ethnography* approach in particular offers us a way to examine the link between the lived experience and what she refers to as the relations of ruling not afforded in theoretical perspectives previously discussed.

Feminism has been a particularly influential perspective in medical sociology. This is perhaps most evident in the spate of studies examining the medicalization of women's bodies and women's lives. This began with criticisms of the medicalization of pregnancy and childbirth, which helped foster an entire social movement toward normalizing birth and in some cases radicalizing it through the home birth movement (Ehrenreich and English 1973; Oakley 1984):

> … we treat childbirth not as a natural event of great significance, but as an illness. We place the expectant mother in a hospital, otherwise assigned to the care of the ill, induce weakness and dependency in her by the use of drugs, straps and soon isolate her from her husband and other children just as we isolate the sick and the dying.… This classification of childbirth with illness has a great variety of repercussions all through our culture, some of which we are now attempting to correct. (F.D. MacGregor, *Social Science in Nursing*, p. 80, as cited in McKinlay 1972: 565)

With similar fervour, Frances McCrea (1983) teased apart the sexual politics involved in the medicalization of the menopause. She describes how menopause was "discovered" as a disease of deficiency in the late 1960s following the development of a synthetic form of estrogen. Estrogen-replacement therapy promised women that they could avoid the menopause completely and stay "feminine forever." McCrea describes four pervasive themes in the medical definitions of the menopause: "1) women's potential and function are biologically destined; 2) women's worth is determined by fecundity and attractiveness; 3) rejection of the feminine role will bring physical and emotional havoc; [and] 4) aging women are useless and repulsive" (1983: 111). Her primary argument, therefore, is that the menopause as disease designation is intricately linked to women's role in society.

Another key focus of feminist medical sociological studies is regarding the predicament of female health care providers. Irene Butter and her colleagues (1987), for example, argue that one of the most notable features of the health care division of labour is its segregation by gender—both within and among professions— assigning a secondary status to women. The subordination of nursing in particular is problematized. In her historical examination of nursing work, Susan Reverby (1987) introduces the concept of the *caring dilemma*, which she describes as the imposition upon nurses of a duty to care in a society that devalues the care that they provide both socially and financially. Caring is considered to be a natural extension of women's roles as wives and mothers and not an esoteric skill worthy of professional status. In *Professions and Patriarchy*, Anne Witz (1990, 1992: 677) argues that there is nothing natural about the subordination of nurses, but rather it is directly related to the "differential access to the tactical means of achieving their aims in a patriarchal society within which male power is institutionalized."

Not only is the subordination of female care providers highlighted in the feminist medical sociology literature but their exclusion as well, most notably the decline of midwifery in North America (Biggs 1983; Wertz and Wertz 1979). These discussions created synergies with the literature problematizing the conceptualization of pregnancy and childbirth as an illness discussed above. For example, Ehrenreich and English (1973) argue that the medicalization of women's bodies—thereby promoting the notion of women's frailty—not only qualified them as natural patients, but also disqualified them as dependable health care practitioners. Many feminists specifically argued that patriarchal society's control over the reproduction process was oppressive (O'Brien 1981) and many called for the legitimation of midwifery as a way for women to have more control over the birth process. That is, as reproductive choice and control became central concerns in the feminist movement, midwifery came to be seen as one component of reproductive choice and as a tool for the liberation of women (Rushing 1993).

Thus, in many ways, feminist medical sociology has at least attempted to connect the social structural aspects of patriarchy to the lived experience of women as both providers and recipients of care more explicitly than other sociological perspectives applied to health, illness, and health care. In so doing, it has afforded particularly important insights to the field as a whole. But medical sociological studies from a feminist perspective have also suffered from some of the limitations of early feminist theory more broadly—namely, that it has tended to neglect the particular concerns of working-class women and women of colour. Patricia Hill Collins (1990), for example, argues that African-American women have a unique perspective to offer. More recently, feminists have begun to take up the challenge of these criticisms and have begun to analyze the ways that the effects of gender intersect with class and race for broader understandings of women's health and health care experiences.[9]

Anti-racism and Post-colonialism

Another key social cleavage that causes us to look beyond the influence of class and gender is a focus on race. Although many scholars who focus on the impact of race on health and health care have drawn from a conflict or materialist perspective, some have begun to develop theories addressing issues specific to the structure and experience of race and racism. Anti-racism is one of these perspectives that attempts to uncover the particular structural determinants of racism within society (Dei

1996).[10] Although we commonly consider racism to be an expression of individual prejudice, it is also structured into the very nature of our society. Thus, just as feminists have argued that social structures, ideology, and our everyday experiences are fundamentally gendered, anti-racism scholars argue that they are also *racialized*. As Canadian race scholar Sheryl Nestel (1996/1997) summarizes:

> The term "racialized" is used … to signal that race is a historically and socially constructed category of differentiation and not in any way a "natural" one. "Racialization" then can be seen as a process through which racial significance comes to be conferred upon a wide range of human attributes. (Nestel 1996/1997: 316)

The ultimate process of racializing groups is for unequal treatment (Dei 1996).

A related perspective to the anti-racism school of thought is *post-colonialism*. The main problematic in post-colonial studies is the broader global and historical relations between societies that have been colonized and the colonizer. The link to anti-racism is due to the fact that the sizable majority of colonized societies are also societies of peoples disproportionately of colour. In fact, post-colonial scholars argue that the concept of race was particularly tied to the colonial and imperial expansion activities of Western European powers in the 17th century (Castagna and Dei 2000), which distanced the colonizer from the colonized and in essence created "the other." Post-colonial studies, therefore, attempt to increase our knowledge about "the other," giving them voice and understanding the effects of displacement.

Anti-racism and post-colonialism perspectives are relative newcomers in comparison to the others discussed here, so their full impact on the field of medial sociology has yet to be determined. Whether explicitly drawing from an anti-racism perspective—as it has come to be defined—or not, there have been an increasing number of studies of race differences in health status and inquiries focusing on the racialized experiences of both recipients and providers of care. This is clearly exemplified in studies of the health status of First Nations peoples in Canada and the decimation of their traditional health practices and systems of care following European contact (c.f. Frideres 1994; Wotherspoon 1994). Specifically, it is consistently found that First Nations Canadians have lower life expectancy, higher infant mortality, and higher mortality rates in general, especially in early ages. Causes of death and illness patterns for First Nations peoples reflect those associated with poverty and inadequate standards of living, but systemic and structured racism is the ultimate cause of these social and economic circumstances.

Colonization has also had an impact on local systems of care. Specifically, some of the "exports" that Europeans brought to the "colonies" were training programs in Western medicine and nursing. This enabled the establishment of health care systems modelled after the colonizing countries. But the "Third World" debt crisis has more recently led to the decimation of these fledgling health care system and massive migrations of local health care professionals to high-income countries.

Ishi (1987), for example, outlines that some of the key factors explaining migration patterns include the demands of the service economy in high-income countries; their cultural, political, military, and economic hegemony over low-income countries; and immigrants' experience of uncertainty over their futures in their native land. He continues to describe how high-income countries benefit from hiring immigrant professional labour both economically (in terms of labour) and politically (in terms of its country's apparent attractiveness). Once in their new countries, immigrant health care providers, particularly those of colour, experience both implicit and explicit forms of racism in terms of barriers to access in practising their profession (Nestel 1996/1997) and status of position (c.f. Calliste 1996).

Postmodernism

Postmodernism, which is alternately referred to by some as *post-structuralism*, is a theoretical perspective developed largely out of French philosophical thought often associated with the works of Jacques Derrida, Jean Baudrillard, and most notably Michel Foucault. Whereas materialists, some feminist, and anti-racist scholars encourage us to look more critically at macro-structural conditions of society, postmodernists critique any attempt to create any macro theory of society. They argue instead for the importance of subjectivism and microsociological analysis and, consistent with symbolic interactionism and social constructionism, stress cultural relativism and a plurality of viewpoints.[11] In line with this argument, these scholars stress that there is no "truth" that can be uncovered or known—only different knowledges that can vary tremendously over time.

In a series of books, *Madness and Civilization* (1971), *The Birth of the Clinic* (1973), *Discipline and Punish* (1977), and *The History of Sexuality* (1979), Foucault traced the historical changes in societal attitudes toward punishment, mental illness, and sexuality stressing the disciplinary nature of knowledge and power (which he referred to as *pouvoir/savoir* to denote that they were one and the same).[12] What is particularly applicable to medical sociology from Foucault's work is his focus on how medical knowledge and discourse have been used to control the body through various systems of surveillance in the supposed broader interests of society (Cockerham and Ritchey 1997) or what Turner (1992) coined "the government of the body." As Bryan Turner (1995) states:

[T]he works of Foucault ha[ve] radical implications for medical sociology. We can no longer regard "diseases" as natural events in the world which occur outside the language with which they are described. A disease entity is the product of medical discourses which in turn reflect the dominant mode of thinking ... within society. For example, homosexuality was regarded as a sin under Christian therapy, as a behavioural disorder by early psychology and as merely sexual preference by contemporary medicine. (Turner 1995: 11)

Intricately connected with the increasing *governance* of the body is the focus of the medical profession. For example, in *The Birth of the Clinic*, Foucault described how medicine shifted its view of the body from patients' descriptions of their maladies toward direct clinical observations and physical examinations or what he referred to as the "clinical gaze." Access to this kind of "scientific" knowledge of the body gave physicians considerable power to define health and illness and by extension measures of moral regulation and social control (Turner 1995). Terence Johnson (1995) has also extended Foucault's notion of governmentality by describing how the medical profession has become constitutive of the state and, because of this institutionalization of expertise, is involved in the government of citizens.

A more focused analysis of the body is thus what a postmodernist perspective can bring to medical sociology—something that many authors argue has been heretofore inadequately addressed and in fact considered potentially threatening (Armstrong 1983). Turner (1995: 3) states emphatically that "an adequate medical sociology would require a sociology of the body, since it is only by developing a notion of social embodiment that we can begin adequately to criticise the conventional divisions between mind and body, individual and society." Indeed, a postmodernist perspective has permeated other perspectives described here, most notably feminism. It is anticipated that through this lens a more thorough understanding of the medicalization and regulation of women's bodies can be afforded.

In spite of the opportunities that postmodernism entails for medical sociology, others have cautioned about its limitations. For example, it is not clear how or where the space for resistance to insidious regulation and governance can occur—as indeed it has (Turner 1995). Materialists also criticize that such a relativist position serves only to obscure the relationship between discourse and the materialist conditions of society in the social constructionist phenomenon.[13]

Conclusions

To conclude this brief overview of the key sociological perspectives on health, illness, and health care, it is important to stress how more recent theory has been built upon earlier theories by both expanding upon and in many cases critiquing their assumptions. Studies of the illness experience and medicalization were in part a response to Parsons's sick role concept and provided a more diverse foil to his portrayal. Materialism and conflict theory were also in direct contrast to the consensus-based assumption of functionalism just as postmodernism later emerged as critical of materialism. This dynamic debate has been the way the discipline has moved forward.

It is also important to garner from this review that the point should not be to debate which level of analysis—macro or micro—is most important as both are and, furthermore, are intricately connected. That is, medical sociology is strongest when it is cognizant of the importance of all levels of analysis. As Coburn and Eakin (1998) noted in their review of Canadian medical sociology:

Much of what sociology is all about as an intellectual enterprise concerns the tension between human actions and social structural constraints and opportunities. The discipline is thus characterized by dichotomy: human agency versus social structure; voluntarism versus determinism; "micro" versus "macro" level phenomena. Yet common to all of these positions is the view that phenomena involving human action, including that regarding health and health care, is the product of social interrelationships. (Coburn and Eakin 1998: 84)

The key approach to take is one that is critical of common and often unquestioned assumptions of how society is and ought to be and in doing so focus on the centrality of power.

References

Armstrong, D. (1983). *Political Anatomy of the Body: Medical Knowledge in Britain in the Twentieth Century.* Cambridge: Cambridge University Press.

Armstrong, P., and H. Armstrong. (2002). *Wasting Away,* 2nd ed. Toronto: Oxford University Press.

Becker, H.S., B. Geer, E.C. Hughes, and A.L. Strauss. (1961). *Boys in White: Student Culture in Medical School.* Chicago: University of Chicago Press.

Berger, P., and T. Luckmann. (1967). *The Social Construction of Reality.* Garden City: Doubleday.

Biggs, C.L. (1983). "The Case of the Missing Midwives: A History of Midwifery in Ontario from 1795–1900." *Ontario History* 65(1): 21–35.

Blane, D. (1985). "An Assessment of the Black Report's Explanation of Health Inequalities." *Sociology of Health and Illness* 7(3): 423–445.

Bloom, S. (2002). *The Word as Scalpel: A History of Medical Sociology.* New York: Oxford University Press.

Brannon, R.L. (1994). *Intensifying Care: The Hospital Industry, Professionalization, and the Reorganization of the Nursing Labor Process.* New York: Baywood.

Bury, M. (1982). "Chronic Illness as Biographical Disruption." *Sociology of Health and Illness* 4: 167–182.

Butter, I.H., E.S. Carpenter, B.J. Kay, and R.S. Simmons. (1987). "Gender Hierarchies in the Health Labour Force." *International Journal of Health Services* 17(1): 133–149.

Calliste, A. 1996. "Antiracism Organizing and Resistance in Nursing: African Canadian Women." *The Canadian Review of Sociology and Anthropology* 33(3): 361–390.

Castagna, M., and G.S. Dei. (2000). "An Historical Overview of the Appliation of the Race Concept in Social Practice." In *Anti-racist Feminism: Critical Race and Gender Studies,* edited by A. Calliste and G.S. Dei, 19–38. Halifax: Fernwood.

Charmaz, K. (1987). "Struggling for a Self: Identity Levels of the Chronically Ill. The Experience and Management of Chronic Illness." In *Research in the Sociology of Health Care,* edited by J.A. Roth and P. Conrad, 283–321. Greenwich: JAI Press.

Coburn, D., and J.M. Eakin. (1998). "The Sociology of Health in Canada." In *Health and Canadian Society: Sociological Perspectives,* 3rd ed., edited by D. Coburn, C. D'Arcy, and G. Torrance, 619–634. Toronto: University of Toronto Press.

Cockerham, W., and F. Ritchey. (1997). *Dictionary of Medical Sociology.* Westport: Greenwood.

Collins, P.H. (1990). *Black Feminist Thought.* New York: Routledge.

Conrad, P. (1975). "The Discovery of Hyperkinesis: Notes on the Medicalization of Deviant Behavior." *Social Problems* 23(1): 12–21.

———. (1987). "The Experience of Illness: Recent and New Directions. The Experience and Management of Chronic Illness." In *Research in the Sociology of Health Care,* edited by J.A. Roth and P. Conrad, 6: 1–31. Greenwich: JAI Press.

Conrad, P., and J.W. Schneider. (1980). "A Theoretical Statement on the Medicalization of Deviance." In *Deviance and Medicalization: From Badness to Sickness,* edited by P. Conrad and J.W. Schneider, 261–276. St. Louis: C.V. Mosby.

Conrad, P. and J.W. Schneider (1992). *Deviance and Medicalization: From Badness to Sickness.* Philadelphia: Temple University Press.

Conrad, P. and V. Leiter (2004). "Medicalization, Markets, and Consumers." *Journal of Health and Social Behaviour* 45 (Supplement 1): 158-176.

Dei, G.J.S. (1996). "Critical Perspectives in Antiracism: An Introduction." *Canadian Review of Sociology and Anthropology* 33(3): 247–267.

Ehrenreich, B., and D. English. (1973). *Witches, Midwives and Nurses.* New York: Feminist Press at CUNY.

Eisenstein, H. (1983). *Contemporary Feminist Thought.* Boston: G.K. Hall & Co.

Foucault, M. (1971). *Madness and Civilization.* New York: Pantheon.

———. (1973). *The Birth of the Clinic.* New York: Pantheon.

———. (1977). *Discipline and Punish.* New York: Pantheon.

———. (1979). *The History of Sexuality: An Introduction.* Harmondsworth: Penguin.

Fox, B. (1988). "Conceptualizing 'Patriarchy.'" *Canadian Review of Sociology and Anthropology* 25(2): 163–181.

Frideres, J.S. (1994). "Racism and Health: Case of the Native People." In *Health, Illness, and Health Care in Canada,* 2nd ed., edited by B. Singh Bolaria and H. Dickinson, 202–220. Toronto: Harcourt Brace.

Goffman, E. (1961). *Asylums: Essays on the Social Situation of Mental Patients and Other Inmates.* Garden City: Anchor.

———. (1963). *Stigma: Notes on the Management of Spoiled Identity.* Englewood Cliffs: Prentice Hall.

Haas, J., and W. Shaffir. (1977). "The Professionalization of Medical Students: Developing Competence and a Cloak of Competence." *Symbolic Interaction* 1: 71–88.

Hughes, E.C. (1971). *The Sociological Eye: Selected Papers on Institutions and Race.* Aldine: Chicago.

Ishi, T. (1987). "Class Conflict, the State, and Linkage: Migration of Nurses from the Philippines." *Berkeley Journal of Sociology* 37(1): 281–312.

Jary, D., and J. Jary. (1991). *The Harper Collins Dictionary of Sociology.* New York: HarperCollins.

Jasso-Aguilar, Waitzkin, Landwehr. (2004) "Multinational Corporations and Health Care in the United States and Latin America: Strategies, Actions, and Effects." *Journal of Health and Social Behaviour* 45(1): 136–157.

Johnson, T.J. (1995). "Governmentality and the Institutionalization of Expertise." *Health Professions and the State in Europe,* edited by T. Johnson, G. Larkin, and M. Saks, 7–24. London and New York: Routledge.

Kaufert, P. (1982). "Myth and the Menopause." *Sociology of Health and Illness* 4(2): 141–166.

Lachmann, R. (1991). *The Encyclopedic Dictionary of Sociology*, 4th ed. Guilford: The Dushkin Publishing Group.

Matcha, D. (2000). *Medical Sociology*. Boston: Allyn and Bacon.

McCrea, F. (1983). "The Politics of Menopause: The 'Discovery' of a Deficiency Disease." *Social Problems* 31(1): 111–123.

McKinlay, J. (1972). "The Sick Role—Illness and Pregnancy." *Social Science and Medicine* 6: 561–572.

Mechanic, D., and E.H. Volkart. (1960). "Illness Behavior and Medical Diagnosis." *Journal of Health and Human Behavior* 1(2): 86–93.

Merton, R.K., G.G. Reader, and P.L. Kendall, eds. (1957). *The Student Physician: Introductory Studies in the Sociology of Medical Education*. Boston: Harvard University Press.

Navarro, V. (1976). *Medicine under Capitalism*. New York: Prodist.

_____. (1986). *Crisis, Health and Medicine: A Social Critique*. London: Tavistock.

Nestel, S. (1996/1997). "'A New Profession to the White Population in Canada': Ontario Midwifery and the Politics of Race." *Health and Canadian Society* 4(2): 315–341.

Novek, J., A. Yassi, and J. Spiegel. (1990). "Mechanization, the Labor Process, and Injury Risks in the Canadian Meat Packing Industry." *International Journal of Health Services* 20(2): 281-296.

Oakley, A. (1984). *The Captured Womb: A History of the Medical Care of Pregnant Women*. Oxford: Basil Blackwell.

O'Brien, M. (1981). *The Politics of Reproduction*. Boston: Routledge and Kegan Paul.

Parsons, T. (1951). *The Social System*. New York: The Free Press.

Reverby, S. (1987). *Ordered to Care*. Cambridge: Cambridge University Press.

Rushing, B. (1993). "Ideology in the Re-emergence of North American Midwifery." *Work and Occupations* 20: 46–67.

Smith, B.E. (1981). "Black Lung: The Social Production of Disease." *International Journal of Health Services* 11(3): 343–359.

Smith, D. (1993). *Texts, Facts and Femininity: Exploring the Relations of Ruling*. London: Routledge.

Strauss, A.L., J. Corbin, S. Fagerhaugh, B.G. Glaser, D. Maines, B. Suczek, and C.L. Weiner. (1984). *Chronic Illness and the Quality of Life*, 2nd ed. St. Louis: Mosby.

Strauss, R. (1957). "The Nature and Status of Medical Sociology." *American Sociological Review* 22: 200–204.

Szasz, J., and M. Hollender. (1956). "The Basic Models of the Doctor-Patient Relationship." *Archives of Internal Medicine* 97: 585–592.

Townsend, P. N. Davidson, and M. Whitehead, eds. (1992). *Inequalities in Health: The Black Report and the Health Divide*. New York: Penguin.

Turner, B. (1995). *Medical Power and Social Knowledge*, 2nd ed. Newbury Park, CA: Sage.

Turner, B.S. (1992). *Regulating Bodies: Essays in Medical Sociology*. London: Routledge.

Twaddle, A.C. (1969). "Health Decisions and Sick Role Variations: An Exploration." *Journal of Health and Social Behavior* 10(2): 105–114.

Waitzkin, H. (1983). *The Second Sickness: Contradictions of Capitalist Health Care*. New York: The Free Press.

Weitz, R. (1996). *The Sociology of Health, Illness and Health Care: A Critical Approach*. New York: Wadsworth Publishing Co.

Wertz, R.W., and D.C. Wertz. (1979). *Lying in: A History of Childbirth in America*. New York: Schocken Books.

Witz, A. (1990). "Patriarchy and Professions: The Gendered Politics of Occupational Closure." *Sociology* 24(4): 675-690.

_____. (1992). *Professions and Patriarchy*. New York: Routledge.

Wotherspoon, T. (1994). "Colonization, Self-Determination, and the Health of Canada's First Nations Peoples." In *Racial Minorities, Medicine and Health*, edited by B.S. Bolaria and R. Bolaria, 247–267. Halifax: Fernwood.

Zola, I. (1972). "Medicine as an Institution of Social Control: The Medicalization of Society." *The Sociology Review* 20(4): 487–504.

Notes

1. www.britannica.com/eb/article?tocId=222951
2. www.changesurfer.com/Hlth/DPReview.html
3. I would like to thank Dorothy Pawluch for her insightful comments on this section.
4. http://web.grinnell.edu/courses/soc/s00/soc111-01/IntroTheories/Symbolic.html
5. It is important to point out that in some instances groups who suffer from a particular ailment seek medical distinction; this has been argued to be the case for alcoholism.
6. Though this term could also be used to denote studies of power from a Weberian perspective (Cockerham and Ritchey 1997).
7. For an expanded discussion of this, see chapter 11 in this volume. See also Brannon (1994) on the intensification of care and the reorganization of the nursing labour force in the U.S.
8. http://home.earthlink.net/~ahunter/RFvSoc/conflict.html
9. http://web.grinnell.edu/courses/soc/s00/soc111-01/IntroTheories/Other.html
10. See also B.S. Bolaria and P.S. Li, "Theories and Policies of Racial Discrimination," in *Racial Oppression in Canada*, 2nd ed., edited by B.S. Bolaria and P. Li, 27–40 (Toronto: Garamond Press, 1988); and G.J.S. Dei, L.L. Karumanchery, and N. Karumanchery-Luik, (eds.) *Playing the Race Card: Exposing White Power and Privilege* (New York: Peter Lang, 2003).
11. www.cfmc.com/adamb/writings/marxpost.htm
12. http://web.grinnell.edu/courses/soc/s00/soc111-01/IntroTheories/Other.html#PoMo
13. www.cfmc.com/adamb/writings/marxpost.htm

• •

Critical Thinking Questions

1. What are some events outside of medical sociology that may have influenced the particular trajectory of perspectives outlined here?
2. What is the difference between the social production and the social construction of disease? Are these two perspectives mutually exclusive?
3. How might we best reconcile micro perspectives on illness experience with macro perspectives on structural influences on health and illness?

4. What are some key questions about the social and structural nature of health, illness, and health care that remain to be uncovered in new emerging perspectives?

Further Readings

Books

Albrecht, G.L., R. Fitzpatrick, and S. Scrimshaw, eds. (2000). *Handbook of Social Studies in Health and Medicine.* Thousand Oaks: Sage.
This is an international reader highlighting the key debates within medical sociology.

Coburn, D., C. D'Arcy, and G. Torrance, eds. (1998). *Health and Canadian Society: Sociological Perspectives*, 3rd ed. Toronto: University of Toronto Press.
This is a key Canadian reader that exemplifies the range of sociological studies of health, illness, and health care undertaken in the Canadian context.

Conrad, P., and R. Kern, eds. (1986). *The Sociology of Health and Illness: Critical Perspectives*, 2nd ed. New York: St. Martin's Press.
This is a key American reader that touches upon the range of medical sociology issues and debates primarily from a U.S. perspective.

Scambler, G., ed. (1987). *Sociological Theory and Medical Sociology.* New York: Tavistock.
This classic links medical sociology and mainstream sociology, and stimulates other social scientists to do the same.

Turner, B. (1995). *Medical Power and Social Knowledge*, 2nd ed. Thousand Oaks, CA: Sage.
An excellent text that covers a range of medical sociological issues from the various perspectives described herein.

_____. (2004). *The New Medical Sociology: Social Forms of Health and Illness.* New York: Norton.
The latest text on medical sociology, which represents the state of the art with a heavy focus on the postmodernist perspective.

Journals

Health and Canadian Society includes key social science and health articles within a Canadian context.
International Journal of Health Services is particularly for studies from a materialist perspective.

Journal of Health and Social Behavior tends to focus on U.S. studies.
Research in the Sociology of Health Care is published once yearly around key themes.
Social Science and Medicine is an international journal incorporating a variety of social scientific perspectives on health, illness, and health care.

Sociology of Health and Illness, the journal of the British Medical Sociology group, leans more toward theoretical articles and those from a critical interactionist or constructionist perspective.
Women and Health focuses on studies of health, illness, and health care organization and provision from a feminist perspective, broadly defined.

Relevant Web Sites

American Sociology Association, Medical Sociology Section
http://dept.kent.edu/sociology/asamedsoc/
    The Medical Sociology Section, one of the ASA's largest sections, brings together social and behavioural scientists from a variety of backgrounds who share an interest in the social contexts of health, illness, and health care. Central topics include the subjective experience of health and illness; political, economic, and environmental circumstances that threaten health; and societal forces that impact on the medical care system and on people's responses to illness.

Faculty of Social Sciences at the University of Amsterdam
http://www2.fmg.uva.nl/sociosite/topics/health.html
    The SocioSite is a project based at the Faculty of Social Sciences at the University of Amsterdam. It presents the resources and information that are important for the international sociological scene. It links students of sociology to many interesting, sociologically relevant locations in cyberspace. The SocioSite is a tool kit for social scientists. It contains high-quality resources and texts that can be used as wheels for the sociological mind.

Health Sociology site of the Australian Sociological Association
www.latrobe.edu.au/telehealth/esochealth/
    This Web site takes advantage of the increasing communications capabilities of the Internet to foster a community of health social scientists whose interests lie in the social and cultural aspects of health and illness and to broaden the resource base of its members. The community is not restricted to Australian members as witnessed by the occasional sections on New Zealand news and contributions from health social scientists abroad.

Medical Sociology Group of the British Sociological Association
www.britsoc.co.uk/bsaweb.php?area=item2&link_id=55
Founded in 1951, the group's members are drawn from a wide range of backgrounds—research, teaching, and students and practitioners in a variety of fields. The BSA provides a network of communication to all who are concerned with the promotion and use of sociology and sociological research.

Glossary

Anti-racism: An analytical perspective that attempts to uncover the structural determinants of racism within society.

Congruence thesis: Argues that the power of the medical profession is derivative from capital due in large part to the congruence between the individualistic focus of Western biomedicine and the ideology of individualism in capitalist society.

Governance: The way that medical knowledge and discourse have been used to control or regulate the body through various systems of surveillance.

Medicalization: The process by which a cluster of symptoms/life events/deviant behaviour comes to be defined, medically, as a disease.

Patriarchy: Denotes an autonomous system of relations between men and women, comparable to an economic system of production.

Sociology in medicine: The study of medical or health-related problems through the application of sociology with an orientation toward improving care or formulating policy.

Sociology of medicine: The study of societal or sociological problems through the lens of health-related issues, medical settings, or the organization of health care with an orientation of advancing sociological theory or concepts.

CHAPTER THREE

HEALTH AND HEALTH CARE

A Political Economy Perspective

David Coburn

Learning Objectives

At the conclusion of this chapter, the reader will be able to
- present a materialist political economy approach to health issues
- analyze the influence of neo-liberalism on health and health care
- explain phases of capitalism and types of welfare state
- identify basic structural causes of health status differences among nations
- explain differences in health care systems between Canada and the United States

Introduction

This chapter is about a critical political economy perspective on health. What does this mean and entail? One way of understanding a political economy approach to health is to see what kinds of questions such a view would pose. Political economists ask such questions as: Why do some people, groups, nations, or groups of nations have better health than others? Why is it that some groups or societies have different kinds of health care systems than others? How much inequality in health and access to health care is there and why are there these inequalities? What is defined as healthy and what is defined as sick in particular kinds of society and what do people do about these states? How do all these things vary historically and across nations or societies? The unique point of view of political economy is that it focuses on the links between health and the economic, political, and social life of different people, regions, or societies.

In this chapter, following the general questions noted above, I ask specific questions regarding health and health care: Why does the United States, one of the richest nations in the world, have one of the poorest health records of any of the developed nations? Why are there increasing health inequalities within and among the developed nations? And why does Canada have a national insurance system and the United States a private system? Illustrative data are provided on health and health care internationally.

The implication of "a" political economy is that there are actually a variety of political economies. The version presented in this chapter is a major stream within political economy, but not the only one. The approach is materialist, in the sense of viewing ideas and institutions as emerging from how a society organizes production, and uses such concepts as mode of production and class. I hope to open a window on the world that can transform the way we see the world and how societies work.

It is a *critical* political economy because inherent in the approach taken is the notion that people within a society may or may not have an accurate idea of how their society actually works. If a political economy approach has validity, it can challenge (be critical about) current perceptions, beliefs, ideologies, and ideas and also contribute to asking questions about how things could be different. Hence, the critical component.

This chapter constitutes a critique of the currently dominant view of how the world works—that is, neo-liberalism. Neo-liberalism arose in the developed world in the 1970s. At its most basic, neo-liberalism asserts that free enterprise policies produce economic growth, which in turn is the basis for all human well-being. Thus, "free" trade both within and among nations will improve human welfare. The contrary view taken here is that free-enterprise politics and policies in fact tend to undercut the social bases for well-functioning economies—economies are embedded within social contexts, hence neo-liberal claims that their policies produce long-run economic growth are suspect. But, in addition, the evidence indicates that high gross national product is not at all highly related to well-functioning societies and to human well-being. The neo-liberal paradigm is simply incorrect. In what follows I will show an alternative way of looking at the world to that of the dominant neo-liberal orthodoxy by pointing to its major problems and by arguing that, in a capitalist world, less "capitalist" (less neo-liberal) systems are better than pure "neo-liberal" ones.

The stream within political economy described here is materialist. Being materialist does not mean examining only the influence of concrete objects, nor does it mean ignoring the role of ideas (idealism being the opposite of materialism). What it does mean is that whereas idealism gives primacy to the role of ideas in history, materialism gives more basic explanatory primacy to the way people live than to the ideas they produce. While materialists believe ideas are important, and may be crucial, they nevertheless think that the world shapes ideas more than ideas shape the world.

Within a materialist point of view, some ideas can simply be "before (or perhaps after) their time" in the sense that these ideas do not resonate with the way people live. Ideas, like seeds being planted, have to find fertile ground and the right conditions before they will thrive. There may be many good reasons for having social housing or a national health care or national health insurance system, but unless these ideas are supported by groups with enough resources to transform them into actual action, they will remain simply ideas.

The emphasis on context is supported by a processual rather than a static view of social life. That is, we who produce ideas are all products of our upbringing in a particular kind of society at a particular time—social structure or society comes first, then our own subjectivities, identities, or "selves." We do not create the societies or institutions within which we find ourselves, we reproduce, modify, or transform already existing structures. Our own most unique ideas and beliefs are, somehow, based on the fact that we were born, brought up, and socialized in a specific family, group, area, society, civilization. Different social formations or nations—Canada, Sweden, China, the United States—produce different (but also somewhat similar) kinds of people. The type of society of which we are a part shapes, enables, and constrains everything within it, including what people want, consider desirable, or worth sacrificing, even dying, for. If we are all shaped by our existing society, and if the social formations of which we are a part also enable and constrain what we do and what is possible, it is important to understand what "type" of society we live in.

The orientation of this chapter is materialist. Historical materialism argues that social formations reflect the predominant way in which goods and services are produced and the social relations that accompany such production. Our present social formation is characterized by a capitalist mode of production, hence, from our materialist perspective, the result is not only a particular way of producing goods and services but also a particular type of distinctively capitalist society.

Capitalism influences everything within a capitalist social formation—from the beliefs people have, to what they consider desirable, to prevalent ideas, to politics, to social life—either very directly or more indirectly. Capitalism is also characterized by the predominant power of those who own and control the means of production. Ownership of the means of production confers power. Ownership not only gives the power to make investments where, when, and with whom owners of capital want, but also to control those who work for them. This power, however, also extends outside of work and the economy to an influence on the media, politics, the state, and the type of society we have generally, but it also fundamentally limits what is possible.

We are reminded, over and over, that "free speech" is a fundamental characteristic of democratic capitalism. Yet the ability to shape the media, through ownership or the power of advertisers, through setting up think-tanks to promulgate a particular point of view, to an influence on political life and political parties that is widely acknowledged, marks owners off from others. For example, I am writing this chapter in British Columbia, the western-most province in Canada. B.C. has two major cities,

Vancouver and Victoria. CanWest Global, a single Canadian corporation with a conservative ideology, not only owns the three major newspapers in these two cities, hence in British Columbia, but also controls one of the two national newspapers and numerous small community newspapers as well as a television network. Incidentally, the "other" national newspaper is also conservative in orientation. The media as much shapes public opinion and events as reflects these. Hence, hundreds of thousands of more progressive people in B.C. have no real public outlet in which to express their interests and ideas. The formal right of free speech is contradicted by vastly unequal access to actually having a public voice.

Thus, there is a tension between capitalism and democracy. While the latter assumes most are approximately equal in opportunities to influence events, the former ensures that some have much more chance of doing so than do others. We may all have one vote, but it is simply not true that I have as much political influence or power as does Bill Gates. Even when we confront the law as citizens, law supposedly being the formal bastion of equality, the idea that I and General Motors are both citizens and therefore on equal terms in court is not really true given GM's ability to hire platoons of expert lawyers, to draw on relatively unlimited funds, etc. While democracy asserts power equality, capitalism produces inequality. *Capitalists preach democracy, but practise power.* We must distinguish formal claims to democracy and equality from the ability to actually enact these claims.

A major tendency within political economy is to see different groups or classes as having inherently contradictory views or interests and capitalism itself as characterized by contradictions and specific trends. A major contradiction is that individual owners want to drive down wages of their own workers, yet capital in general needs workers to have purchasing power to buy the goods they produce. In this instance what is good for individual owners is not good for owners as a whole. And, ironically, while capitalists preach the virtues of competition, the inherent tendency of markets is for owners to enact monopolies or oligopolies in particular market sectors. These contradictions and tendencies, and the way work is organized into huge enterprises, facilitates groups, workers, and others with interests in opposing capitalist power and, eventually, the capitalist system itself.

Capitalists are not just people who own consumer goods. Possessing a house, televisions, etc., does not a capitalist make. Capitalists are those people who make most of their money through the labour of others—they employ others and make money from their work—they pay their workers less than the amounts for which they can sell the goods or services that these workers produce. They appropriate societal surplus, but in a different and somewhat more hidden manner than the way feudal lords appropriated the surplus produced by their serfs. Thus, the division of society into classes of people who have different interests—capitalists and others. Yet the ideology of capitalism is supremely individualist rather than class or collectivity oriented. We are, according to neo-liberalism, our own products; what happens to us is entirely due to our own efforts and the greatest good is that which frees individuals from any constraints. But, as we have noted, markets ensure that, in fact, those with more money and power are much more equal than those without such resources—the ideology is contradicted by life's realities. Moreover, the notion that capitalists are all self-made is not compatible with the inheritance of capacities and resources, or with the fact that much of what helps or enables people to do things—education, transportation, communications, infrastructure—are collectively rather than individually constructed. While capitalists have power both within the economy and outside it, they do not want to acknowledge either their reliance on social resources as the foundation of their enterprises and profits, nor the effects their own policies have on society at large. Whether social problems arise from low wages, unemployment, or pollution from which some make profits while others suffer health effects, capitalists have wide powers but narrow accountability.

A good example of power inequalities is regarding the role of the state. A neo-liberal or pluralist interest group analysis views states or governments as more or less equally responsive to many different organized groups. But a political economy approach argues that many important decisions are not even within state purview—for example, the decision to invest in a particular area or industry or not (decisions taken by private business owners). The state is much more responsive to business groups than to others. The state has an inherent bias toward business because states must ensure a well-functioning (and in a capitalist society, capitalist) economy to ensure their own success, but also because state personnel move back and forth between the state and business enterprises and because current societal ideology is overwhelmingly market- and business-oriented. If a crucial labour union went on strike, the immediate reaction is to force workers back to work—when there is a "capital strike" (that is, periods of low investment), the immediate "solution" is to make sure that owners of capital make more money. The state is influenced through functionalist, instrumental, political, and ideological channels in favour of business groups more than others.

Phases and Types of Capitalism and the Rise of Neo-liberalism

Capitalism is a particular type of social formation dominated by a free-enterprise economy that shapes everything embedded within it. But, the capitalism of today is different from the capitalism in Britain in the 17th and 18th centuries. The capitalism of today in most of the developed nations is also different from the capitalism of 1945–1970 during the welfare state era. In fact, many contend that we are now in a new phase of capitalism, global capitalism, in which business and corporate power has been overwhelmingly reasserted.

There are also different forms of capitalism in the contemporary world. The capitalism of India differs from that of Japan, which in turn differs from that of Sweden and from that of the United Kingdom, the United States, or Canada. Within the developed world—that is, countries in Europe, North America, and the English-speaking world generally—nations have been categorized as displaying particular types of capitalism according to the way they organize the provision of care for their citizens, that is, types of welfare-state regimes. These different regimes are consequences of varying class structures and class conflict—the balance of class power and class coalitions.

An adequate political economy account has to help explain this historical change and contemporary variation. In what follows I use the idea of global capitalism as a new phase of capitalism replacing earlier forms (from Ross and Trachte 1990) to analyze historical change and welfare regime types (from Esping-Andersen 1990, 1999) in accounting for health inequalities within and among nations and the existence of societies (Canada and the United States) with different types of health care systems.

To sketch an explanation, capitalism moves through entrepreneurial, monopoly, and, most recently, global phases. Each of these phases has its own set of class, economic, and political characteristics. Economic globalization, as a real force and as ideology, brought the re-emergence of business on national and international levels to a dominant class position from the previous phase of a nationally focused monopoly capitalism in which capital and labour had arrived at various forms of accommodation. Contemporary business dominance, and its accompanying neo-liberal ideology and policies, led to attacks on working-class rights in the market (e.g., undermining unions) and to citizenship rights as expressed even in the market-dependent weak versions of the welfare state enacted in the Anglo-American nations after the Second World War. Labour's lessened market power and fragmentation, and the shredding of the welfare state also led to major increases in social inequality, poverty, income inequality, and social fragmentation. The relative autonomy of the state (from business) decreased. The dominance of the United States internationally was a prime factor in the spread of neo-liberal doctrines and policies.

Neo-liberalism has doctrinal affinities with inequality and with lowered social cohesion (Coburn 2000). Neo-liberal philosophy and policies are either unconcerned with or positively endorse inequalities (as encouraging work motivation, participation in markets, etc.). Moreover, they are particularly individualistic in attacking various forms of collective or state action, insisting that we face markets only as individuals or families, that we provide for ourselves. I argue that the forceful enactment of neo-liberal ideologies and politics exacerbates differences among rich and poor within the market, and increases socially determined health inequalities. Neo-liberalism both undermines those social factors that promote good health while diminishing forms of health care designed to cure illness and disease or that might buffer the influence of declining social infrastructure supports on health.

Neo-liberal economic globalization undermined the welfare state. But alternative national forms of welfare regime, based on varying national class and institutional structures (Esping-Andersen 1990, 1999), differentially resisted international trends toward the dominance of market-based inequalities. Nations develop specific patterns of political and social institutions and policies. Welfare regimes can be categorized according to the extent to which they decommodify citizens'

> ### Box 3.1: Corporate Concentration and Social Inequalities
>
> Global changes in production technologies and in the organization of production have also taken place, with fewer and fewer corporations controlling such critical sectors as information, energy, transport, and communication.... Thus, around 100 Transnational Corporations control 33% of the world's productive assets, account for one-third of world production and employ only 5% of the global workforce. At the same time, the state sector in Third World countries, which was the only sector large enough to enable investment for wider development, has been pushed into a much less significant role. Such measures as the sale of public assets (often to TNCs), and fiscal policies that combined decreasing taxation of the richer segments of the population with decreasing subsidies to weaker segments, essentially meant a widening of income disparities. It is not surprising that income inequalities within countries have significantly increased.
>
> *Source*: M. Rao and R. Loewenson, "The Political Economy of the Assault on Health" (2004). Available on-line at www.phmovement.org/about/background1 People's Health Movement.

relationships to the market. Decommodification refers to the degree to which citizens have an alternative to complete dependence on the labour market (or working for money), in order to have an acceptable standard of living (for example, welfare, unemployment insurance, pensions, and labour market policies). Esping-Andersen notes three major types of welfare state: the social democratic welfare states, showing the greatest decommodification and emphasis on citizenship rights; the liberal welfare state, which is the most market dependent and emphasizes means and income testing; and an intermediate group, the conservative, corporatist, or familist welfare states, which are characterized by class and status-based insurance schemes and a heavy reliance on the family to provide support.

Among the developed nations the major examples of the social democratic welfare states are the Scandinavian countries such as Sweden, Norway, and Finland. The liberal welfare states include the Anglo-American nations particularly the United Kingdom and the United States (at one time the U.K. was close to social democratic status). The corporatist/familist states include such countries as Germany, France, and Italy. These nations represent differing ways of approaching *both* market and state welfare phenomena based on differing class structures and class coalitions — they constitute distinct socio-political entities and not only welfare state regimes (O'Connor and Olsen 1998).

A major explanation for differences in welfare regimes is a class or class coalitional perspective. Greater working-class strength and/or upper-class weakness and various combinations of class coalitions, degrees of class cohesion/organization (e.g., the formation of a working class-based political party), produce stronger welfare regimes or help preserve these in the face of attack. Welfare regimes not only have causes but they also have consequences for the class and stratification structure. For example, it has been found that universalist welfare measures, those that apply to everyone, are more likely to receive continued political support than those that are targeted only at the poor. Though the latter policy might seem more "efficient," it is actually less effective because almost inevitably, measures to help the poor become more and more stringent and stingy because most people are not benefiting from them. More universalistic programs tend to be more politically robust.

Globalization is, however, enacted partly through regional trade pacts or alliances. Thus, in Europe there is the E.U. and, in North America, the North America Free Trade Agreement (NAFTA). When analyzing events in Canada or the United States, we are already discussing highly developed historical inter-country relationships (in which Canada and Mexico are more influenced by, and dependent on, the United States than vice versa). NAFTA was enacted during a time of a highly neo-liberal (Progressive Conservative) federal government. NAFTA constrains and limits what might be done in health and health care. In health care—for example, in Canada—new areas cannot be brought within government control from the private area without the possibility of the U.S. taking countervailing measures in other areas, and corporations can sue for possible lost business. There is a bias in NAFTA toward the provision of services in the private sphere; reform of health care in a more collective direction is made extremely difficult.

But Canada–U.S. relationships go much deeper and broader than simply NAFTA. All of Canada's history in the latter half of the 20th century can be described in terms of seeking to prevent Canada's absorption by the United States. Living beside the world's hegemonic power has meant that Canada has been highly influenced economically, politically, culturally, and militarily by the United States. This relationship provides great support for neo-liberal economic and political forces within Canada, at the same time as the influence of the United States has, at times, provided a foil for the institution or promotion of factors that "make Canada different." The fact that Canada still has somewhat more of a welfare state than the United States, which influences health status in Canada, and the enactment of Medicare, or national health insurance in Canada, are part of these differences. Indeed, Medicare is often noted whenever the United States and Canada are compared.

Health Status within and among Nations

The cause of global neo-liberal capitalism is driven by dominant business groups within nations; by the most powerful nation, the United States; and by emerging international organizations reflecting the interests of powerful nations and corporations—the International Monetary Fund, the World Bank, and the World Trade Organization (though the World Bank now is showing much more concern with social cohesion, literacy, and poverty than it did previously). At the global level, corporations, and states that they influence, are the only actors; citizens are completely absent and have no voice, except indirectly. Indeed, nationally based corporations and business interests perceive international treaties and international organizations as constraining what they view as an "excess" of democracy on the national level. An "excess" in this case means that citizens at the national level were actually making their voices heard. International treaties, supposedly simply about trade, are actually much more. They are a way of entrenching, at the international and national level, the rule of corporations and business. The latter have many rights but few obligations under international treaties while these treaties limit the ability of national states to organize their own societies to protect and enhance the lives of their own citizens. *What neo-liberals, conservative parties, and corporate interests cannot get in the ballot box, they seek to ensure through international trade agreements.*

Much of the analysis in this chapter pertains to the developed nations, countries for which we have good data. But the main health problems in the world today lie in the underdeveloped nations and the stark health discrepancies in the world. Some nations have so much wealth and food that obesity is the major issue, while in other parts of the world millions die or are stunted by starvation and hundreds of millions more have no chance to develop their human capacities. We live in a world in which the amount spent on armaments could feed, clothe, and educate everyone. We are not living in a world of scarcity, but in a world in which resources are radically maldistributed relative to need. This international picture directly contradicts the claim of neo-liberals that free markets can best meet human needs. As we note in what follows, in fact, *the wants of the wealthy trump the needs of the poor*. Capitalist enterprises follow profit. If the poor—nations, groups, or individuals—have little money, then markets are not at all interested in their needs.

Box 3.2: Increasing Global Inequality

In 1960, the 20% of the world's people living in the richest countries had 30 times the income of the poorest 20%. Now they command 74 times more. The richest 20% of the world's population command 86% of the world GDP while the poorest 20% command merely 1%. More than 80 countries now have per capita incomes lower than they had a decade ago: 55 countries, mostly in sub-Saharan Africa, Eastern Europe and the Commonwealth of Independent States (CIS), have had declining per capita incomes. Although the world today is richer than ever before, nearly 1.3 billion people live on less than a dollar a day and close to 1 billion cannot meet their basic consumption requirements.

Source: M. Rao and R. Loewenson, "The Political Economy of the Assault on Health" (2004). Available on-line at www.phmovement.org/about/background1 People's Health Movement.

In respect to the social determinants of health regarding adequate nutrition, clean water, employment, housing, and education, and regarding what societies generally do about people showing disease or ill health—that is, develop some form of health care—the less-developed nations are deficient. On the latter point, to return to the "wealthy get all the attention in capitalism" argument, the case of health care research is instructive since that area, including the development of drugs and pharmaceuticals, is characterized by the term 90/10. That is, 90 percent of the research is focused on the issues affecting the 10 percent of world health problems shown in the affluent nations. Why? Because in the developed nations there is a market for such products as blood pressure- or cholesterol-lowering medications while there is little market for much more immediately serious conditions in the less developed world. It is no accident the World Health Report (2003) notes: "Of the 4.1 million people in sub-Saharan Africa in urgent need of antiretroviral drugs fewer than 2% have access to them" (Jong-Wook 2003: 2083). This is not to argue that medications are the solution to the health problems of the underdeveloped world. General living conditions are the crucial determinants of health in such regions.

The distribution of health in the world in the early 21st century is shocking. While the healthiest nations have overall longevity rates ranging around 80, the unhealthiest nations show rates of half that—around 40–45 years. Similarly, regarding the proportion of children per 1,000 dying under the age of five, mortality rates in the developed nations are around five or six for males and four and five for females—with the most deprived nations showing rates 20 times those totals. As the *World Health Report* of 2003 notes: "A baby born today in Afghanistan is 75 times more likely to die before age 5 years than a child born in Iceland or Singapore. Life expectancy at birth in Sierra Leone is less than half that in Japan" (Jong-Wook 2003: 2083). The *World Health Report* also indicates that of all the regions of the world, sub-Saharan Africa shows by far the worst health. On a global scale, the life expectancy of the 642 million people in sub-Saharan Africa is 51 years, 27 years less than that of those who live in rich countries. Life expectancy at birth in 2002 ranged from 78 years for women in developed countries to less than 46 years for men in sub-Saharan Africa.

Most of the unhealthiest nations are also the poorest. In the case of the less developed world there is a correlation between GNP/capita (a measure of national wealth) and overall health status. In this respect the world seems to be broken into two groups: those with less than about U.S. $5,000/year GNP/capita and those with more; the latter, the developed world, we will examine in more detail later. The important point about the correlation between GNP/capita and health status for the poorer nations, however, is that there are wide disparities in health for nations at similar levels of GNP/capita. "Life expectancy at birth is about a year longer in Sri Lanka than in Malaysia, even though the latter is more than twice as wealthy as the former. Similarly, life expectancy in Costa Rica is 25 years longer than in Gabon, although both are at a similar economic level" (McKee 2001: 130). The lesson is that, *for the less developed world, high GNP/capita is neither a sufficient nor a necessary condition for a country to show good average levels of health.* Some poor nations have relatively good health and some rich nations have relatively poor health. And among the developed nations, as we will see, GNP/capita is unrelated to a nation's health.

The major issue is that the current forms of "development" pushed by dominant nations such as the United States and Britain, and by international agencies such as the IMF, are based on a neo-liberalism that has impaired health improvements and raised rather than reduced inequalities. *Some types of economic growth—of "development"—are better than others.* Compared with the era preceding the onset of neo-liberal politics and policies, a period of rapid economic growth and health improvements, in the past two decades, health improvements have slowed and health inequalities have vastly increased.

The chief differences among developing nations accounting for the wide differences in the health status these nations show seem to be government or civil society activism or some form of corporatist state-labour-business relationships to facilitate the more equal spread of power and resources. Government action to support welfare state-like measures or to provide controlled economic growth and a degree of independence of the state from business elites may well be the source of better health in poor nations and also the link between improved economic performance and human health and well-being in the more developed states. Yet the bias of international institutions is toward lesser government and more markets, a corporate-dominated agenda—the opposite of what the well-being literature suggests is good for the health of the citizens of the less developed nations.

We can explore the suggestions of an economic growth–welfare state–health linkage more closely regarding the nations on which we have the best data—the 20 to 30 nations of the Organisation for Economic Co-operation and Development (OECD). The position taken here is that the onset of neo-liberalism within the past few decades has produced increased social inequalities within nations. More neo-liberal nations show greater social inequalities and also greater health inequalities and poorer overall health status than do more social democratic nations. The main focus in what follows is on the two contrasting types of welfare regime: those nations exemplifying a "strong" welfare regime (the least neo-liberal, i.e., the social democratic nations) and the most neo-liberal welfare state countries (i.e., the liberal nations).

Neo-liberalism, Income Inequalities, and Health Inequalities within Nations

In the developed nations the onset of neo-liberalism has been associated with increasing within-nation inequalities. Increases in inequality have been particularly pronounced in those nations adopting more stringent neo-liberal or market-oriented politics and policies. In the early 1990s the United States, Australia, Canada, and the United Kingdom stood at the top of the income inequality ladder, while Norway,

Sweden, and the Netherlands were the lowest (although by 1994 Canada had moved more toward the middle). Table 3.1 shows the data on income inequalities. Social democratic nations (or the most decommodified nations) are indicated by double asterisks. Clearly neo-liberal nations are the most unequal regarding income distributions. Since many of these are market societies in which family incomes define access to resources, as opposed to many social democratic nations in which the state provides many forms of access to resources, citizens in neo-liberal societies are doubly disadvantaged.

Table 3.1: Ratio of the Top 10 Percent of Income Earners to the Bottom 10 Percent and the Gini Index of Inequality (the higher the ratio and the Gini, the worse the inequality)

Country	Decile Ratio 90/10	Gini Index
Finland 1991**	2.75	.233
Sweden 1992**	2.78	.229
Belgium 1992	2.79	.230
Norway 1995**	2.85	.242
Denmark 1992**	2.86	.239
Luxembourg 1994	2.93	.235
The Netherlands 1991	3.05	.249
Italy 1991	3.14	.255
Taiwan 1995	3.38	.277
Switzerland 1982	3.43	.311
New Zealand 1987/1988*	3.46	NA
Germany 1994	3.84	.300
Canada 1994*	3.93	.287
Spain 1990	4.04	.306
France 1989	4.11	.324
Israel 1992	4.12	.305
Japan 1992	4.17	.315
Ireland 1987*	4.18	.328
Australia 1989*	4.30	.308
United Kingdom 1995*	4.56	.346
United States 1994*	6.44	.368

** Social democratic or encompassing regimes
*Liberal (neo-liberal) or basic security regimes
Source: P. Gottschalk and T.M. Smeeding, "Empirical Evidence of Income Inequality in Industrialized Countries," in *The Handbook of Income Distribution*, vol. 1 (Amsterdam: Elsevier, 2000): Figure 2.

Two examples of increasing income and health inequalities associated with the politics of neo-liberalism are the U.K. and U.S. Beginning with the Reagan and Thatcher regimes, the United States and the United Kingdom demonstrate particularly high and ever-increasing rates of inequality. Prior to the neo-liberal era, income inequality in the United States and the United Kingdom had been relatively low and declining since the Second World War—the welfare state, such as it was in those two nations, actually did what it was supposed to do. From about 1968 in the U.S. and 1977/1978 in the U.K., income inequality began a steep and rapid rise that continued into the 1990s.

Box 3.3: In the United States, It's Good at the Top

Another way to look at this [inequality] is how much we pay our CEO's—the heads of our corporations. In 1980, we paid them 40 times what an entry-level worker made. By 1999, they were being paid 478 times what an entry-level worker made, and in 2001, for the Fortune 100 companies, the CEO's made a thousand times what an entry-level worker made.

Source: S. Bezrucha, keynote address, "Poverty Is Bad for the Health of Americans" (2003). Available on-line at www.fremontpublic.org/SPAN/summit_keynote. Statewide Poverty Action Movement.

Even during times of economic expansion, inequality increased in the United States. The lowest 60 percent of households in that country actually experienced a *decrease* in after-tax income between 1977 and 1999. During the same period, incomes of the top 5 percent of households grew by 56 percent and the top 1 percent mushroomed by 93 percent (Bernstein, Mishel, and Brocht 2001: 7). In fact, despite being one of the richest nations on earth, in 1991 the United States had one of the highest rates of *absolute* (as well as relative) poverty among the developed nations; of 15 countries, only Italy, Ireland, Australia, and the U.K. had higher rates (Kenworthy 1999).

Different welfare regimes and rising inequalities of various kinds have important implications for health inequalities. In general, within nations, the higher a group's socio-economic status (SES), the higher its health status. Within nations, SES differences in health (however measured) are substantial and have been widely reported. Illustrative comparisons indicate that the health differences between high and low SES areas in U.S. metropolitan areas were equivalent to "the combined loss of life from lung cancer, diabetes, motor vehicle crashes, HIV infections, suicide and homicide" (Lynch et al. 1998: 1074). Mortality would be reduced by 139.8 deaths per 100,000 if the SES differences noted were eliminated. In the U.S. people in the very poorest households were four to five times more likely to die in the next 10 years than were those in the richest (Kaplan 2000). In Britain in 1996 the differences in longevity between the highest SES group and the lowest (of five groups) were 9.5 years for men and 6.4 years for women. In Canada there are similar, but perhaps a little less extreme, health differences between those high and low in income (Humphries and van Doorslaer 2000).

Despite expanding economies, health inequalities have increased. Americans living in low SES areas have much worse mortality rates than those living in high SES areas. These mortality inequalities had increased by at least 50 percent between 1969 and 1998 (Singh and Siahpush 2002). A commentator on Britain, a nation that experienced a prolonged period of neo-liberal politics, noted that "the inequalities in health between social classes are now the greatest yet recorded in British history"(Yamey 1999: 1453). Simply reducing current wealth inequalities in Britain to their 1983 level would save 7,500 deaths among people younger than 65 (Dorling 1997; Mitchell, Shaw, and Dorling 2000; Shaw et al. 1999).

Of course, there are many forms of health inequalities. Males suffer a major "mortality deficit" since among 18 OECD nations in 2000, longevity rates favoured females by from 4.6 years (in Sweden) to 7.5 years (in France). On the other hand, females are more likely to suffer various forms of morbidity or disability. In the United States and Canada, infant mortality rates and longevity rates are highly related to geographical region and to race and Aboriginal status. In the U.S., for example, the White/Black longevity rates in 2002 favoured Whites by 5.2 years. And within the U.S., those states with better welfare measures showed much better health status than many of the southern states lower in welfare assets. In Canada, First Nations groups show much worse health than do other Canadians. These differences, however, are part of SES differences in general and are not necessarily attributable to something unique to Blacks or Aboriginal populations per se.

National Differences in Health Status

The United States is a striking outlier with respect to inequalities and health. Whereas the U.S. is one of the highest-ranked nations in the world in terms of GNP/capita, it has a dismal inequality and health record. For example, in 2002 the United States ranked 25th in the world and the United Kingdom 24th in longevity. These two countries, characterized for many years by neo-liberal policies during the Reagan/Bush and Thatcher eras, thus ranked worse, for example, than Italy, Greece, Spain, and Ireland. Regarding the probability of dying before age five, the U.S. ranked 35th for males and 31st for females below the best-performing nations—this even though the United States spends more money per capita on health care than any other nation on earth.

Canada shows lower income inequality than does the United States (Ross et al. 2000), but higher inequality than many European countries. And, concomitantly, Canada can boast of relatively high longevity rates, lower infant mortality rates, and lower SES or income-related health differences than does the United States (or the

U.K). In the case of infant mortality, in 1996 the infant mortality rates in the poorest neighbourhoods in Canada were better than the national rate of infant mortality in the U.S., yet the rates in the richest Canadian neighbourhoods were not much better than the national average rates in Sweden (Statistics Canada 2000). There are fears, however, that Canadian government social cutbacks will soon begin to have their detrimental health effects.

Welfare State Regimes and Health Differences

Infant Mortality

Welfare regime type (countries more or less neo-liberal) is highly related to infant mortality (infant mortality refers to the number of deaths under one year/1,000 live births). The social democratic nations (Austria, Sweden, Denmark, Norway, Finland) show better infant mortality rates than do the liberal nations (U.S., U.K., Canada, Ireland) for all decades from 1960 to 2000. While all nations show decreasing infant mortality rates between 1960 and 2000, the percentage differences between the mean infant mortality rates for the two contrasting regime types—the social democratic and the liberal—are substantial. Moreover, in a startling development, in the early years of the 21st century, both Canada and the United States showed *increases* in their infant mortality rates. Moreover, within Canada, in one of the wealthiest, albeit highly conservative, provinces, Alberta, the infant mortality in 2002 increased to a shocking 7.3 per 1,000 live births, reaching levels not seen since 1994 (Statistics Canada, *The Daily*, September 27, 2004).

If welfare regime arguments are correct, one might expect increasing differences over time in the relative standing of nations regarding infant mortality (Navarro 1998; Navarro and Shi 2001). Given greater movements toward neo-liberalism shown by the liberal nations, one would expect them to drop in the World League tables of infant mortality as compared to the social democratic countries, which is what the rank order of infant mortality rates shows. For example, while in 1960 the U.K. and the U.S. were ranked 7th and 8th in infant mortality (of 18 nations with number one being the nation with the best infant mortality rate), by 2000 they were 15th and 18th out of the same 18 nations. Canada ranked 9th in 1960 and 12th in 2000. That is, relative to other nations, the infant mortality rates in these Anglo-American liberal regime nations are not improving as quickly as they are in other nations. Comparing extreme cases, the United States has over twice the infant mortality rates of Sweden, a telling loss of life between the best- and worst-case scenarios.

General Health Status

Most measures of health to some degree reflect infant mortality and there is great overlap among measures; they are not independent estimates of health. The measures are also highly influenced by latency effects—that is, infant mortality is more likely to show the effects of current societal conditions whereas overall health

Table 3.2: Mean Infant Mortality Rates (deaths/1000 live births) 1960–2000 by Welfare Regime Type[a] (18 nations)

	1960	1970	1980	1990	2000[b]
Social democratic	23.1	15.4	9.1	6.8	4.3
Christian democratic	29.2	20.1	11.2	7.4	4.9
Liberal	26.3	19.2	11.6	8.0	5.9
Ex-fascist	53.8	37.0	18.2	9.4	5.4
Liberal minus social democratic mean infant mortality rate	3.2	3.8	2.5	1.2	1.7
Liberal mean as a percentage of the social democratic mean	114%	125%	127%	118%	140%

Sources:
(a) Adapted from V. Navarro and L. Shi, "The Political Context of Social Inequalities and Health," *Social Science and Medicine* 52(2001): Table 7.
(b) 2000 from OECD Health Data, 2003.

Social democratic: Austria, Sweden, Denmark, Norway, Finland.
Christian democratic: Belgium, Germany, Netherlands, France, Italy, Switzerland.
Liberal: United Kingdom, Ireland, United States, Canada
Ex-fascist: Spain, Portugal, Greece

younger.

Using data from the OECD, in all cases the social democratic nations show better general measures of health than do the liberal nations, although in some instances the differences are small. Comparing the relative standing of Canada, the United States, and the United Kingdom (for comparison purposes), the U.S. and the U.K. did not improve their health status as much as many of the other 18 OECD nations regarding both life expectancy and potential years of life lost (a measure that calculates the number of years death occurs before age 70). For example, the United States ranked seventh best in life expectancy of the 18 nations noted in 1960 and 15th in the year 2000. Interestingly, Canada tended to rise in the hierarchy or League Tables of Health in Life Expectancy from sixth to third. Apart from the relatively better welfare system of Canada than the U.S., one possible explanation for Canada's good performance might be that Canada has experienced very high rates of recent immigration—18 percent of Canadians were born elsewhere, and

Table 3.3: Rank Order of Infant Mortality Rates, 1960–2000, by Welfare Regime Type[a]

(18 nations; results for the Christian democratic and ex-fascist nations omitted for ease of comparison)

(– = worse position; + = better position; 0 = the same rank in 2000 as in 1960)

	(1 = Low Infant Mortality)		*(Rank Order in 2000 Relative to 1960)*[b]
	1960	**2000**	
Social democratic			
Austria	14	7	+7
Sweden	1	1	0
Denmark	6	12	–6
Norway	3	2	+1
Finland	4	2	+2
Christian democratic			
Belgium, Germany,			
Netherlands, France, Italy,			
Switzerland.			
Liberal			
United Kingdom	7	15	–8
Ireland	11	16	–5
United States	8	18	–10
Canada	9	12	–3
Ex-fascist: Spain, Portugal,			
Greece			

Sources:
(a) Welfare regime classification from V. Navarro and L. Shi, "The Political Context of Social Inequalities and Health," *Social Science and Medicine* 52 (2001): 481–491.
(b) 2000 infant mortality rates from OECD Health Data, 2003.

rates of recent immigration—18 percent of Canadians were born elsewhere, and immigrants tend to be in better health than native-born Canadians.

One health measure used by the World Health Organization calculates the proportions of people from an original cohort of 100,000 living to various ages, based on current age/sex-adjusted mortality rates. The difference in proportions of people alive at age 65 for specific countries are considerable. For example, in 1994 the United States had an estimated 74,710 males and 85,460 females per 100,000 population born still alive at age 65; Sweden has 83,525 males and 90,075 females (World Health Organization 1998). Again, Canada is closer to Sweden than to the U.S.; Costa Rica shows better rates than the U.S.; and Cuba, a chronically underdeveloped nation suffering under a decades-long trade boycott by its neighbour, the United States, keeps about as many people alive until age 65 as does the U.S.! Extrapolating to total populations, there are literally millions of "missing Americans" and, to a lesser extent, Canadians, who would have been alive if they had been born and brought up in Sweden.

Health Care Systems: The United States and Canada

Although much of the attention regarding health status today focuses on the broader social determinants of health rather than on health care, nevertheless this attention should not be overplayed. At various stages of development health care is important. In the less developed world, basic human needs for pure water, adequate nutrition, basic sanitation, education, and access to work are vital. Nonetheless, medical care in these circumstances also has a part to play, particularly regarding primary care. Health care also contributes to the health of people in the developed nations, although the exact impact of health care on population health status is difficult to estimate.

For OECD nations, health care forms part of the development of welfare state measures (Korpi and Palme 1998). In this respect the United States is the exception in not having some form of national health service or national health insurance. Explanations for the development of health care insurance or systems parallels analyses of the introduction of other types of welfare state measures and have been viewed as having somewhat the same underlying causes. The presence of an organized working class and its institutionalization in a labour or left political party is seen as crucial as is, as an alternative, the concatenation of the state, with peak and organized business and labour groups in some form of corporatist arrangement.

Regarding the difference in health systems between the United States and Canada, a variety of factors have been said to play a part. In Canada, the formation of a socialist or social democratic party, which attained power in Saskatchewan at the end of the Second World War, was crucial. This party first introduced hospital insurance, and later health insurance for hospital and doctor care. This example haunted the federal government and the other provinces. Pressure from various sources—many but not all of these originating with working-class movements—eventually led to its enactment on the federal level. However, even when Medicare did finally come about across Canada in 1971, this was not a national health service, as in Britain, in which doctors and facilities were directly employed by the state; rather, it is a national government-sponsored insurance system in which everyone is insured for all medically necessary hospital and doctors services through a provincial plan, which is partially underwritten from general revenues by the federal government and partially by the provinces. There are significant omissions in this plan, including, for example, prescription drugs, home care, care for the elderly (care not involving hospitals or doctors), etc. Many of the costs excluded under Medicare are, however, covered by public plans in some of the provinces (for example, drugs for the elderly, or some forms of home care) and/or by private insurance plans.

The United States, many commentators like to remark, has a "non-system." That is, it includes federally sponsored plans for the poor and the elderly, but not much, other than private plans, for those in between. Hence the problem that about 40 million Americans lack any medical care insurance at all and millions more have plans with more or fewer restrictions on the amount that will be paid in the event of illness, deductibles, and services covered.

Medical care occupies a unique place in the political economy of nations. It has been claimed that education and medical care are functional for capital, hence that big capital or big corporations at least are not necessarily opposed to some form of national health insurance. In Canada, for example, the fact that automobile manufacturers in Canada do not have to help pay for the health costs of their employees is an advantage in their trade with the United States. Ideologically, however, national health services or insurance are total anathema to neo-liberals. Small employers, major carriers of the ideology of free enterprise, view the privatization of health care as necessary and desirable. So, there are divisions about state-supported health care within the business community. These divisions probably aided the implementation of health insurance in Canada as did the lesser opposition to state involvement by the Canadian than by the American medical profession. In the United States, there does seem to be an incipient state/business coalition to control the costs of care, although business in the United States is much more united in its opposition to any form of government involvement in the financing of care than is business in Canada.

Some analysts feel that the political system in the United States, which institutionally discourages the formation of third or regional parties, encompassing left dissidents within a broad coalition in the Democratic Party, hindered the formation of alternative parties on the left, which might have pushed for health insurance or a health service. Moreover, the congressional system contains many more veto points and opportunities for lobbying by powerful organized groups than does the Canadian system. In the Canadian system party, discipline is firm and dissidents have to leave or be expelled (Maioni 1998). At all levels—the class level, the state or neo-institutional level, and the interest-group politics level—Canada had an advantage regarding forces supporting health care than did the United States.

Health care systems, then, are inversely tied to the strength of neo-liberal politics and policy and to the same forms of class struggles and class coalitions on which welfare state developments relied. State health care systems are, however, not as vulnerable to general welfare state clawbacks as are such measures as unemployment insurance and welfare measures for the poor, since the latter two are much more closely and directly tied to the labour market interests of business than are health and education. However, within any form of capitalist social formation there are continuous pressures toward the "commodification" of health care. No matter how popular government-provided health services or health-financed services are, individual private firms continually push to convert collectively provided health care into private markets for care. Corporations see the potential for enormous profits in the provision of care. Powerful interests in Canada—in business, politics, and the media—want to create enough crisis in public health care that private care becomes attractive. Alternatively, conservative governments claim to want to "save" Medicare by introducing policies (beginning with alternative private services) that will actually undermine it.

There is a continuous strain within capitalism to privatize everything, including anything, such as land, water, and other goods that were once part of the "commons." Neo-liberalism produces a vast "enclosure" movement similar to that in 18th- and 19th-century Britain at the time when landowners fenced off collective land in order to raise sheep. Today, the push toward privatization ranges everywhere from the commodification of knowledge, including knowledge about health, previously commonly held in universities, to privatization even of specific human gene pools. All of this has profound implications for the provision of health care. It is a daily struggle within neo-liberalism to preserve any form of collective benefit.

Overall, the quality of care in the two nations is probably not too different, although the very best private care for those Americans who can afford it may be better than Canadian care. In the past, Canadians generally tended to be more satisfied than Americans with their health care, although this is changing (incidentally, on a recent television program asking audiences to name the most important Canadian, Tommy Douglas, the socialist premier of Saskatchewan who first introduced Medicare, ranked number one). In addition to "real" problems with the delivery of care in Canada under Medicare, it is in the interests of private health interests to make Canadians dissatisfied with public health care and to create a "crisis."

The challenges for the Canadian health care system are to reduce or avoid waiting lists, to make the system more responsive to patients, and to have a more geographically equal distribution of access. The major challenge in the United States is to get access to care more equally distributed—that is, the problem of health care inequalities (particularly related to income and race)—and the huge administrative and other costs.

Though Canadians have fewer financial barriers to access to care, this does not guarantee equality in actual usage. Aboriginal peoples in Canada, those in isolated areas, and the poor receive less adequate or appropriate care than the less isolated and those higher in SES, but nevertheless health care is more equally provided and accessible than in the United States, and more equitably provided than before Medicare. The point is that financial accessibility is just the first step to the provision of adequate care for everyone. But health care cannot make up for socially produced illness and disease. In Canada, as elsewhere, it remains the case that the wealthy live longer, healthier lives than do the poor (I owe this felicitious phrase to Richard Sandbrook), yet health care is "rationed" everywhere. Not everything that is medically possible or desirable is done for every person. In Canada, the implicit rationing is due to constraints on available personnel and equipment; in the United States, it is rationing by income.

A joint survey in Canada and the U.S. indicated that the poor in Canada were less likely than those in the U.S. to state that they had "unmet health needs." The most often expressed reasons for "unmet health needs" stated by respondents was "waiting too long" in Canada and "costs" in the U.S. In fact, a recent study of personal bankruptcies in the U.S. found that 46 percent of the bankruptcies studied were caused by medical bills. Extrapolating from those surveyed to the total American population, it was estimated that there were about two million "medical bankruptcies" in the U.S. (CBConline, February 3, 2005).

Examining publicly provided or financed care generally, public systems, and/or those with a single or few payers, are more efficient and cheaper—they are more effective at controlling costs generally than are private systems. In 2001, the United States paid a greater proportion of its GNP for health care (13.9 percent or U.S. $4,887 per person) than did any other nation. By comparison Canada pays 9.7 percent and Sweden and Japan (nations with the highest longevity in the world) 8.7 and 8.0 percent respectively (Reinhardt, Hussey, and Anderson 2004). The U.S. totals had risen to 14.9 percent of GDP and U.S. $5,440 by 2002 (Hellander 2004). Contrary to free-market ideology, the market-oriented health system in the United States has much more waste in the form of administrative costs than does the simpler payment system of the Canadian version. In 1999 administrative costs for health care were U.S. $1,059 per capita in the United States and U.S. $307 in Canada (Woolhandler, Campbell, and Himmelstein 2003). While Americans might pay less money through taxes for health care, they pay much more overall through taxes, plus private payments for health care, for fewer services on a population-wide basis. The United States seems to have the worst of both worlds—high health care costs and poor average levels of health.

Conclusions
The examples given indicate that the prevailing form of political, economic, and social policy—that of neo-liberalism—has profoundly negative effects on societies generally, and on health and health care specifically. The arguments and data presented also indicate that there are alternatives to a purely neo-liberal view of the world. Nations or societies that support their citizens in times of crisis may not only do better economically but certainly do produce higher overall health. The

United States is a striking instance showing that economic wealth is not a sufficient cause of better national health. The instances of Kerala, Costa Rica, Cuba, Finland, and the Netherlands at various levels of GDP/capita suggest that economic wealth is not even a necessary condition for health.

A materialist political economy approach can, better than alternative theoretical perspectives, help us to understand and explain the existence of these health and health care similarities and differences.

References

Bernstein, J., L. Mishel, and C. Brocht. (2001). "Anyway You Cut It: Income Inequality on the Rise Regardless of How It's Measured." Briefing paper. Washington, DC: Economic Policy Institute.

Coburn, D. (2000). "Income Inequality, Social Cohesion and the Health Status of Populations: The Role of Neoliberalism." *Social Science and Medicine* 51: 135–146.

Dorling, D. (1997). "Death in Britain: How Local Mortality Rates Have Changed: 1950s to 1990s." Joseph Rowntree Foundation. Available on-line at www.jrf.org.uk.

Esping-Andersen, G. (1990). *The Three Worlds of Welfare Capitalism.* Princeton: Princeton University Press.

_____. (1999). *Social Foundations of Postindustrial Economies.* Oxford: Oxford University Press.

Gottschalk, P., and T.M. Smeeding. (2000). "Empirical Evidence of Income Inequality in Industrialized Countries." In *The Handbook of Income Distribution,* vol. 1, edited by A.B. Atkinson and F. Bourguignon, 261-308. Amsterdam and Holland: Elsevier.

Hellander, I. (2004). "A Review of Data in the U.S. Health Sector, March, 2004." *International Journal of Health Service* 34(4): 729–750.

Humphries, K.H., and E. van Doorslaer. (2000). "Income-Related Health Inequality in Canada." *Social Science and Medicine* 50: 663–671.

Jong-Wook, L. (2003). "Global Health Improvement and WHO: Shaping the Future" *The Lancet* 362: 2083-2088.

Kaplan, G.A. (2000). "Economic Policy Is Health Policy." Paper presented at the Income Inequality, Socioeconomic Status, and Health conference, April, Washington, D.C.

Kenworthy, L. (1999). "Do Social-Welfare Policies Reduce Poverty? A Cross-National Assessment." *Social Forces* 77(3): 1119–1139.

Korpi, W., and J. Palme. (1998). "The Paradox of Redistribution and Strategies of Equality: Welfare State Institutions, Inequality and Poverty in the Western Countries." *American Sociological Review* 63(5): 661–687.

Lynch, J.W., G.A. Kaplan, F.R. Pamuk, R.D. Cohen, K.E. Heck, J.L. Balfor, and I.H. Yen. (1998). "Income Inequality and Mortality in Metropolitan Areas of the United States." *American Journal of Public Health* 887: 1074–1080.

Maioni, A. (1998). *Parting at the Crossroads: The Emergence of Health Insurance in the United States and Canada.* Princeton: Princeton University Press.

McKee, M. (2001). "Global Health Inequalities: The Challenge to Epidemiology." *NSW Public Health Bulletin* 12(5): 130–133.

Mitchell, R., M. Shaw, and D. Dorling. (2000). *Inequalities in Life and Death: What If Britain Were More Equal?* The Joseph Rowntree Foundation. Cambridge, UK: The Polity Press.

Navarro, V. (1998). "Neoliberalism, Globalization, Unemployment, Inequalities, and the Welfare State." *International Journal of Health Services* 28(4): 607–682.

Navarro, V., and L. Shi. (2001). "The Political Context of Social Inequalities and Health." *Social Science and Medicine* 52: 481–491.

O'Connor, J.S., and G.M. Olsen, eds. (1998). *Power Resources Theory and the Welfare State: A Critical Approach.* Toronto: University of Toronto Press.

Reinhardt, U.E., P.S. Hussey, and G.F. Anderson. (2004). "U.S. Health Care Spending in an International Context." *Health Affairs* 23(3): 10–25.

Ross, N.A., M.C. Wolfson, J.R. Dunn, J.-M. Berthelot, G.A. Kaplan, and J.W. Lynch. (2000). "Relations between Income Inequality and Mortality in Canada and in the United States," *British Medical Journal* 320(1): 898–902.

Ross, R.J.S., and K.C. Trachte. (1990). *Global Capitalism: The New Leviathan.* Albany: University of New York.

Shaw, M., D. Dorling, D. Gordon, and G. Davey Smith. (1999). *The Widening Gap: Health Inequalities and Policy in Britain.* Bristol: The Policy Press.

Singh, G.K., and M. Siahpush. (2002). "Increasing Inequalities in All-Cause and Cardiovascular Mortality among U.S. Adults Aged 25–64 Years by Area Socioeconomic Status, 1969–1998." *International Journal of Epidemiology:* 31(3): 600–613.

Statistics Canada. (2000). "Health Reports: How Healthy Are Canadians?" *The Daily* (March 31). Statistics Canada cat. no. 11-001E.

Woolhandler, S., T. Campbell, and D.U. Himmelstein. (2003). "Costs of Health Care Administration in the United States and Canada." *The New England Journal of Medicine* 349(8): 768–775.

World Health Organization. (1998). *World Health Statistics Annual.* Life Tables.

Yamey, G. (1999). "Study Shows Growing Inequalities in Health in Britain." *British Medical Journal* 319: 1453.

• •

Critical Thinking Questions

1. What has been said in the media about the health status of Americans or about health inequalities in the U.S. and Canada? Anything? How do the statements align with some of the sources listed in the Further Readings?

2. What are the differences and similarities or relationships between a social class view of health and health care and an SES view?

3. What kinds of political and economic policies do you think would help the less developed nations improve their average levels of well-being?

4. Are the media biased regarding their reporting of political, economic, and health issues and the way these are related? In what way and why?

5. Could you now offer an alternative "political economy" view to key issues or events described and analyzed in the newspaper or on television news?

Further Readings

Armstrong, P., H. Armstrong, and D. Coburn, eds. (2001). *Unhealthy Times: Political Economy Perspectives on Health and Health Care in Canada.* Toronto: Oxford University Press.
A series of articles on a political economy perspective applied to health in the Canadian context.

Coburn, D. (2004). "Beyond the Income Inequality Hypothesis: Globalization, Neo-liberalism and Health Inequalities." *Social Science and Medicine* 58(1): 41–56.
This article reports on a class model of viewing health rather than simply an income inequality model.

Drache, D., and T. Sullivan, eds. (1999). *Health Reform: Public Success, Private Failure.* London and New York: Routledge.
A collection of articles describing and comparing public and private health care systems, including some U.S. and international material.

Gordon, C. (2003). *Dead on Arrival: The Politics of Health Care in Twentieth-Century America.* Princeton: Princeton University Press.
This book provides an overview of the various factors influencing the American health care system.

Hofrichter, R., ed. (2004). *Health and Social Justice.* San Francisco: Jossey-Bass.
Most of the numerous articles in this volume touch on the U.S. experience with some coverage of international health issues.

Navarro, V., ed. (2002). *The Political Economy of Social Inequalities.* Amityville: Baywood Publishing.
Many of these articles describe the U.S. experience with some articles also touching on the experience in other countries and international health issues generally. Contains articles on the WHO and the IMF, among other institutions.

Relevant Web Sites

Note: All Web sites have to be approached in a critical vein. That is, none should be accepted at face value. The *International Journal of Health Services* often contains various critiques of prominent reports or organizations.

Luxembourg Income Studies Project
www.lisproject.org/

This site describes the Luxembourg Income Studies Project, the most thorough examination of income and other inequalities. The most useful part is listed under "Publications" in which hundreds of downloadable working papers are available on topics related to welfare state dynamics and income inequality.

Organisation for Economic Co-operation and Development
www.oecd.org

Clicking on "Health" in the subject index brings up numerous publications related to health and welfare state issues. There are downloadable files of selected data from some of the OECD Health Data series issued annually.

United Nations Millennium Goals
www.un.org.milleniumgoals/

This site describes the United Nations Millennium Goals, the latest version of which was issued in February 2005. Numerous background papers are available.

World Bank
www1.worldbank.org/hnp/

The World Bank lists dozens of world health and world poverty reports and papers.

World Health Organization
www.who.int/whr/en/

Available on this site are copies of the *World Health Report*, published annually by the World Health Organization, as well as many other studies related to poverty and health.

Glossary

Decommodification: Commodification means the production of goods or services for sale in the marketplace. Decommodification regarding welfare state issues means the degree to which individuals can live a reasonable life without relying on market wages. Can older people or the unemployed—those not earning a market wage—live a reasonable life?

Historical materialism: This concept means that people's ideas are a product of their social existence rather than their social existence being the result of their consciousness. Related to this is the hypothesis that history can be viewed as a succession of differing modes of production—differing mechanisms for producing the means of existence and of reproducing human beings and society. Capitalism emerged from feudalism and, in turn, capitalism is expected to be succeeded by another mode of production.

Phases of capitalism, entrepreneurial, monopoly, and global capitalism: These refer, not to different modes of production, but to different phases within capitalism itself. It is assumed that each of these phases have different class structures and display different types of class conflict. Monopoly capitalism is characterized by somewhat increased power for the working class and somewhat less resistance to working-class demands for wage increases or benefits through the "social wage" or welfare state. Globalization strengthens the power of capital because capital is more mobile and can threaten governments with leaving their jurisdiction if their demands are not met.

Socio-economic status (SES): A person's position or socio-economic status is usually measured in terms of educational level, occupational status, income, or some combination of these. There are no real social relationships among people at different levels and there is no necessary antagonism among those lower or higher. From our perspective, class factors (classes determined by their relationship to the means of production) determine SES differences. A focus on SES is thus not necessarily wrong, simply radically incomplete.

Welfare state: Welfare regimes refer to the different ways in which different nations or societies provide for the well-being of their citizens or compensate for the failures of markets to do so. Social democratic welfare regimes tend to provide more resources, and on a more universalistic basis, than do liberal welfare regimes, which tend to target welfare measures to the poor and to provide fewer benefits to those less eligible for such benefits. The conservative-corporatist-familist regime provides benefits as a side benefit of working or relies on the family to provide support.

....

CHAPTER FOUR

THE RIGHT TO HEALTH

Human Rights Approaches to Health

Marcia Rioux

....

Learning Objectives

At the conclusion of this chapter, the reader will be able to
- distinguish the right to health and its parameters, including particular elements that comprise the right to health
- identify the major international human rights instruments that define a right to health
- recognize the difference between health good practice and the right to health good practice
- have an understanding of the right to health in practice—its application to HIV/AIDS, reproductive health, and disability

---

Introduction

> A table, which distances them from the litigants, the "third party" that is the judges.... Now this idea that there are people who are neutral in relation to others, that they can make judgments about them on the basis of ideas of justice which have absolute validity, and that their decisions must be acted upon, I believe that all this is far removed from and quite foreign to the very idea of modern justice. (Foucault and Gordon 1980: 8)

How many people must feel like they are in front of such judges every time they need health care or every time they feel the influences of societies that do not provide justice in the context of the right to health? For people who are concerned with health, where judgments are the nature of the business for health care providers, for hospital administrators, for social and policy makers, for social policy analysts, for economists, for scientists, and for individuals, the who, how, and why of judgments are important. Judgments are made about which diseases take precedence in research, which determinants of health are addressed, about who will be vulnerable to ill health, about which populations and individuals have access to drugs, just to suggest a few.

A recent development in understanding health is to contextualize it from the perspective of human rights—that is, to put it in the framework of justice as a way to approach it. "Health is influenced by a variety of social, economic and environmental factors, and not just by access to health care…. The extensive empirical literature on social determinants of health—and inequalities in health—has yet to be matched by an appreciation of the normative underpinnings of health equity …" (Anand et al. 2004: 2). Moreover, health equity expresses a commitment of public health to social justice (Anand et al. 2004). A rights-based approach to health means using human rights as a framework for health development. It means making principles of human rights integral to the design, implementation, and evaluation of policies and programs. And it means assessing the human rights implications of health policy, programs, and legislation.

Box 4.1: Human Rights Principles

- Universal inherence
- Inalienability
- Inherent self-worth of each individual
- Autonomy and self-determination
- Equality for all
- Preservation of freedom of individual through social support

---

A human rights and social justice approach enables the use of various categories of rights and recognizes how rights have to be a concern in thinking about approaches to health and social policy that enhance, rather than diminish, the well-being of all people. These include political and civil rights, such as the right to life, freedom of opinion, a fair trial, and protection from torture and violence. These are the rights that are the most common concern of nations, particularly in the North and West. Human rights also include economic, social, and cultural rights, such as the right to work, social protection, an adequate standard of living, the highest possible standards of physical and mental health, education, and enjoyment of the benefits of cultural freedom and scientific progress. Finally, human rights include the right of nations to development, economic autonomy, and security of their citizens.

UN human rights documents describe what governments and societies should not do, including engaging in torture, slavery, and violence against women and

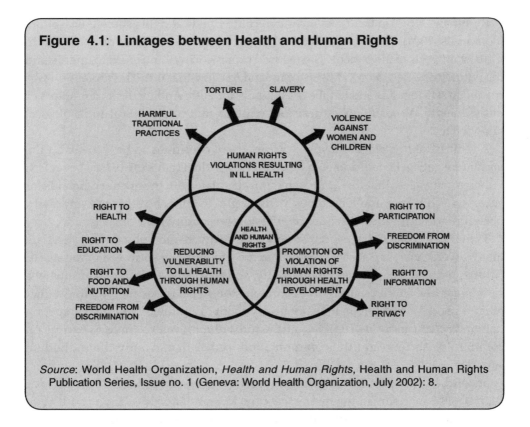

Figure 4.1: Linkages between Health and Human Rights

Source: World Health Organization, *Health and Human Rights*, Health and Human Rights Publication Series, Issue no. 1 (Geneva: World Health Organization, July 2002): 8.

children. They also describe what should be ensured for all people, including providing health, education, food, nutrition, and freedom from discrimination. There are complex links between health and human rights.

Health as Ethics

Health is not a business like other businesses. Despite arguments to the contrary, health is not a matter of statistics and bottom lines. Decisions about health are related to how we see ourselves as individuals and societies. It is about our fundamental values and beliefs. It raises issues about the very notion of life and its meaning and an understanding of how to be humane and caring. It raises questions of illness, dependence, and mortality. And it raises questions of how we determine which values will take precedence, who will be entrusted as the gatekeepers to health care, what guidelines are used to make decisions, and whose understanding of health and its etiology will have primacy. There is an ever-present tension among differing perspectives on these issues.

Health, law, and ethics are inextricably intertwined. The surprise is how little attention has been given to putting a human rights lens on health despite the obvious importance of this to ensuring that people have access to this fundamental right.

Rights and ethics in health were, until recently, medical rights and medical ethics (Somerville 2004). They relied on the physician to "do good" or to do what was in the best interests of the patient. The medical profession was entrusted to understand the nature of what was good health care and to carry that out. The profession was trusted to self-regulate and to follow a Hippocratic oath. And medical committees or individuals made health policy decisions within a context of medical and biological knowledge.

A shift is taking place, however. While there continues to be a focus on the individual patient benefit and on questions of individual rights to medical benefits, it is increasingly clear that this approach is not adequate with the greater demands for access to technology, and it becomes increasingly clear that health is not singularly, nor even primarily, the consequence of biological conditions.

Things have changed. First, our society is more diverse and pluralistic—there are many diverse views in society, views that are grounded in socio-economic status, culture, religion, sexual orientation, ability, and race. This diversity means that we cannot assume shared values or a common story. This raises the possibility that what is good for one person may not be of benefit to another. There are competing demands that cannot be resolved at the individual level, so there is a focus on community, society, and the common good, rather than simply the individual situation.

Second, science and biotechnology are progressing at a rapid rate. For example, the mapping of the human genome in a matter of 15 years, a result of an internationally financed biological research collaboration, has opened up whole new areas of scientific knowledge that raise questions of ethics and rights and the allocation of health dollars that is unparalleled. The Human Genome Project has been termed by many as a "major new science" and the findings as the "most significant intellectual discovery in humanity's scientific evolution" (Cahill 1996: 21). Science and technology can be characterized as both a promise and a threat. Patients can die from the side effects of drug protocols, such as chemotherapy, that are supposed to cure them. The definition of death has changed in response to modern transplantation and other medical interventions. Gene therapy can be performed involving both administering replacement genes even in utero and regulating genes by replacing command sequences. This has led to predictions about the possibility of an era of "designer babies" as a consequence of the genetic ability to choose the characteristics of children and cloning (Shakespeare 1996; Somerville 1996).

Third, there are obvious inequities in the way in which health care, health status, biotechnology, and drugs are made available to people. These cannot be ignored. Included among the dilemmas raised are issues related to the unequal access to technology and drugs; the way in which resources are allocated; the public outcry about patients suffering and even dying because of inadequate care; the burden on families made responsible for medical and health care; the responsibility of corporations for health conditions that are avoidable; and the preference for health care that addresses the individual medical condition rather than the social determinants of ill health.

Good Health Is Social Justice

Health, then, is not a condition that is set apart from issues of social justice, social values, or citizenship. It is affected by cultures, laws, and values.

Health is connected to international agreements relating to human rights. It is linked to the national constitutional and legal protection of individuals.[1] These guarantees are intrinsic to the defence of equal access to treatment and an equal right to well-being. Notions of economic efficiency (Deber 1999) and evidence-based quality of practice cannot be relied upon to provide a basic guarantee to good health, and even democratic political mandates and ethical standards do not do so. Hospital ethics committees and self-regulating professions are not replacements for the equality guarantees in health. While an ethics committee will make sure that valid consent is assured for all patients in a hospital, they are not in a position to ensure that drug protocols that are not used in that hospital become available to patients. Medical care and health care decisions cannot be isolated from our basic social contract, as though medical ethics and law are a mysterious, exclusive domain comprehensible only to professional practitioners. Instead, it is important to apply existing rules of non-discrimination and human rights to health policy decisions as we are in fact required to do by human rights policy, standards, and ethics.

A Social Imperative

Using human rights is a means to making equitable health outcomes a social imperative. It would be naïve to suggest that such an approach could provide a clear map through the minefields of decision making, but it does give us a single standard against which we can measure our health priorities at the international level, the national level, and in individual treatment decisions. For example, it does hold us to a norm of non-discrimination in the provision of health care services so that a person with an income of less than $20,000 is not less likely to get a heart bypass than someone with an income over $100,000.

What are the building blocks of health and human rights? The right to "the highest attainable standard of health" was first articulated in the World Health Organization constitution, which was adopted by the World Health Conference in 1946 (World Health Organization 1948). It was reiterated in the 1978 *Declaration of Alma Atal*[2] (World Health Organization 1978) and in the *World Health Declaration* adopted by the World Health Assembly in 1998[3] (World Health Organization 1998). It has been affirmed in a wide range of international and regional human rights instruments.

Box 4.2: **Selected International Instruments Incorporating a Right to Health**

Universal Declaration of Human Rights (1948)
Article 25 (1): "Everyone has a right to a standard of living adequate for the health of himself and his family, including food, clothing, housing and medical care and necessary social services."

International Covenant on Economic, Social, and Cultural Rights (1966)
Article 12 (1): States parties recognize "the rights of everyone to the enjoyment of the highest attainable standard of physical and mental health."
Article 12 (2): Illustrates the breadth of areas that needed to be addressed and other human rights that have be addressed "to achieve the full realization of this right."

International Convention on the Elimination of All Forms of Racial Discrimination (1963)
Article 5(e)(iv): States undertake to prohibit and eliminate racial discrimination and equality before the law, in respect to "The right to public health, medical care, social security, and social services."

Convention on the Elimination of All Forms of Discrimination against Women (1979)
Article 12 (1): "States Parties shall take all appropriate measures to eliminate discrimination against women in the field of health care in order to ensure, on a basis of equality of men and women, access to health care services, including those related to family planning."

Convention on the Right of the Child (1989)
Article 24 (1): "States Parties recognize the right of the child to the enjoyment of the highest attainable standard of health and to facilities for the treatment of illness and rehabilitation of health. States Parties shall strive to ensure that no child is deprived of his or her right of access to such health care services."

The United Nations' *International Covenant on Economic, Social, and Cultural Rights*[4] (ICESCR) (UN General Assembly 1966), which has been ratified by 145 countries (2002), is the most authoritative international instrument. In 2000, the committee for that covenant adopted a General Comment on the right to health (UN Committee on Economic, Social, and Cultural Rights 2000), clarifying[5] the meaning of this right. Most important, the General Comment recognized the relationship of the right to health to other rights, including the right to food, housing, work, education, participation, the enjoyment of the benefits of scientific progress and its application, life, non-discrimination, equality, the prohibition against torture, privacy, access to information, and freedom of association, assembly, and movement. It recognized that the right to health was dependent on these other rights. In other words, the right to health is more than access to health care and applies equally to other social determinants of health. The General Comment further set out four criteria for evaluating the right to health:

- availability
- accessibility
- acceptability
- quality

Table 4.1: The Recognition of the Right to Health Internationally

Countries that ratified the ICESCR 142

Countries that ratified regional treaties with a right to health 83

Countries that recognize a right to health in their national constitutions 109

Source: Eleanor D. Kinney, "The International Human Right to Health: What Does This Mean for Our Nation and World?" *Indiana Law Review* 34 (2001): 1465.

Availability includes adequate public health (including sanitation and safe drinking water) and health care facilities, including hospitals and clinics as well as sufficient trained personnel and essential unexpired drugs. Under accessibility are the four categories of non-discrimination, physical accessibility, economic accessibility, and information accessibility. Evaluated on the basis of acceptability means that health care is provided with attention to criteria of medical ethics, cultural sensitivity, gender and life cycle needs, and confidentiality. Health facilities, and goods and services are expected to be scientifically and medically appropriate and of good quality.

Taken together, these international instruments outline a normative standard for the right to health. Most states have national constitutions that incorporate the key principles of respect for human rights and many states have signed regional and international standards and treaties that specify the particular human rights they protect. The right to health is a comprehensive right extending to timely, affordable and appropriate health care and to the basic determinants of health, including safe and potable water and adequate nutrition, healthy occupational and environmental conditions, and access to health-related information and education. It is also the right to the enjoyment of a variety of facilities, goods, and services necessary for the realization of the highest standard of health. And, finally, the facilities, goods and services, and the underlying social determinants of health have to be available, accessible, acceptable, and of good quality.

Measuring the Right to Health

The UN Special Rapporteur on the right to health (UN Economic and Social Council 2003: 7) recommends the following categories of right to health indicators: Structural indicators, process indicators, and outcome indicators. He includes in structural indicators those structures, systems, and mechanisms that are necessary to the realization of the right. By way of example, he includes constitutions and policies that incorporate the right to health, lists of essential medicines, and national pharmaceutical policies. Process indicators in this schemata measure the degree to which "activities that are necessary to attain certain health objectives are carried out, and the progress of those indicators over time. They monitor, as it were, effort, not outcome" (UN General Assembly 2003: 9). Some examples of process indicators would be the number of times a person sees a skilled health professional during a time of medical need; the number of available health care facilities available per population needing it; numbers of people with a particular condition receiving the needed drugs (e.g., people with HIV/AIDS receiving anti-retroviral combination therapy). Finally, outcome indicators measure the results achieved by health-related policies. This would include examples of measures such as maternal mortality rate; perinatal deaths per number of births; number of teens with HIV/AIDS; disease patterns disaggregated by income level, and so on. These outcome indicators are influenced by the wide variety of interrelated factors that affect health status.

The United Nations Special Rapporteur on health has proposed that a clear distinction needs to be made between health good practices and right to health good practices. He has identified an initial set of criteria for this distinction and has challenged others to examine the adequacy of those criteria. Thus, he has opened the debate for recognizing that a new framework on right to health requires a new taxonomy and new criteria to enable the measure of compliance with a human rights approach to health nationally and under international norms and standards.

Paul Hunt (the UN Special Rapporteur on health) proposes the following as categories for taxonomy to classify initiatives:

- the *availability* of health facilities, goods, and services within the jurisdiction
- the accessibility without discrimination in law or fact of health facilities, goods, and services
- the *physical accessibility* of health facilities, goods, and services
- the *economic accessibility* of health facilities, goods, and services
- the *accessibility of health information*

***

Box 4.3: Health Good Practice ▢ Right to Health Good Practice

Three criteria needed:
1. demonstrably enhances an individual's or group's enjoyment of one or more elements of the right to health, e.g., by:
   - improving access to essentials medicines
   - enhancing quality of the workplace environment
   - reducing discriminatory health practices
   - improving participation of all in health policy-making
   - strengthening right to health accountability mechanisms, etc.
2. pays attention to vulnerable groups, including those living in poverty
3. in process and outcome, the good practice is consistent with the enjoyment of all rights

Source: UN General Assembly, *Human Rights Situations: Human Rights Situations and Reports of Special Rapporteurs and Representatives*, 58th Session, October 10, UN Doc. A/58/427: 13.

***

- the *cultural acceptability* of health facilities, goods, and services
- the *quality* of health facilities, goods, and services
- the *active and informed participation* of individuals and groups, especially the vulnerable and disadvantaged, including those living in poverty, in relation to health polices, programs, and projects
- the right to health *monitoring and accountability* mechanisms that are effective, transparent, and accessible

These provide a way to monitor good right to health practice at the national and international level and to measure the degree to which states are in compliance with human rights standards in their policies and programs. The realization of human rights as an indicator of well-being may prove to be a more accurate indicator than traditional health status indicators (Mann 1999a). "Information and statistics are a powerful tool for creating a culture of accountability and for realizing human rights" (UN Development Programme 2000: 10).

Differential Access to Health and Well-being

The right to health cannot be viewed in isolation. It is closely related to the enjoyment of other human rights, including non-discrimination and equality. A disproportional degree of compromised health is borne by those who are marginalized and vulnerable in society.

It is one of the greatest of contemporary social injustices that people who live in the most disadvantaged circumstances have more illnesses, more disability and shorter lives than those who are more affluent. (Benzeval, Judge, and Whitehead 1995: xxi)

This is a result of a number of factors that can include direct discrimination, as has been the case when individuals with disabilities are not given the same priority for transplants, for example. In other cases, people's well-being is compromised when they live in institutional settings in which their health needs are not met or when their access to good health services is restricted.

More often even than the direct discrimination are the instances of indirect or covert discrimination faced by people who are marginalized, and the failure of governments and others to put in place policies and programs that would address the inequalities in health and illness. These are conditions that may be both national and international. For example, governments' failure to monitor national industries so that they meet at least the minimum legal environmental standard in their home country when they are operating in developing countries is an omission that leads to inequity in health and disease patterns. Similarly, governments' failure to address income inequities results in differential patterns of disease based on socio-economic status.[6]

The *Declaration on the Elimination of the Violence against Women* (UN General Assembly 1993) recognizes the link between violence against women and the historically unequal power relations between men and women.

With respect to health and health care, it is now generally recognized that the prohibition of discrimination includes:

> … any discrimination in access to health care and the underlying determinants of health, as well as to means and entitlements for their procurement, on the grounds of race, colour, sex, language, religion, political or other opinion, property, birth, physical or mental disability, health status (including HIV/AIDS), sexual orientation, civil, political, social or other status, which has the intention or effect of nullifying or impairing the equal enjoyment or exercise of the right to health. (UN Committee on Economic, Social, and Cultural Rights 2000)

There are many examples of discrimination in health. A recent case in Canada helps to underline the way in which systemic discrimination can occur.

In October 1997, the Canadian Supreme Court delivered a decision in *Eldridge v. British Columbia*, which involved a claim by three deaf applicants that the legislation governing health care services and hospitals in the province was discriminatory because it neither included sign language interpreter services as an insured service, nor required hospitals to provide sign language interpreter services. The court ruled that the government had violated the equality provisions of the Canadian Charter of Rights and Freedoms in its implementation of the provincial medical services plan. The court held that, in order for deaf people to receive the benefit of medical services, they required communication with their doctors. Interpreters were not an ancillary service but an integral part of medical care. In providing a benefit scheme, the state was obliged to provide the benefit in a non-discriminatory manner. "Failure to provide interpreters meant that deaf people would receive an inferior quality of health care to hearing persons" (Mosoff and Grant 1999: 42).

This decision is important for a number of reasons. First, it is the court's holding that "once the state provides a benefit, it is obliged to do so in a non-discriminatory manner" (*Eldridge v. British Columbia*, Ministry of Health (1997) 3 S.C.R. 624). Second, it is important because of the interpretation of equality that the Charter protects. The denial of equality in *Eldridge* arose from the government's failure to take action (rather than the imposition of a burden). The discrimination arose from the adverse effects of a public benefit scheme that failed to provide the same level of service (adverse impact discrimination). The court held that

> [t]o argue that governments should be entitled to provide benefits to the general population without ensuring that disadvantaged members of society have the resources to take full advantage of those benefits bespeaks a thin and impoverished vision of S 15(1). It is belied, more importantly, by the thrust of this Court's equality jurisprudence. (*Eldridge v. British Columbia*, Ministry of Health (1997) 3 S.C.R. 624)

The key principle here is that the government has an obligation to remedy inequality notwithstanding that the health benefit scheme appeared neutral and the remedy meant that the government had to spend money. The third issue of importance is the court's holding that effective communication is an indispensable component of the delivery of a medical service. This is important to recognizing the systemic nature of the discrimination against people with disabilities and recognizing that the discrimination cannot be redressed without changes to the definition of the health services that the government provides (Degener 1995).

Disability and the Right to Health

The *Standard Rules on the Equalization of Opportunities for Persons with Disabilities* (UN General Assembly, High Commission for Human Rights, 1993) are important in interpreting ICESCR rights in the context of disability, particularly because the ICESCR explicitly acknowledged the interpretative value of the *Standard Rules* in General Comment no. 5.[7] Two of the *Standard Rules* relate directly to health: Rule 2 on medical care and Rule 3 on rehabilitation. Rule 2 focuses on equal quality of medical services for people with disabilities and access to treatment or medicines necessary to improve levels of functioning, as well as adequate training of medical professionals. Rule 3 addresses the accessibility, design, and content of rehabilitation programs to meet the actual needs of people with disabilities.

Box 4.4: Food for Thought

Should one deny medical care to a person solely on the grounds of his or her disability?

The right to health for people with disabilities is often infringed because of their limited access to health services. They are commonly unable to take advantage of available medical services because of assumptions about their quality of life and whether it is beneficial to them or to others to provide medical and health benefits that others receive. There was a recent example of a young boy with Down syndrome being denied a place on a waiting list for a kidney transplant. It was purported by the hospital that, because of his quality of life—that is, because he had Down syndrome—he would not benefit as greatly from a kidney transplant as someone without a disability, so they argued solely on the basis of his disability that he should not be placed on the list. Triaging is not uncommon in medical care, and widely held prejudices against people with disabilities often result in discrimination in their access to the benefits of medical treatment. Health needs of people with disabilities are regularly limited to curing or improving their impairments, rather than improving their health. The reported incidences of selective non-treatment of people with disabilities suggest that medical standards are differentially applied, a practice that infringes on the right to health and rehabilitation. People with disabilities are also particularly vulnerable to standards of living that affect health: poverty, poor housing, unemployment, lack of services, and literacy.

The *Principles for the Protection of Persons with Mental Illness and the Improvement of Mental Health Care* address issues related to the right to health in principles 6–14 and 22 (UN General Assembly 1991). These principles cover confidentiality; the role of the community and culture; standards of care, treatment, medication, consent to treatment; notice of rights, rights and conditions in mental health facilities; and resources for mental health facilities.[8]

The Committee on Economic, Social, and Cultural Rights (CESCR) General Comment no. 5 on people with disabilities quotes the *Standard Rules* in indicating that the same level of medical care within the same medical system for those with disabilities and those without disabilities is a key element of the right to health. ECOSOC interprets Article 12 of the ICESCR as a guarantee "to have access to, and to benefit from, those medical and social services ... which enable persons with disabilities to become independent, prevent further disabilities and support social integration." The paragraph continues:

Similarly, such persons should be provided with rehabilitation services which would enable them to reach and sustain their optimum level of independence and functioning. All such services should be provided in such a way that the persons concerned are able to maintain full respect for their rights and dignity. (UN Committee on Economic, Social, and Cultural Rights 1994: General Comment no. 5, para. 34)

Both the Mental Health Care Principles and the ECOSOC approach to the right to health in the context of disability are important because they recognize the social determinants of health—that is, determinants of health that originate from the exercise of other rights including self-determination and control over one's own lifestyle and surroundings, autonomy, human dignity, active participation in the community, and non-discrimination. This connection between health status and the exercise of rights has significant implications for people with disabilities.

Box 4.5: International Instruments Recognizing a Right to Health

Regional Instruments Recognizing a Right to Health
European Social Charter (1961)
African Charter on Human and Peoples' Rights (1981)
Additional Protocol to the American Convention on Human Rights in the Area of Economic, Social and Cultural Rights (1988)

Other United Nations Affirmations of the Right to Health
Commission on Human Rights proclaimed the right to health (2000)
Vienna Declaration and Programme of Action (1993)

The ICESCR's General Comment no. 14 on the right to health lays out the core obligations and elements of the right: "availability, accessibility, acceptability and quality" (UN Committee on Economic, Social, and Cultural Rights 2000: General Comment no. 14, para. 12). Non-discrimination is a key element of accessibility and the ICESCR highlights the accessibility needs of vulnerable groups, including people with disabilities. It stresses "the need to ensure that not only the public health sector but also private providers of health services and facilities comply with the principle of non-discrimination in relation to persons with disabilities." Both physical and mental disability are specifically included as prohibited grounds for discrimination (UN Committee on Economic, Social, and Cultural Rights 2000: General Comment no. 14, para. 14).

The UN's *Convention on the Elimination of All Forms of Discrimination against Women* General Recommendation no. 24 on women and health[9] refers to the need to give special attention to the health needs and rights of women who belong to vulnerable and disadvantaged groups, including women with physical or mental disabilities (UN General Assembly 1979: General Recommendation no. 24, para. 6). The General Recommendation also refers specifically to the needs of women with disabilities:

Women with disabilities, of all ages, often have difficulty with physical access to health services. Women with mental disabilities are particularly vulnerable, while there is limited understanding, in general, of the broad range of risks to mental health to which women are disproportionately susceptible as a result of gender discrimination, violence, poverty, armed conflict, dislocation and other forms of social deprivation. States parties should take appropriate measures to ensure that health services are sensitive to the needs of women with disabilities and are respectful of their human rights and dignity. (UN General Assembly 1979: General Recommendation no. 24, para. 14)

The Committee on the Rights of the Child (CRC) has issued General Comment no. 4 on adolescent health and development. The committee requires states to "adopt special measures to ensure the physical, sexual and mental integrity of adolescents with disabilities, who are particularly vulnerable to abuse and neglect" (UN Committee on the Rights of the Child 2003: General Comment no. 4, para. 12). The committee notes that systematic collection of data is necessary to monitor the right to health, including data on adolescents with disabilities (UN Committee on the Rights of the Child 2003: General Comment no. 4, para. 13). The committee reaffirms that those adolescents with mental and/or physical disabilities "have an equal right to the highest attainable standard of physical and mental health." This obligates states parties to

(a) ensure that health facilities, goods and services are available and accessible to all adolescents with disabilities and that these facilities and services promote their self-reliance and their active participation in the community; (b) ensure that the necessary equipment and personal support are available to enable them to move around, participate and communicate; (c) pay specific attention to the special needs relating to the sexuality of adolescents with disabilities; and (d) remove barriers that hinder adolescents with disabilities in realizing their rights. (UN Committee on the Rights of the Child 2003: General Comment no. 4, para. 35)

There are some particular rights that need to be protected for people with disabilities. These include[10] the quality and accessibility of services as well as the availability of a range of services, particularly rights related to:

- free and informed consent; prevention of unwanted medical and related interventions and corrective surgeries from being imposed on people with disabilities
- protection of the privacy of health and rehabilitation information
- participation in legislative and policy development as well as in the planning, delivery, and evaluation of health and rehabilitation services

Finally, and perhaps most importantly, the "highest attainable standard of health" for people with disabilities is related to the recognition that they are entitled to the same human rights, citizenship, and social inclusion as others. The presumption in public health and in the biomedical sciences that the goal of health policies is to reduce illness, death, *and disability* is to fundamentally deny the nature of disability as a social condition and to stigmatize people with disabilities in a way that drives an irresolvable wedge between health and disability.

Defining disability as a contingent part of ill health is, in itself, the most fundamental barrier to the right to health for people with disabilities.

Reproduction and the Right to Health

Reproductive health refers to people being able to have satisfying and safe sexual expression and to make decisions about whether and when they want to reproduce. It is an area of health that is fraught with an overlay of norms and values about sexuality, responsibility, and prejudice. It involves the enjoyment of sexuality and choice in pregnancy; protection against abuse, coercion, and harassment; and safety from sexually transmitted diseases. Two international conferences in the 1990s focused attention on the promotion and protection of human rights in reproductive and sexual health. The *Convention on the Elimination of All Forms of Discrimination against Women* (1979) also specifically mentioned women's rights related to reproductive planning.

In the *Programme of Action* developed at the International Conference on Population and Development in Cairo in 1994 (UN Department of Economic, Social Information, and Policy Analysis 1995) and subsequently at the International Conference on Women in Beijing in 1995, reproductive health was defined in the context of the WHO definition of health as a "state of complete physical, mental and social well-being and not merely the absence of disease or infirmity in all matters relating to the reproductive system and to its functions and processes" (UN Department of Public Information 1996: para. 94).

The *Programme of Action* laid out the way in which reproductive rights are incorporated in the scope of human rights:

> These rights rest on the recognition of the basic right of all couples and individuals to decide freely and responsibly the number, spacing and timing of their children, and to have the information and means to do so; and the right to attain the highest level of sexual and reproductive health. It also includes their right to make decisions concerning reproduction free of discrimination, coercion and violence, as expressed in human rights documents. (UN Department of Economic, Social Information, and Policy Analysis 1995: para. 7.3)

How are these rights expressed? A woman's right to free choice in decisions concerning her body and her reproductive options have been in the forefront of the reproductive rights movement. Some specific human rights that can contribute to reproductive and sexual health and well-being include rights relating to: life, survival, security and sexuality; reproductive self-determination and free choice of maternity; health and the benefits of scientific progress; non-discrimination and due respect for difference; and information, education, and decision making (Cook, Dickens, and Fathalla 2003).

In practice, these rights have been protected by courts (Cook and Dickens 2003; Cook, Dickens, and Fathalla 2003: 159–161, 164, 170, 187–209; Cook, Dickens, Ngwena, and Plata 2001) in cases involving rights to basic services necessary for the reproductive and sexual health (rights to life, survival, security, and sexuality). These would include such examples as the right of women to go through pregnancy and childbirth safely and to protect the confidentiality of people seeking reproductive health services.

Reproductive rights are an area of health in which examples of inequity are widespread. Not only is this inequity found between men and women in reproductive rights, but it is also clear that there are significant inequities among countries. In particular, the differential is evident between high-income countries and low-income countries and between countries in which the rights of women are respected and in those in which they are not. The ability of individuals to control their own fertility and safety from sexually transmitted communicable diseases is of particular concern for inequities and the contravention of human rights. "Inability of individuals, and particularly of women, in developing countries to regulate and control their fertility is not only affecting the health of the people immediately concerned, but has implications for global stability and for the balance between population and natural resources and between people and environment, and is a violation of women's human rights" (Cook, Dickens, and Fathalla 2003: 13).

HIV/AIDS and the Right to Health

The transmission of communicable diseases is another important and pressing issue in ensuring the right to health on an international basis (UN Office of the High Commissioner for Human Rights 1998). Some 42 million people around the world now live with HIV and thousands die every day. It is estimated that treatment reaches fewer than 5 percent of those affected. As access to health care is one of the fundamental instruments of the right to health, it is of particular concern. People who are not receiving drugs are those in low-income countries and marginalized populations in high-income countries. For many people in low-income countries, the cost of treatment remains intolerably high. This type of discrimination is a human rights violation[11] that is a barrier both to prevention efforts and access to treatment and care.

The United Nations issued comprehensive, detailed, and specific guidelines in 1998 based on the recognition that there is a fundamental relationship between human rights and the HIV/AIDS epidemic: "In the context of HIV/AIDS, an environment in which human rights are respected ensure that vulnerability to

HIV/AIDS live a life of dignity without discrimination and the personal and societal impact of HIV infections is alleviated" (Cohen 2002: 5). The guidelines have three broad and interrelated approaches:

> ... improvement of governmental capacity for acknowledging the government's responsibility for multisectoral coordination and accountability; widespread reform of laws and legal support services, with a focus on anti-discrimination, protection of public health, and improvement of the status of women, children and marginalized groups; and support for increased private sector and community participation in the response to HIV/AIDS .... (Cohen 2002: 5)

An important issue here, as with reproductive health and disability, is how to understand and address the social determinants of vulnerability. Also, it is how to address the discrimination resulting from the subordination of women and girls; hostility toward gay, lesbian, bisexual, and transgendered people; the subordination of Aboriginal peoples; the dependency of prisoners on others to prevent the spread of disease in prisons; and a disproportionate emphasis on controlling drug use and sex work through criminal and public health law.

This coercive use of law, added to demands to curtail the conventional notion of confidentiality of medical testing, makes clear the ease with which people's human rights can so easily be disregarded in the area of public health. It exposes the fundamental importance of using human rights as a framework if people are to realize their health and well-being.

Increasingly since 1988 there have been efforts to "add and integrate a societal dimension with the previous individually centered, risk-reduction approach" (Mann 1999b: 218). The conventional notion that disease is a dynamic event taking place in a static environment as the basis for education and services has been challenged as the answer to the AIDS/HIV epidemic. Mann argues that while "risk-reduction is necessary it is not sufficient to control the pandemic" (Mann 1999b: 219).

In this context, access to information about the transmission of HIV is important as a means to prevent transmission; adequate medical care and treatment, nutrition, shelter, and income are necessary to reduce the susceptibility of people with HIV to ill health and disease; people with HIV/AIDS have to be engaged in the design and implementation of prevention programs and support services; and the stigma associated with HIV/AIDS, which results in discrimination in the workplace, housing, immigration, and access to health and social services, has to be addressed.

These conditions are similar to those that apply in cases of other marginalized populations and result in the failure to be able to exercise the right to health. The enforcement of basic human rights—as outlined in international human rights treaties and instruments as well as in national law—is broad enough to address these pressing issues in health.

Health Research and the Right to Health

The expenditure on health research—which results in the vast majority of health research and development being expended on health problems that affect only a small proportion of the world's population—has significant right-to-health implications. The World Health Organization calls certain diseases (for example, leprosy and dengue fever) the "neglected diseases,"[12] which it says affects more than one billion people worldwide. "Neglected diseases are hidden diseases as they affect almost exclusively extremely poor populations living in remote areas beyond the reach of health services. Their low mortality despite high morbidity places them near the bottom of mortality tables and, in the past, they have received low priority" (Kindhauser 2003: 6). They are also neglected because, confined to poor populations, there has been a lack of incentives to develop drugs and vaccines for markets that cannot pay. And, thirdly, they are neglected because even where effective and low-cost drugs are available, the inability to pay results in little or no demand for them. In other words, there is no effective market and no effective incentive for health research and development for new drugs, vaccines, or other medical interventions.[13]

Impact of Globalization on the Right to Health

Globalization and the flow of capital have created new types of human rights issues for health (Fidler 2000), many of which have been ignored until now. The flow of capital can create new employment opportunities in some areas, but the consequence of those new jobs may be conditions that are harmful to the health of the people who work in those jobs or live in proximity. For example, child labour is well documented in some parts of the majority world (i.e. India, China, and other areas where the majority of the world's population lives) and clearly is hazardous to the health of children; environmental hazards may also be a consequence of some types of industry that are in areas where people's right to health is already compromised by poverty, poor nutrition, and unsanitary conditions generally.

A further impact of globalization is its potential to stimulate the spread of disease and pandemics because of the increased mobility of people; this was evidenced with the pattern of transmission of SARS. SARS moved from country to country, airport to airport, and town to town non-contiguously. The failure to see the right to health in its international context can lead to unintended consequences. Globalization can lead to worldwide marketing of harmful substances. Fast food, tobacco, and alcohol are examples of such marketing. In some cases, it has been suggested that as the market for tobacco has decreased in high-income countries, promotion of cigarettes has increased in the majority world. The right to health information has arguably been contravened with the marketing of fast foods both in high-income countries and evidently in the majority world. In these cases, relatively low-cost, overprocessed, high-calorie, and minimum-nutrition food is made available in heavily marketed outlets, appealing in many cases to children and people with limited incomes. The impact of consumption of this food on health is not made clearly available to the consumer, nor are the environmental impacts of the type of packaging divulged to the consumer.

Increasingly, those engaged with globalization are big business, biomedical research firms, pharmaceutical companies, health management organizations, and health insurance companies. They are non-government and multinational, the consequence of which is that legal control is limited and international human rights law does not directly apply to them.

Conclusions

Globalization has led to greater recognition of health as a matter of human rights. States and courts are increasingly bringing health within the ambit of social, economic, cultural, political, and civil rights. This has had real effect. For example, the court has interpreted state neglect of an individual's basic health needs as a denial of the right of security of the person, and the court has argued the right to non-discrimination as a reason to ensure equitable access to health care. The recognition that controlling HIV/AIDS through criminal and public health law was not as effective as looking at health promotion strategies is an example of the effect of a human rights approach. Each legal precedent and public policy of this nature is an important step forward.

Human rights are another way to understand the problem of poor health status globally, regionally, and locally. They provide a new lens by which to decide how to address health and well-being. It is a move away from translating data describing risk and distribution of health conditions being defined primarily or exclusively in individual terms, to uncovering the societal dimensions that influence and constrain individual behaviour.

A sustainable human rights framework for health recognizes, at a minimum, that health is a result of social, legal, and economic status and that a broad set of factors contribute to exclusion and the loss of human rights, which in turn leads to poor health status. It underscores that respect for diversity contributes to well-being. It recognizes that people must be supported in exercising their rights, and that people need a sense of fairness in their communities and societies to reach the highest attainable standard of health. A human rights framework forces governments to address health disparities and holds governments accountable for the societal barriers to good health.

There is still a long way to go, but some progress in recognizing health as a human right is being made. Martin Luther King, the leader of another great movement for social justice, once said: "The arc of history is long, but it always bends towards justice." The urgency felt by those marginalized outside the boundaries of justice is palpable. But as they push, we can see the direction in which the arc is bending.

References

Anand, S., F. Peter, and A. Sen. (2004). *Public Health, Ethics and Equity*. Oxford: Oxford University Press.

Benzeval, M., K. Judge, and M. Whitehead. (1995). *Tackling Inequalities in Health: An Agenda for Action*. London: King's Fund.

Cahill, G. (1996). "A Brief History of the Human Genome Project." In *Morality and the New Genetics: A Guide for Students and Health Care Providers*, edited by B. Gert et al., 1–27. Boston: Jones and Barlett Publishers.

Canadian Charter of Rights and Freedoms, Part I of the Constitution Act, 1982, being schedule B to the Canada Act 1982 (U.K.), 1982, c. 11.

Cohen, J.C. (2002). "Developing States' Response to the Pharmaceutical Imperatives of the TRIPS Agreement." In *The Economics of Essential Medicines*, edited by B. Granville, 115–136. London and Washington: Royal Institute of International Affairs.

Cook, R.J., and B.M. Dickens. (2003). "Access to Emergency Contraception." *Journal of Obstetrics and Gynecology Canada* 25(11): 914–916.

Cook, R.J., B.M. Dickens, and M.F. Fathalla. (2003). *Reproductive Health and Human Rights: Integrating Medicine, Ethics, and Law*. Oxford and New York: Clarendon Press. Available on-line at www.loc.gov/catdir/toc/fy043/2003270259.html.

Cook, R.J., B.M. Dickens, C. Ngwena, and M.I. Plata. (2001). "The Legal Status of Emergency Contraception." *International Journal of Gynecology and Obstetrics* 75(2): 185–191.

Deber, R. (1999). "The Use and Misuse of Economics." In *Do We Care?: Renewing Canada's Commitment to Health: Proceedings of the First Directions for Canadian Health Care Conference*, edited by M.A. Somerville and J.R. Saul, 53–68. Montreal and Ithaca: McGill-Queen's University Press.

Degener, T. (1995). "Disabled Persons and Human Rights: The Legal Framework." In *Human Rights and Disabled Persons: Essays and Relevant Human Rights Instruments*, edited by T. Degener and Y. Koster-Dreese, 9–39. Dordrecht and Boston: M. Nijhoff.

Eldridge v. British Columbia, Ministry of Health (1997) 3 S.C.R. 624.

Fidler, D.P. (2000). "The Globalization of Public Health." In *International Law and Public Health: Materials on and Analysis of Global Health Jurisprudence*, edited by D.P. Fidler, 16–23. Ardsley: Transnational Publishers.

Foucault, M., and C. Gordon. (1980). *Power/Knowledge: Selected Interviews and Other Writings, 1972–1977*. New York: Pantheon Books.

Kindhauser, M.K. (2003). *Communicable Diseases Cluster, Communicable Diseases 2002: Global Defence against the Infectious Disease Threat*. Geneva: World Health Organization. Available on-line at www.who.int/infectious-disease-news/cds2002/index.html.

Mann, J.M. (1999a). "Health and Human Rights." In *Health and Human Rights: A Reader*, edited by J.M. Mann, S. Gruskin, M. A. Grodin, and G.J. Annas, 7–20. New York: Routledge.

_____. (1999b). "Human Rights and AIDS: The Future of the Pandemic." In *Health and Human Rights: A Reader*, edited by J.M. Mann, S. Gruskin, M.A. Grodin, and G.J. Annas, 216–226. New York: Routledge.

Mosoff, J., and I. Grant. (1999). *Intellectual Disability and the Supreme Court: The Implications of the Charter for People Who Have a Disability*. Toronto: Canadian Association for Community Living.

Shakespeare, T. (1996). "Disability, Identity and Difference." In *Exploring the Divide: Illness and Disability*, edited by C. Barnes and G. Mercer, 94–113. Leeds: Disability Press.

Somerville, M.A. (1996). "Genetics, Reproductive Technologies, Euthanasia and the Search for a New Societal Paradigm." *Social Science and Medicine* 42(12): ix–xii.

———. (2004). *The Ethical Canary: Science, Society and the Human Spirit*. Montreal: McGill-Queen's University Press.

UN Ad Hoc Committee on a Comprehensive and Integral International Convention on the Protection and Promotion of the Rights and Dignity of Persons with Disabilities. (2004). *Report of the Working Group to the Ad Hoc Committee, Annex 1: Draft Comprehensive and Integral International Convention on the Protection and Promotion of the Rights and Dignity of Persons with Disabilities, New York, 5–16 January.* UN Doc. A/AC.265/2004/WG.1.

UN Committee on Economic, Social, and Cultural Rights (CESCR). (1994). *11th Session, General Comment no. 5, Persons with Disabilities.* UN Doc. E/1995/22.

———. (2000). *22nd Session, Geneva, 25 April–12 May, General Comment no. 14.* UN Doc. E/C.12/2000/4.

UN Committee on the Rights of the Child (CRC). (2003). *Convention on the Rights of the Child, 33rd Session, 19 May–6 June, General Comment no. 4.* UN Doc. CRC/GC/2003/4.

UN Department of Economic, Social Information, and Policy Analysis. (1995). *Population and Development: Programme of Action Adopted at the International Conference on Population and Development, Cairo, 5–13 September 1994.* New York: United Nations, Dept. for Economic, Social Information, and Policy Analysis.

UN Department of Public Information. (1996). *The Beijing Declaration and the Platform for Action: Fourth World Conference on Women, Beijing, China, 4–15 September 1995.* New York: Dept. of Public Information, United Nations.

UN Development Programme. (2000). *Human Development Report 2000: Human Development and Human Rights.* New York and Oxford: Oxford University Press.

UN Economic and Social Council (ECOSOC), Commission on Human Rights. (2003). *Report of the Special Rapporteur, 59th Session, 13 February.* UN Doc. E/CN.4/2003/58.

UN General Assembly. (1966). *International Covenant on Economic, Social, and Cultural Rights (ICESCR), 21st session, resolution 2200A/21.*UN Doc. A/6316.

———. (1979). *Convention on the Elimination of All Forms of Discrimination against Women (CEDAW), 18 December, Resolution 34/180.*

———. (1991). *Principles for the Protection of Persons with Mental Illness and the Improvement of Mental Health Care, 75th Plenary Meeting, 17 December, Resolution 46/119.* UN Doc. A/RES/46/119. From www.un.org/documents/ga/res/46/a46r119.htm

———. (1993). *Declaration on the Elimination of Violence against Women (UNDEVW), 85th Plenary Meeting, Preamble, 20 December, Resolution 48/104.* UN Doc. A/RES/48/104.

———. (2003). *Human Rights Situations: Human Rights Situations and Reports of Special Rapporteurs and Representatives, 58th Session, 10 October.* UN Doc. A/58/427.

UN General Assembly, High Commission for Human Rights. (1993). *Standard Rules on the Equalization of Opportunities for Persons with Disabilities, 48th Session, 85th Mtg., Resolution 48/96.* UN Document A/RES/48/96.

UN Office of the High Commissioner for Human Rights. (1998). *HIV/AIDS and Human Rights, International Guidelines: Second International Consultation on HIV/AIDS and Human Rights, Geneva, 23–25 September 1996.* New York: United Nations, UN Doc. HR/PUB/98/1.

World Health Organization. (1948). *Preamble to the Constitution of the WHO, as Adopted by the International Health Conference, New York, 19–22 June, 1946; Signed on 22 July 1946 by the*

Representatives of 61 States (Official Records of the World Health Organization, no. 2, p. 100)
and Entered into Force on 7 April 1948. Geneva: World Health Organization.

_____. (1978). *Declaration of Alma-Ata, International Conference on Primary Health Care,*
Alma-Ata, USSR, 6–12 September. Available on-line at www.who.int/chronic_conditions/
primary_health_care/en/almaata_declaration.pdf.

_____. (1998). *World Health Declaration, 51st World Health Assembly, Annex 7.* WHO Doc.
WHA 51.7.

_____. (2002). *Health and Human Rights Publication Series* 1(July). Geneva: World Health
Organization.

Notes

1. In Canada there is a constitutional commitment to reasonable, equal access to essential services, and equitable taxation and equality before and under the law. This commitment is the basis for all equality rights in Canada and these constitutional guarantees are intrinsic to the defence of equal access to treatment and an equal right to well-being.

2. The *Declaration* called on national governments to ensure the availability of the essentials of primary health care, including: education concerning health problems and the methods for preventing and controlling them; promotion of food supply and proper nutrition; adequate supply of safe water and basic sanitation; child and maternal health care, including family planning; immunization against major infectious diseases; prevention and control of locally endemic diseases; appropriate treatment of common diseases and injuries, and provision of essential drugs.

3. The WHO Assembly reaffirmed the original WHO constitution and stressed the "will to promote health by addressing the basic determinants and prerequisites for health [and] to pay the greatest attention to those most in need, burdened by ill health, receiving inadequate services for health or affected by poverty"(World Health Organization 1998, 51st World Health Assembly, Annex 7).

4. International human rights treaties are binding on governments that ratify them. Two central UN treaties are the UN *International Covenant on Civil and Political Rights* (1966) and the UN *International Covenant on Economic, Social, and Cultural Rights* (ICESCR) (1966). The most important Declarations are non-binding, although in many cases, the norms and standards laid out in them reflect principles that are binding in customary international law.

5. General Comments in UN instruments clarify the nature and content of individual rights and the obligations of the states who have ratified the treaty.

6. See Dennis Raphael's work (Chapter 5) in this volume.

7. The Rules relevant to social and cultural rights are Rules 2, 3, 5, 6, 10, and 11.

8. Reference to Mary Wiktorowitz's work (Chapter 10) in this volume.

9. See also the next section of this paper on reproductive health.

10. The UN *Draft Comprehensive and Integral International Convention on the Protection and Promotion of the Rights and Dignity of Persons with Disabilities,* Article 21 (UN Ad Hoc Committee on a Comprehensive and Integral International Convention on the Protection and Promotion of the Rights and Dignity of Persons with Disabilities 2004), identifies key human rights issues related to the health and rehabilitation of people with disabilities as well as these areas.

11. The UN Declaration on HIV/AIDS emphasizes that the full realization of human rights and fundamental freedoms for all, including the right to the highest attainable standard of health, is an essential element of the global response to the HIV/AIDS pandemic. The WHO passed the TRIPS agreement to promote public health and to promote access to medicines for all. For further discussion of the TRIPS agreement, see Cohen (2002).

12. The WHO includes in this category of diseases: onchocerciasis, leprosy, guinea worm disease, lymphatic filariasis, schistosomiasis and soil-transmitted helminthiasis, African trypanosomiasis, human rabies, dengue and dengue haemorrhagic fever, leishmaniasis, and buruli ulcer (World Health Organization 2002).

13. For a more comprehensive discussion of the implications of international drug policy, see Chapter 14 by Joel Lexchin.

••••••••••••••••••••••••••••••••••••

Critical Thinking Questions

1. What is meant by a rights-based approach to health?
2. The United Nations have claimed that health is an issue of human rights. Reframing health as a rights issue rather than an issue of social development changes its context. Why has it taken so long for this to happen? What are the particular circumstances surrounding health that have acted as barriers to this recognition?
3. Why is it not enough simply to provide more and better medical services for marginalized groups if the goal is to improve health?
4. How would you explain the differences in health between the rich and poor countries?
5. If you could rewrite the *United Nations Declaration of Human Rights*, what clauses would you put in that are not there?

Further Readings

Anand, J., F. Peter, and A. Sen. (2004). *Public Health, Ethics and Equity*. Oxford: Oxford University Press.
This book explores the foundations of health equity from the perspectives of philosophers, anthropologists, economists, and public health experts. It is organized around five major themes: health equity; health, society and justice; responsibility for health and health care; ethical and measurement problems in health evaluation; and equity and conflicting perspectives on health evaluation.

Cook, R.J., B.M. Dickens, and M.F. Fathalla. (2003). *Reproductive Health and Human Rights*: *Integrating Medicine, Ethics and Law*. Oxford: Oxford University Press.
This book explores a unique and important area of study within the umbrella of health and human rights. It provides the different perspectives of medicine, ethics, and law toward human reproduction as a way of understanding how human rights values can interact to improve reproductive and sexual health.

Mann, J.M., S. Gruskin, M.S. Grodin, and G.J. Annas. (1999). *Health and Human Rights*. New York: Routledge.
This is an essential work in this field. The authors argue that public health, ethics, and human rights are integrally connected and motivated by the value of human well-being. Human rights violations adversely affect the community's health, coercive health policies violate human rights, and the two fields are mutually reinforcing.

Office of the High Commissioner for Human Rights. (1998). *Basic Human Rights Instruments*. Geneva: Office of the High Commission for Human Rights.
This is a compilation of the texts of the seven major international human rights treaties and the *Universal Declaration of Human Rights*.

Quinn, G., and T. Degener, eds. (2002). *Human Rights and Disability: The Current Use and Future Potential of United Nations Human Rights Instruments in the Context of Disability*. Geneva: Office of the High Commission for Human Rights. Available on-line at http://193.194.138.190/disability/study.htm.

Relevant Web Sites

Canadian HIV/AIDS Legal Network
www.aidslaw.ca
   The Canadian HIV/AIDS Legal Network is a national, community-based, charitable organization working in the area of policy and legal issues raised by HIV/AIDS. It was formed in November 1992 and has over 250 members across Canada and internationally. The Web site provides a wealth of information on current policies and links to other Web sites, policy documents, and international action.

Disability Rights Promotion International (DRPI)
www.yorku.ca/drpi
   DRPI is a collaborative human rights project working to establish an international monitoring system for disability rights. The site provides detailed information about the ongoing monitoring in the areas of individual violation focus, system focus—including legislative frameworks, disability case law, and government policies and programs—and media focus.

United Nation Office of the High Commissioner for Human Rights
www.ohchr.org/english

The High Commissioner is the principal UN official with responsibility for human rights. This site provides both general information about the high commissioner's office as well as details about the most recent meetings and activities of the commission.

www.unhchr.ch/tbs/doc.nsf.

This makes available all international treaties and treaty body documents for easy reference.

UN Special Rapporteur on Health
www.ohchr.org/english/issues/health/right/standards.htm

This site provides the mandate of the UN Special Rapporteur on health and also links to a number of sites about his current activities and special initiatives on health within the framework of the UN High Commission on Human Rights office.

World Health Organization
www.who.int/hhr/news/en

This site follows the specific issues of World Health Organization on health and human rights. It provides international news, activities, information resources, databases and key instruments, and provides updates on health emergencies around the world.

Glossary

Biotechnology: The official definition of biotechnology (European Federation of Bio-technology 1989) is "the integration of natural sciences and engineering sciences in order to achieve the application of organisms, cells, parts thereof and molecular analogues for products and services." In non-technical terms, it is the use of biological processes to solve problems or make useful products.

Ethics: Is the study of human conduct from the perspective of moral principles, which incorporate the body of obligations and duties that a particular society requires of its members. The field of ethics, sometimes called moral philosophy, involves understanding concepts of right and wrong behaviour.

Health: Is a "state of complete physical, mental and social well-being, and not merely the absence of disease or infirmity" (World Health Organization 1946). The enjoyment of the highest attainable standard of health is one of the fundamental rights of every human being and is inseparable from the enjoyment of other human rights such as right to food, housing, adequate income, education, participation, privacy, freedom from torture, and freedom from discrimination.

Health equity: Is a term that contextualizes health from a social justice perspective. It is a commitment of public health to social justice and is the absence of systemic disparities in health among groups with different levels of social advantage or disadvantage.

Non-discrimination: Is where no different or unequal treatment has occurred on a categorical basis that is unjust. The principle of non-discrimination requires that all rights be guaranteed to everyone without distinction, exclusion, or restriction based on disability or based on race, colour, sex, language, religion, political or other opinion, national or social origin, property, birth, age, or any other status.

PART II

SOCIAL DETERMINANTS OF HEALTH

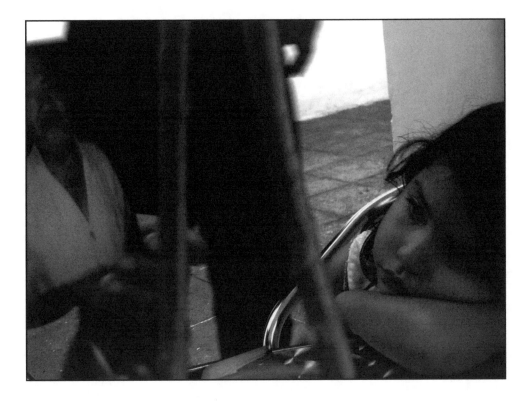

There is increasing recognition that the mainsprings of health are to be found in the manner in which societies are organized and resources distributed among the population. The concept of the social determinants of health is an illustration of how the various paradigms by which health, illness, and health care can be examined contribute to furthering our understanding of these issues.

A focus upon society and its characteristics as a source of health is clearly a subordinate approach to these issues. Governmental, public, and the media's concerns are firmly entrenched within a medical model of health whereby the body is a machine that is either running well or in need of repair. If the body is free of illness, the person is healthy. If it is either infected with pathogens or afflicted with system or organ-malfunctioning disease, illness occurs. The remedy for such disease and illness is found in medical or curative care, which is located in the health care system and administered by doctors and nurses.

The allocation of government spending to the health care system, research activities, and disease foundations reflects this commitment to the medical model. The preoccupation of all key players—the public, the media, and governments—with the medical model ensures that issues related to health and health care will receive primary attention. These strong tendencies are reinforced by increasing governmental adherence to public policy approaches associated with neo-liberalism: the belief that the marketplace is the best arbiter of societal resources and that citizens are best viewed as individual consumers rather than members of a communal whole. Individualism focuses attention on people and their bodies rather than the societal structures and the political, economic, and social forces that create either health or disease.

In Chapter 5, Dennis Raphael defines and identifies the social determinants of health. He provides evidence that factors such as the distribution of income, the provision of housing and food security, and the security of employment and the quality of working conditions are the primary determinants of health. These social determinants of health help explain increases in health in countries such as Canada over the past century, differences among Canadians, and why Canadians are healthier than Americans, but less healthy than citizens of nations of northern Europe. Despite this evidence governments and the media pay little attention to these determinants. Raphael shows how each of the perspectives identified in Part I of this volume contributes to understanding these issues and identifies key questions that need to be considered.

In Chapter 6, Carles Muntaner and colleagues explore social class inequalities in health. They provide an overview of social class and note that there is little research in Canada that considers why social class appears to be such an important social determinant of health. Social class represents relations of ownership or control over productive resources (i.e., physical, financial, and organizational) that have important consequences for the lives of individuals. They then provide findings from a comparative study that considers whether social class differences in health are similar across nations with different welfare state regimes. Their findings raise questions about the nature of class relations in capitalist nations and how these relations influence health status among citizens.

In Chapter 7, Ann Pederson and Dennis Raphael explore the interactions of gender and race with health. Sex and gender are seen as influencing health status, whether and how health care is used, and the differences between men's and women's experiences of health and illness. Research on race in Canada is focused on two primary areas: Aboriginal health and immigrant health. Reasons for the very poor health status of Aboriginal peoples are considered. Recent evidence is provided that the health of non-European immigrants to Canada appears to deteriorate over time and that this can be traced to their experience of the poor quality of a variety of social determinants of health. Their findings reinforce the importance of integrating gender and diversity concepts into health research and health policy.

Finally, in Chapter 8, Toba Bryant shows how the quality of various social determinants of health is influenced by governments' public policies. She compares the public policies of Canada, the U.S., the United Kingdom, and Sweden and their differential impact on health determinants. She traces the political, economic, and social influences that lead governments to take one public policy position rather than another. Political ideology and political and social organization are strong influences upon public policy. Policies developed and implemented in nations oriented toward neo-liberal approaches such as Canada, the U.S., and the United Kingdom are not as supportive of health as those of social democratic nations. The public policies taken in the U.S. in particular lead to greater incidence of poverty, larger income and wealth gaps between rich and poor, and poorer population health than what is seen in Canada.

································

CHAPTER FIVE

SOCIAL DETERMINANTS OF HEALTH

An Overview of Concepts and Issues

Dennis Raphael

································

Learning Objectives

At the conclusion of this chapter, the reader will be able to
- define and provide examples of the social determinants of health
- provide evidence of how social determinants of health impact health
- present emerging themes in the field
- raise issues suggested by each of the perspectives presented in this text
- identify areas of needed inquiry in the social determinants of health

---

Introduction

A main theme of this chapter and other chapters in this volume is that the health of individuals and populations and the organization of health care are strongly determined by the organization of societies and how these societies distribute material resources among its members. This idea is shared—in varying degrees—by each of the epidemiological, sociological, political economy, and human rights approaches to understanding health, illness, and health care. The concept of the social determinants of health—that economic and social factors are the primary determinants of health—provides an illustration of how sociological inquiry can inform our understanding of these issues and identify areas of needed inquiry.

The idea that societal factors are important determinants of health is not new. During the 19th century, Rudolph Virchow and Frederich Engels outlined the political, economic, and social forces that threaten health and well-being and spawn disease and early death (Engels [1845] 1987; Virchow [1848] 1985). More recently, renewed Canadian and international interest in the social determinants of health has led to a refocusing upon the non-medical and non-behavioural precursors of health and illness. While this approach is well developed in many European nations and has been integrated into their development and application of public policy, in North America the approach remains subordinate to traditional medical and behavioural paradigms of health, illness, and health care (see Chapters 8 and 15 in this volume).

Box 5.1: Rudolph Virchow and the Social Determinants of Health

German physician Rudolph Virchow's (1821–1902) medical discoveries were so extensive that he is known as the "Father of Modern Pathology." But he was also a trailblazer in identifying how societal policies determine health. In 1848, Berlin authorities sent Virchow to investigate the epidemic of typhus in Upper Silesia. His *Report on the Typhus Epidemic Prevailing in Upper Silesia* argued that lack of democracy, feudalism, and unfair tax policies in the province were the primary determinants of the inhabitants' poor living conditions, inadequate diet, and poor hygiene that fuelled the epidemic.

Virchow stated, "Disease is not something personal and special, but only a manifestation of life under modified (pathological) conditions." Arguing that "medicine is a social science and politics is nothing else but medicine on a large scale," Virchow drew the direct links between social conditions and health. He argued that improved health required recognition that "if medicine is to fulfil her great task, then she must enter the political and social life. Do we not always find the diseases of the populace traceable to defects in society?" (Virchow [1848] 1985).

The authorities were not happy with the report and Virchow was relieved of his government position. But he continued his pathology research within university settings and went on to a parallel career as a member of Berlin City Council and the Prussian Diet where he focused on public health issues consistent with his Upper Silesia report. Virchow also bitterly opposed Otto Von Bismarck's plans for national rearmament and was challenged to a duel by the said gentleman. Virchow declined participation.

What Are Social Determinants of Health?

The term "social determinants of health" grew out of researchers' search for the specific mechanisms by which members of different socio-economic groups come to experience varying degrees of health and illness. Individuals of different socio-economic status everywhere show profoundly different levels of health and incidence of disease (Wilkinson and Marmot 2003).

Another stimulus to investigating social determinants of health was the findings of national differences in population health. For example, the health status of Americans—using indicators such as life expectancy, infant mortality, and death by childhood injury rates—compares unfavourably to citizens in most industrialized nations (Navarro et al. 2004). In contrast, the health status of Scandinavians is generally superior to that seen in most nations. The same factors that explain health differences among groups within nations also explain differences seen among national populations.

A variety of approaches to the social determinants of health exist and all of these are concerned with the organization and distribution of economic and social resources (see Figure 5.1). The *Ottawa Charter for Health Promotion* identifies the *prerequisites for health* as peace, shelter, education, food, income, a stable ecosystem, sustainable resources, social justice, and equity (World Health Organization 1986). Health Canada outlines various *determinants of health*—some of which are social determinants—of income and social status, social support networks, education, employment and working conditions, physical and social environments, biology and genetic endowment, personal health practices and coping skills, healthy child development, gender, culture, and health services (Health Canada 1998). A British

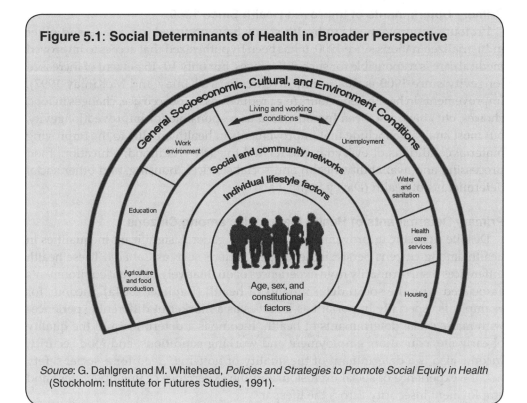

Figure 5.1: Social Determinants of Health in Broader Perspective

Source: G. Dahlgren and M. Whitehead, *Policies and Strategies to Promote Social Equity in Health* (Stockholm: Institute for Futures Studies, 1991).

working group charged with the specific task of identifying *social determinants of health* named the social (class health) gradient, stress, early life, social exclusion, work, unemployment, social support, addiction, food, and transport (Wilkinson and Marmot 2003).

Canadian workers recently synthesized these formulations to identify 11 key *social determinants of health*: Aboriginal status, early life, education, employment and working conditions, food security, health care services, housing, income and its distribution, social safety net, social exclusion, and unemployment and employment security (Raphael 2004b). These determinants are especially relevant to understanding and improving the health of Canadians.

What Is the Evidence Concerning the Social Determinants of Health?

Research based on the social determinants of health provides explanations for: (a) general improvement in health among citizens in developed nations over the past 100 years; (b) health differences observed among populations within nations; and (c) differences in overall health among Canadians and citizens in other developed nations.

Primary Determinants of Improved Health Since 1900

Profound improvements in health status have occurred in Canada and other industrialized nations since 1900. It has been hypothesized that access to improved medical care is responsible for such differences, but only 10–15 percent of increased longevity since 1900 is due to improved care (McKinlay and McKinlay 1997). Improvements in health behaviours (e.g., reductions in tobacco use, changes in food choices, etc.) have also been hypothesized as responsible for improved longevity, but most analysts conclude that improvements in health are due to the improving material conditions of everyday life related to early childhood, education, food processing and availability, health and social services, housing, and other social determinants of health (Davey Smith 2003).

Primary Determinants of Health Inequalities among Citizens

Despite dramatic improvements in health in general, significant inequalities in health among citizens persist in developed nations such as Canada. These health differences result primarily from experiences of qualitatively different environments associated with the social determinants of health (Raphael 2004a). Income, for example, is especially important as it serves as a marker of different experiences with many social determinants of health. Income is a determinant of the quality of early life, education, employment and working conditions, and food security. Income also is a determinant of the quality of housing, need for a social safety net, the experience of social exclusion, and the experience of unemployment and employment insecurity across the lifespan.

Box 5.2: Which Tips for Better Health Are Consistent with Research Evidence?

The messages given to the public by governments and health workers are influenced by the ways in which health issues are understood. Contrast the two sets of messages provided below. The first set assumes individuals can control the factors that determine their health. The second set assumes the most important determinants of health are beyond the control of most individuals. Which set of tips is most consistent with the evidence provided in this book?

The Traditional 10 Tips for Better Health
1. Don't smoke. If you can, stop. If you can't, cut down.
2. Follow a balanced diet with plenty of fruit and vegetables.
3. Keep physically active.
4. Manage stress by, for example, talking things through and making time to relax.
5. If you drink alcohol, do so in moderation.
6. Cover up in the sun, and protect children from sunburn.
7. Practice safer sex.
8. Take up cancer-screening opportunities.
9. Be safe on the roads: follow the Highway Code.
10. Learn the First Aid ABCs: airways, breathing, circulation.

Source: L. Donaldson, *Ten Tips for Better Health* (London: Stationary Office, 1999).

The Social Determinants 10 Tips for Better Health
1. Don't be poor. If you can, stop. If you can't, try not to be poor for long.
2. Don't have poor parents.
3. Own a car.
4. Don't work in a stressful, low-paid manual job.
5. Don't live in damp, low-quality housing.
6. Be able to afford to go on a foreign holiday and sunbathe.
7. Practice not losing your job and don't become unemployed.
8. Take up all benefits you are entitled to, if you are unemployed, retired or sick or disabled.
9. Don't live next to a busy major road or near a polluting factory.
10. Learn how to fill in the complex housing benefit/asylum application forms before you become homeless and destitute.

Source: D. Gordon, *Ten Tips for Better Health*, 1999. Message posted on the Spirit of 1848 Listserv.

Income levels associated with socio-economic position during early childhood, adolescence, and adulthood are all independent predictors of who develops and eventually succumbs to heart disease, diabetes, respiratory diseases, and some cancers (Davey Smith 2003). As just one illustration of the importance of socio-economic position and related factors, Statistics Canada recently examined the predictors of life expectancy, disability-free life expectancy, and the presence of fair or poor health among residents of 136 regions across Canada (Shields and Tremblay 2002).

The health predictors included socio-demographic factors (percentage Aboriginal population, percentage visible minority population, unemployment rate, population size, percentage of population aged 65 or over, average income, and average number of years of schooling). Other health predictors were rates of daily smoking, obesity, infrequent exercise, heavy drinking, high stress, and depression. Behavioural factors were weak predictors of health status as compared to socio-demographic measures. While obesity rate predicted 1 percent of the variation and smoking rate 8 percent of the variation among communities in life expectancy, socio-demographic factors predicted 56 percent of variation in life expectancy. Concerning reports of fair or poor health, obesity predicted 10 percent, and smoking rate predicted 4 percent of variation among communities. But socio-demographic factors predicted 25 percent of the differences among communities.

Incidence of, and mortality from, heart disease and stroke, and adult-onset or type 2 diabetes are especially good examples of the importance of the social determinants of health (Raphael, Anstice, and Raine 2003; Raphael and Farrell 2002). While governments, medical researchers, and public health workers continue to emphasize the importance of traditional adult risk factors (e.g., cholesterol, diet, physical activity, and tobacco use), it is well established that these are relatively poor predictors of heart disease, stroke, and type 2 diabetes rates.

Primary Determinants of Health Differences among Nations

Profound national differences exist among nations in life expectancy, infant mortality, incidence of numerous diseases, and death from injuries (Raphael 2003b). Differences in social determinants of health—such as income and its distribution, quality of early childhood, and employment and working conditions—explain much of the differences in health among citizens of Canada and other nations (see Chapter 8 in this volume). Poverty is an especially important indicator of how various social determinants of health combine to influence health. Canada does not fare well in relation to European nations (Figure 5.2).

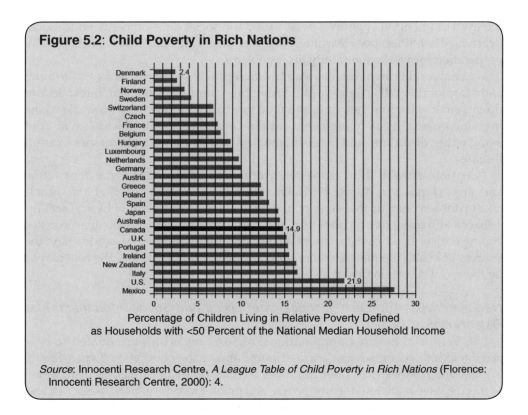

Figure 5.2: Child Poverty in Rich Nations

Percentage of Children Living in Relative Poverty Defined
as Households with <50 Percent of the National Median Household Income

Source: Innocenti Research Centre, *A League Table of Child Poverty in Rich Nations* (Florence:
Innocenti Research Centre, 2000): 4.

Emerging Themes in the Study of the Social Determinants of Health

Social Determinants and Health

Recent theoretical thinking considers how social determinants of health "get under the skin" to influence health. The three dominant frameworks are (a) materialist, (b) neo-materialist, and (c) psychosocial comparison.

Materialist Approach: Conditions of Living as Determinants of Health

This argument is that individuals experience varying degrees of positive and negative exposures over their lives that accumulate to produce adult health outcomes (Shaw, Dorling, Gordon, and Smith 1999). Overall wealth of nations is a strong indicator of population health. But within nations, socio-economic position is a powerful predictor of health as it is an indicator of material advantage or disadvantage over the lifespan. Material conditions of life determine health by influencing the quality of individual development, family life and interaction, and community environments. Material conditions of life lead to differing likelihood of physical (infections, malnutrition, chronic disease, and injuries), developmental (delayed or impaired cognitive, personality, and social development), educational (learning disabilities, poor learning, early school leaving), and social (socialization, preparation for work, and family life) problems.

Material conditions of life also lead to differences in psychosocial stress (Brunner and Marmot 1999). The fight-or-flight reaction—chronically elicited in response to threats such as income, housing, and food insecurity, among others—weakens the immune system, leads to increased insulin resistance, greater incidence of lipid and clotting disorders, and other biomedical insults that are precursors to adult disease.

Adoption of health-threatening behaviours is a response to material deprivation and stress (Jarvis and Wardle 1999). Environments determine whether individuals take up tobacco, use alcohol, have poor diets, and have low levels of physical activity. Tobacco and excessive alcohol use, and carbohydrate-dense diets are means of coping with difficult circumstances. Materialist arguments help us understand the sources of health inequalities among individuals and nations and the role played by the social determinants of health.

Neo-materialist Approach: Conditions of Living and Social Infrastructure as Determinants of Health

Differences in health among nations, regions, and cities are related to how economic and other resources are distributed among the population (Lynch, Smith, Kaplan, and House 2000). American states and cities with more unequal distribution of income have more low-income people and greater income gaps between rich and poor. They invest less in public infrastructure such as education, health and social services, health insurance, supports for the unemployed and those with disabilities, and spend less on education and libraries. Such unequal jurisdictions have much poorer health profiles.

Canada has a smaller proportion of lower-income people, a smaller gap between rich and poor, and spends relatively more on public infrastructure than the U.S. (Ross et al. 2000). Not surprisingly, Canadians enjoy better health than Americans as measured by infant mortality rates, life expectancy, and death rates from childhood injuries. Neither nation does as well as Sweden where distribution of resources is much more equalitarian, low-income rates are very low, and health indicators are among the best in the world.

The neo-materialist view directs attention to both the effects of living conditions on individuals' health and the societal factors that determine the quality of the social determinants of health. How a society decides to distribute resources among citizens is especially important.

Social Comparison Approach: Hierarchy and Social Distance as Determinants of Health

This argument is that health inequalities in developed nations are strongly influenced by citizens' interpretations of their standings in the social hierarchy (Kawachi and Kennedy 2002). There are two mechanisms by which this occurs.

At the individual level, the perception and experience of personal status in unequal societies lead to stress and poor health. Comparing their status, possessions, and other life circumstances to others, individuals experience feelings of shame, worthlessness, and envy that have psychobiological effects upon health. These comparisons lead to attempts to alleviate such feelings by overspending, taking on additional employment that threaten health, and adopting health-threatening coping behaviours such as overeating and using alcohol and tobacco.

At the communal level, widening and strengthening of hierarchy weakens social cohesion, a determinant of health. Individuals become more distrusting and suspicious of others, thereby weakening support for communal structures such as public education, health, and social programs. An exaggerated desire for tax reductions on the part of the public weakens public infrastructure.

This approach directs attention to the psychosocial effects of public policies that weaken the social determinants of health. To what extent are material aspects of society—described in the materialist and neo-materialist approaches—the prime determinants of these psychosocial processes?

The Importance of a Life-Course Perspective

Traditional approaches to health and disease prevention have a here-and-now emphasis upon adoption of "healthy" behaviours. In contrast, life-course approaches emphasize the accumulated effects upon health of experience across the lifespan. Exposures to adverse economic and social conditions have a cumulative effect upon health.

Hertzman outlines three health effects that have relevance for a life-course perspective (Hertzman 2000). *Latent effects* are biological or developmental early life experiences that influence health later in life. Low birth weight, for instance, is a reliable predictor of incidence of cardiovascular disease and adult-onset diabetes in later life. Experience of nutritional deprivation during childhood has lasting health effects.

Pathway effects are experiences that set individuals onto trajectories that influence health, well-being, and competence over the life course. As one example, children who enter school with delayed vocabulary are set upon a path that leads to lower educational expectations, poor employment prospects, and greater likelihood of illness and disease across the lifespan. Deprivation associated with poor-quality neighbourhoods, schools, and housing sets children off on paths that are not conducive to health and well-being.

Cumulative effects are the accumulation of advantage or disadvantage over time that manifests itself in poor health. These involve the combination of latent and pathways effects. Adopting a life-course perspective directs attention to how social determinants of health operate at every level of development—early childhood, childhood, adolescence, and adulthood—to both immediately influence health and provide the basis for health or illness later in life.

The Importance of Policy Environments

The quality of many social determinants of health is determined by approaches to public policy. The organization of health care is also a direct result of governments' policy decisions. These key issues are related to the distribution of societal resources (see Chapter 8 in this volume). Some important policy issues are provision of adequate income; family-friendly labour policies; active employment policies involving training and support; provision of social safety nets; and the degree to which health and social services and other resources are available to citizens.

What Key Issues Are Suggested by Each Perspective?

Epidemiological Perspectives: Providing the "Hard" Evidence

Epidemiologists are concerned with identifying the determinants of individual and population health. Much of this is concerned with identifying individual biomedical and behavioural risk factors associated with disease such as cholesterol and glucose levels, weight, tobacco and alcohol use, diet, and sedentary behaviour. Individual-oriented approaches can also focus upon characteristics of individuals such as income, educational levels, occupational classification, individual control and empowerment, or attitudes and values and how these come to be related to health.

Social epidemiologists have expanded their analysis to broader concerns with environments, social conditions, and even the political context within which environments are created and sustained (Berkman and Kawachi 2000). Within these frameworks the key issues are the nature of environmental structures that influence health and the pathways by which these environmental structures come to influence health. These structural approaches are concerned with how societal structures mediate the social determinants and health relationship.

Horizontal Structures That Influence Health

Horizontal structures are the more immediate factors that shape health and well-being. Some horizontal structures, for example, are the quality of childhood and family environments; the nature of work and workplace conditions; the quality and availability of housing; the availability of resources for food, recreation, and educational resources. Similarly, a neighbourhood with few economic resources may have low levels of social organization or community cohesion.

Vertical Structures That Influence Health

Vertical structures are the more distant macro-level issues that influence health and well-being. Vertical structures are the political, economic, and social forces that determine in large part the quality of the horizontal structures described above. These forces are manifested in a jurisdiction's approaches to employment, training, income, social welfare, and tax policies. There are clear national, regional, and municipal differences in how these policy issues are addressed.

Pathways and Mechanisms

How do social determinants of health get "under the skin" to influence health? How do differences in conditions of living come about in the first place? These are questions about the pathways between environmental conditions and health. A recent study of how Canadian researchers conceptualize a prime social determinant of health—income and its distribution—and its relationship to health found that much of the research failed to take account of perspectives concerned with horizontal and vertical social structures (Raphael et al., 2005). Among 241 studies about income and health, only 16 percent focused on horizontal structures and 10 percent on vertical structures. An additional 14 percent focused on both kinds of structures, leaving 60 percent of studies neglecting these issues.

Concerning pathways linking income to health, 29 percent of studies simply noted that social class or education-related group memberships were related to income and health, and 28 percent were focused on behavioural risk factors. Only 33 percent were concerned with materialist or neo-materialist interpretations of the relationship between income and health, and only 22 percent were concerned with political-economic pathways. What are the reasons that epidemiologists limit themselves to these narrow analyses?

Sociological Perspectives: Understanding the Gap between Knowledge and Action

Considering what we know about the social determinants of health, why is there so little action on these issues in Canada? Sociological perspectives offer us some insights into these issues.

Psychological Constructs and Issues

Sociologists have explored how we come to understand our world (see Chapter 2 in this volume). The view that reality is socially constructed—that is, our understandings of the world are not given by nature but are chosen—is important for understanding how health and the determinants of health are conceptualized and, once so conceptualized, acted upon. Why is it that the social determinants of health are not the primary understandings held by the public, health workers, and government policy makers? What are the political, economic, and social forces that shape our understandings of the world? Who benefits from our holding certain world views of the causes of illness?

Disciplinary Approaches: Professions

Professions differ profoundly on how they address issues of health, illness, and health care. Labonte suggests that health and health care can be viewed within three general frameworks: the biomedical, lifestyle, and socio-environmental (Labonte 1993). In the biomedical approach, emphasis is on high-risk groups, screening of one sort or another, and health care delivery. The behavioural approach focuses on high-risk attitudes and behaviours and developing programs that educate and support individuals to change behaviours. The socio-environmental approach focuses on risk conditions and considers how individuals adjust to these conditions or move to change them.

Clearly, the dominant paradigm among health care workers and researchers is the biomedical. Public health is focused on the behavioural, and the socio-environmental is underemphasized and the domain of only a handful of health researchers. The concept of the social determinants of health resides in the last category and continues to be subordinate. Why is this the case and what can be done to rectify this neglect?

Concepts from sociology, political economy, and human rights have had little penetration into traditional health sciences training (Muntaner 1999). In addition, there are numerous barriers to having issues such as social inequalities and social determinants of health addressed in professional training.

> I suggest that lay world views legitimating social inequalities are often in conflict with explanations arising from social epidemiology and medical sociology. The dominance of medicine in public health, through its often implicit assumptions about the biological determinants of human behaviour, is also identified as a barrier to teaching social inequalities in health. Educational elitism, which restricts higher education to members of the upper middle class, is identified as another barrier to teaching social inequalities in health. (Muntaner 1999: 161)

Institutional Mandates and Political Issues

Why do health care and public health organizations downplay the social determinants of health? Is it because these agencies are funded by governments that are responsible for policy decisions that either strengthen or weaken the social determinants of health? Given this relationship, how can public health agencies act objectively on the broader determinants of health?

Political Economy Perspectives: Identifying the Political and Economic Context

While sociological approaches direct attention to broader political and economic structures that influence health, it is the field of political economy that is devoted to exploring these issues and their influence upon health. It is an undeveloped area with few active health researchers. Particularly important issues are power relationships, government ideology and public policy, and welfare state typologies. Also of increasing interest is the role played by economic globalization and trade agreements.

Power Relationships

Hofrichter's recent volume contains an excellent overview of how issues of class, gender, and race come to influence health in developed nations (Hofrichter

2003). Chapters 6 and 7 in this volume consider how class, gender, and race come to influence health in Canada. In these analyses, class, gender, and race are not simply indicators of individuals' characteristics as much as markers of the power individuals within particular groups have within society.

It has also been pointed out that power relationships within a society are more equalized when labour unions and the "left" within a nation have more influence. Canadians who are members of unions have higher incomes, an important determinant of health (Table 5.1). One way in which power is more equally distributed is through adoption of proportional representation in elections. Nations in which this is established show greater commitment to income distribution and provision of public services to their citizens (see Chapter 8 in this volume).

Governmental Ideology and Public Policy

Coburn has pointed out how social determinants of health such as income and income inequality as well as housing, food security, and health and social services are heavily influenced by the ideology of the government of the day (Coburn 2000, 2004). He considers how neo-liberalism—through its emphasis on the market as the arbiter of societal values and resource allocations—supports regressive political and economic forces. Implementing neo-liberal economic policies fosters income and wealth inequalities, weakens social infrastructure, dissipates social cohesion, and threatens civil society.

Raphael considers how one aspect of neo-liberal ideology—the emphasis on reducing taxes—directly benefits the wealthy and translates into increasing income inequality and the weakening of communal institutions that support citizens (Raphael 1999). This raises the question of what is the best means of shaping health policy. Should we focus on presenting research evidence to effect policy change or should we focus on political activity to create more progressive public policy?

Welfare States and Their Variants

Esping-Andersen has identified what he calls the three worlds of welfare capitalism: social democratic, conservative, and liberal (Esping-Andersen 1990, 1999). The social democratic welfare states (Finland, Sweden, Denmark, and Norway) emphasize universal welfare rights and provide generous benefit entitlements. The conservative welfare states (France, Germany, Spain, and Italy) also offer generous benefits, but provide these based on employment status with emphasis on male primary breadwinners. The liberal Anglo-Saxon economies (the U.K., the U.S., Canada, and Ireland) provide only modest benefits and step in only when the market fails to provide adequate supports. These liberal states depend on means-tested benefits targeted to only the least well off. There are many differences in public policy among these types (see Table 5.2 and Chapter 8 in this volume).

Table 5.1: The Union Wage Advantage in 2002

Median Hourly Wage of All Paid Employees

	Union Covered	Non-union	Union Wage Advantage	Union Advantage as %
All	$19.60	$13.80	$5.80	42.0%
Men	$20.63	$15.50	$5.13	33.1%
Women	$18.29	$12.00	$6.29	52.4%
Public sector	$21.07	$18.76	$2.31	12.3%
Private sector	$17.50	$13.33	$4.17	31.3%
Selected occupations				
Natural/applied sciences	$25.00	$23.45	$1.55	6.6%
Clerical	$17.84	$13.22	$4.62	34.9%
Retail sales and cashiers	$10.76	$8.25	$2.51	30.9%
Chefs/cooks	$13.50	$8.85	$4.65	52.5%
Protective services	$21.68	$12.00	$9.68	80.7%
Child care/ home support	$15.31	$10.00	$5.31	53.1%
Construction trades	$23.00	$15.00	$8.00	53.3%
Machine operators/ assemblers	$17.73	$13.50	$4.23	31.3%

Note: Half of the group makes more, and half make less than the median wage.
Source: Andrew Jackson, In Solidarity: The Union Advantage (Ottawa: Canadian Labour Congress, 2003): 7.
Original Source: Statistics Canada, Labour Force Survey.

Health Impacts of Globalization and Trade Agreements

Teeple sees increasing income and wealth inequalities and the weakening of infrastructure within Canada and elsewhere as resulting from the ascendance of concentrated monopoly capitalism and corporate globalization (Teeple 2000). Transnational corporations apply their increasing power to oppose aspects of the welfare state to reduce labour costs. With such a power shift, business has less need to develop political compromises with labour and governments. Important

Table 5.2: 25 Key Indicators of Social Development

Legend: GOLD   SILVER   BRONZE

	Canada	U.S.	Sweden
INCOME AND POVERTY			
Income per person (% U.S.)	79%	100%	70.2%
Poverty rate	10.3%	17.0%	6.4%
Child poverty rate	15.5%	22.4%	2.6%
JOBS			
Employment rate	71.1%	74.1%	74.2%
Unemployment rate	6.8%	4.0%	5.9%
Working long hours	22.0%	26.0%	17.0%
Low-paid jobs	20.9%	24.5%	5.3%
Earnings gap	3.7	4.6	2.2
EMPLOYMENT SECURITY			
UI benefits as % of earnings	28.0%	14.0%	29.0%
Job supports	0.5 %	0.2%	1.8%
Unionized rate	36.0%	18.0%	89.0%
SOCIAL SUPPORTS			
Health care (public share)	69.6%	44.7%	83.8%
Tertiary education (public share)	60.0%	51.0%	91.0%
Private social spending	4.5%	8.6%	3.0%
HEALTH			
Life expectancy (men)	75.3	72.5	75.9
Life expectancy (women)	81.3	79.2	81.3
Infant mortality/100,000	5.5	7.2	3.5
CRIME			
Homicides per 100,000	1.8	5.5	N/A
Assault/threat per 100,000	4.0	5.7	4.2
Prisoners per 100,000	118	546	71
EDUCATION			
Adults/post-secondary ed.	38.8%	34.9%	28.0%
High literacy (% adults)	25.1%	19.0%	35.5%
Low literacy (% adults)	42.9%	49.6%	25.1%
Grade 12 math score	519	461	552
CIVIC PARTICIPATION			
Voter turnout	56.2%	49.1%	83.2%

Final Medal Standings	U.S.	SWE	CAN
GOLD	2	20	4
SILVER	3	2	19
BRONZE	20	2	2

Source: Andrew Jackson, *Canada Beats U.S.A.—But Loses Gold to Sweden* (Ottawa: Canadian Council on Social Development, 2000).

questions raised by this perspective include: To what extent is the weakening of the welfare state inevitable? What is the role that trade agreements play in the weakening of the welfare state?

Human Rights Perspectives: Providing the Legal and Moral Justifications for Action

Canada is signatory to many international covenants that guarantee the provision of citizen supports that show commonalities with the social determinants of health. The *Universal Declaration on Human Rights* states:

> Everyone has the right to a standard of living adequate for the health and well-being of himself and of his family, including food, clothing, housing and medical care and necessary social services, and the right to security in the event of unemployment, sickness, disability, widowhood, old age or other lack of livelihood in circumstances beyond his control. (United Nations 1948: 7)

Similarly, the 1995 *Declaration of the International Summit for Social Development* identified the following commitments:

> Achieving specified target dates which have been agreed previously at the international level for meeting basic human needs such as food, shelter, water, sanitation, health care, and education, and in relation to areas such as South Asia which have substantial concentrations of people in poverty.
>
> Ensuring adequate economic and social protection during periods of vulnerability such as unemployment, ill health, maternity, child-rearing and old age. (United Nations 1995)

Non-governmental organizations consistently report that Canada does not live up to its commitments to these international agreements (Raphael and Bryant 2004). Indeed, conditions either continue to deteriorate or stagnate, yet governments do little in response to these negative reports.

Social Justice and Health Equity

Issues of health equity and the role played by social determinants of health that lead to such inequity are rooted in concepts of social justice (Braveman and Gruskin 2003). The equity issue plays itself out in use of different terms to describe health differences. "Health disparities" is a value-neutral term favoured by epidemiologists. For example, the U.S. government states: "Health disparities are differences in the incidence, prevalence, mortality, and burden of diseases and other adverse health conditions that exist among specific population groups."

For those who wish to make the point more dramatically, Kawachi et al. offer:

"*Health inequality* is the generic term used to designate differences, variations, and disparities in the health achievements of individuals and groups" (Kawachi, Subramanian, and Almeida-Filho 2002: 647). And to introduce the values aspect into the discussion they provide: "*Health inequity* refers to those inequalities in health that are deemed to be unfair or stemming from some form of injustice." The term "health inequities" implies something is wrong in a society with profound health differences among citizens. This introduces the concept of social justice. There are two reasons why a concept of social justice is important in considering the roots of differences in health:

> First, social justice demands an equitable distribution of collective goods, institutional resources (such as social wealth), and life opportunities.... Second, social justice calls for democracy—the empowerment of all social members, along with democratic and transparent structures to promote social goals. This is another way of describing political equality. (Hofrichter 2003: 13)

The focus on justice and fairness in discussions of health, illness, and health care is an important contribution of the human rights approach. What role can moral, legal, and human rights arguments play in promoting the quality of the social determinants of health? How useful can these arguments be in provoking the public to advocate for more public policies that support health?

What Are Areas of Needed Inquiry?
In addition to the questions raised in the sections above, there are some key areas that could benefit from inquiry applying a social determinants of health framework.

- *Recovery from illness and rehabilitation*: While it is well established that social determinants of health are excellent predictors of illness and diseases, we know little about how these same health determinants lead to recovery from illness.
- *Organization and activities of public health units*: Public health units in Canada are focused upon behavioural approaches to disease prevention; only a handful take seriously the social determinants of health (Raphael 2003a). Why is it that some health units are able to undertake a broader approach to health determinants while others appear unable or unwilling to do so?
- *Concept representation and the media*: There has been virtually no penetration of the social determinants of health into the media (Hayes 2002). The overwhelming proportion of coverage in the written press, radio, or television is on biomedical research and behavioural risk factors (Commers, Visser, and De Leeuw 2000; Westwood and Westwood 1999).

We need to understand why the press is so limited in its health-related coverage. What are the barriers to fostering reporters' understanding of the social determinants of health?

- *Public understanding and action*: Considering media coverage of health, we should not be surprised to find the public has little understanding of the social determinants of health (Eyles et al. 2001). A recent study asked 601 residents of Hamilton, Ontario, to identify up to seven causes of heart disease (Paisley, Midgett, Brunetti, and Tomasik 2001). In response to this open-ended question, only one respondent of 601—and only one of 4,200 potential responses—identified poverty as a cause of heart disease. Yet polls consistently show that Canadians favour reducing poverty and income inequality, reducing homelessness and food bank use, and increasing program spending to improve Canadians' quality of life (Adams 2003). Yet, in spite of these views, governments have acted in the opposite manner, reducing spending and reducing taxes. How can Canadian values be applied to influence government policy making?
- *Links between evidence and policy (in)action*: Lavis concludes that social determinants of health continue to be a marginalized approach to developing public policy (Lavis 2002). While there is policy maker awareness of the importance of these concepts, governments do not institute health-promoting social policies. Is the creation of healthy public policy primarily about health? Or is healthy public policy primarily about politics?

Conclusions

The social determinants of health offers a window into both the micro-level processes by which social structures lead to individual health or illness and the macro-level processes by which power relationships and political ideology shape the quality of these social structures. The epidemiological approach directs attention to the pathways that link these social structures to health and illness.

The sociological approach directs attention to how we develop explanations and actions to address the causes and treatment of disease and illness. The political economy perspective forces us to ask questions about power and politics and how economics shapes the organization of society and the distribution of wealth and other resources. Finally, the human rights approach asks about the values that determine the type of society we live in and our commitments to providing every citizen with the resources necessary to realize health, well-being, and achieve our full human potential. The social determinants of health is a rich area for both sociological inquiry and political and social action to improve health, health care services, and society in general.

References

Adams, M. (2003). *Fire and Ice: The United States, Canada and the Myth of Converging Values.* Toronto: Penguin Books Canada.

Berkman, L., and I. Kawachi, eds. (2000). *Social Epidemiology.* New York: Oxford University Press.

Braveman, P., and S. Gruskin. (2003). "Defining Equity in Health." *Journal of Epidemiology and Community Health* 57: 254–258.

Briggs, A. (1961). "The Welfare State in Historical Perspective." *European Journal of Sociology* 2: 251–259.

Brunner, E., and M.G. Marmot. (1999). "Social Organization, Stress, and Health." In *Social Determinants of Health,* edited by M.G. Marmot and R.G. Wilkinson, 17–43. Oxford: Oxford University Press.

Coburn, D. (2000). "Income Inequality, Social Cohesion and the Health Status of Populations: The Role of Neo-liberalism." *Social Science and Medicine* 51(1): 135–146.

_____. (2004). "Beyond the Income Inequality Hypothesis: Globalization, Neo-liberalism, and Health Inequalities." *Social Science and Medicine* 58: 41–56.

Commers, M.J., G. Visser, and E. De Leeuw. (2000). "Representations of Preconditions for and Determinants of Health in the Dutch Press." *Health Promotion International* 15(4): 321–332.

Davey Smith, G., ed. (2003). *Inequalities in Health: Life Course Perspectives.* Bristol: Policy Press.

Engels, F. [1845] (1987). *The Condition of the Working Class in England.* New York: Penguin Classics.

Esping-Andersen, G. (1990). *The Three Worlds of Welfare Capitalism.* Princeton: Princeton University Press.

_____. (1999). *Social Foundations of Post-industrial Economies.* New York: Oxford University Press.

Eyles, J., M. Brimacombe, P. Chaulk, G. Stoddart, T. Pranger, and O. Moase. (2001). "What Determines Health? To Where Should We Shift Resources? Attitudes towards the Determinants of Health among Multiple Stakeholder Groups in Prince Edward Island, Canada." *Social Science and Medicine* 53(12): 1611–1619.

Gordon, D., and P. Townsend, eds. (2000). *Breadline Europe: The Measurement of Poverty.* Bristol: The Policy Press.

Hayes, M. (2002). "Media Suffering from 'Tunnel Vision,' Says Health Researchers." Simon Fraser University. Retrieved October 12, 2005. Available on-line at www.sfu.ca/mediapr/sfu_news/sfunews03210202.html.

Health Canada. (1998). "Taking Action on Population Health: A Position Paper for Health Promotion and Programs Branch Staff." Health Canada. Retrieved August 2002. Available on-line at www.hc-sc.gc.ca/hppb/phdd/pdf/tad_e.pdf.

Hertzman, C. (2000). "The Case for an Early Childhood Development Strategy." *Isuma* (Autumn): 11–18.

Hofrichter, R. (2003). "The Politics of Health Inequities: Contested Terrain." In *Health and Social Justice: A Reader on Politics, Ideology, and Inequity in the Distribution of Disease,* edited by R. Hofrichter, 1–56. San Francisco: Jossey Bass.

Jarvis, M.J., and J. Wardle. (1999). "Social Patterning of Individual Health Behaviours: The Case of Cigarette Smoking." In *Social Determinants of Health*, edited by M.G. Marmot and R.G. Wilkinson, 340–255. Oxford: Oxford University Press.

Kawachi, I., and B. Kennedy. (2002). *The Health of Nations: Why Inequality Is Harmful to Your Health*. New York: New Press.

Kawachi, I., S.V. Subramanian, and N. Almeida-Filho. (2002). "A Glossary for Health Inequalities." *Journal of Epidemiology and Community Health* 56(9): 647–652.

Labonte, R. (1993). *Health Promotion and Empowerment: Practice Frameworks*. Toronto: Centre for Health Promotion and ParticipAction.

Lavis, J. (2002). "Ideas at the Margin or Marginalized Ideas? Nonmedical Determinants of Health in Canada." *Health Affairs* 21(2): 107–112.

Lynch, J.W., G.D. Smith, G.A. Kaplan, and J.S. House. (2000). "Income Inequality and Mortality: Importance to Health of Individual Income, Psychosocial, Environment, or Material conditions. *British Medical Journal* 320: 1220–1224.

McKinlay, J., and S.M. McKinlay. (1997). "Medical Measures and the Decline of Mortality." In *Sociology of Health and Illness*, 5th ed., edited by P. Conrad, 10–28. New York: St. Martin's Press.

Muntaner, C. (1999). "Teaching Social Inequalities in Health: Barriers and Opportunities." *Scandinavian Journal of Public Health* 27: 161–165.

Navarro, V., C. Borrell, J. Benach, C. Muntaner, A. Quiroga, M. Rodrigues-Sanz, N. Verges, J. Guma, and M.I. Pasarin. (2004). "The Importance of the Political and the Social in Explaining Mortality Differentials among the Countries of the OECD, 1950–1998." In *The Political and Social Contexts of Health*, edited by V. Navarro, 11–86. Amityville: Baywood Press.

Paisley, J., C. Midgett, G. Brunetti, and H. Tomasik. (2001). "Heart Health Hamilton-Wentworth Survey: Programming Implications." *Canadian Journal of Public Policy* 92: 443–447.

Raphael, D. (1999). "Health Effects of Economic Inequality." *Canadian Review of Social Policy* 44: 25–40.

_____. (2003a). "Barriers to Addressing the Determinants of Health: Public Health Units and Poverty in Ontario, Canada." *Health Promotion International* 18: 397–405.

_____. (2003b). "A Society in Decline: The Social, Economic, and Political Determinants of Health Inequalities in the USA." In *Health and Social Justice: A Reader on Politics, Ideology, and Inequity in the Distribution of Disease*, edited by R. Hofrichter, 59–88. San Francisco: Jossey Bass.

_____. (2004a). "Introduction to the Social Determinants of Health." In *Social Determinants of Health: Canadian Perspectives*, edited by D. Raphael, 1–18. Toronto: Canadian Scholars' Press.

_____, ed. (2004b). *Social Determinants of Health: Canadian Perspectives*. Toronto: Canadian Scholars' Press.

Raphael, D., S. Anstice, and K. Raine. (2003). "The Social Determinants of the Incidence and Management of Type 2 Diabetes Mellitus: Are We Prepared to Rethink Our Questions and Redirect Our Research Activities?" *Leadership in Health Services* 16: 10–20.

Raphael, D., and E.S. Farrell. (2002). "Beyond Medicine and Lifestyle: Addressing the Societal Determinants of Cardiovascular Disease in North America." *Leadership in Health Services* 15: 1–5.

Raphael, D., and T. Bryant. (2004). "The Welfare State as a Determinant of Women's Health: Support for Women's Quality of Life in Canada and Four Comparison Nations." *Health Policy* 68: 63–79.

Raphael, D., J. Macdonald, R. Labonte, R. Colman, K. Hayward, and R. Torgerson. (2005). "Researching Income and Income Distribution as a Determinant of Health in Canada: Gaps between Theoretical Knowledge, Research Practice, and Policy Implementation." *Health Policy* 72: 217–232.

Ross, N., M. Wolfson, J. Dunn, J.M. Berthelot, G. Kaplan, and J. Lynch. (2000). "Relation between Income Inequality and Mortality in Canada and in the United States: Cross-sectional Assessment Using Census Data and Vital Statistics." *British Medical Journal* 320(7239): 898–902.

Shaw, M., D. Dorling, D. Gordon, and G.D. Smith. (1999). *The Widening Gap: Health Inequalities and Policy in Britain*. Bristol: The Policy Press.

Shields, M., and S. Tremblay. (2002). "The Health of Canada's Communities." *Health Reports* Supplement 13(July): 1–25.

Teeple, G. (2000). *Globalization and the Decline of Social Reform: Into the Twenty-First Century*. Aurora: Garamond Press.

United Nations. (1948). *Universal Declaration of Human Rights*. New York: United Nations.

_____. (1995). *Commitments of the U.N. World Summit on Social Development*. Copenhagen: United Nations.

Virchow, R. [1848] (1985). *Collected Essays on Public Health and Epidemiology*. Cambridge: Science History Publications.

Westwood, B., and G. Westwood. (1999). "Assessment of Newspaper Reporting of Public Health and the Medical Model: A Methodological Case Study." *Health Promotion International* 14(1): 53–64.

Wilkinson, R., and M. Marmot. (2003). "Social Determinants of Health: The Solid Facts." World Health Organization, European Office. Retrieved October 12, 2005. Available on-line at www.euro.who.int/document/e81384.pdf.

Wolf, R. (2005). *What Is Public Policy?* Queen's University. Retrieved October 12, 2005. Available on-line at www.ginsler.com/html/toolbox.htp.

World Health Organization. (1986). "Ottawa Charter for Health Promotion." World Health Organization. European Office. Retrieved October 12, 2005. Available on-line at www.who.dk/policy/ottawa.htm.

• •

Critical Thinking Questions

1. Review the health-related stories of your local newspaper over the next five days. If you based your understanding of the determinants of health on these stories, what would be your views of what makes some people healthy and others ill?

2.   What evidence is available concerning the extent of housing, food, employment, and income insecurity in your area? Have conditions been improving or declining?

3.   To what extent is the discipline in which you are studying addressing issues related to the social determinants of health? What could be done to increase your discipline's emphasis in this area?

4.   What could be done to improve the public's understanding of the importance of the social determinants of health? What should be the role of your local public health unit or health care professionals?

5.   To what extent is public policy in your nation, region, or city appear concerned with improving the quality of various social determinants of health? Why are other nations more concerned with integrating the social determinants of health into public policy?

Further Readings

Bartley, M. (2003). *Health Inequality: An Introduction to Concepts, Theories and Methods.* Cambridge: Polity Press.
Large differences in life expectancy exist between the most privileged and the most disadvantaged social groups in industrial societies. This book assists in understanding the four most widely accepted theories of what lies behind inequalities in health: behavioural, psychosocial, material, and life-course approaches.

Davey Smith, G. (2003). *Health Inequalities: Life-Course Approaches.* Bristol: Policy Press.
The life-course perspective on adult health and health inequalities is an important development in epidemiology and public health. This volume presents innovative, empirical research that shows how social disadvantage throughout the life course leads to inequalities in life expectancy, death rates, and health status in adulthood.

Hofrichter, R. (2003). *Health and Social Justice: Politics, Ideology, and Inequity in the Distribution of Disease.* San Francisco: Jossey Bass.
This volume offers a collection of articles written by contributors from the fields of sociology, epidemiology, public health, ecology, politics, and advocacy. Each article explores a particular aspect of health inequalities and demonstrates how these are rooted in injustices of racism, sex discrimination, and social class.

Marmot, M., and R.G. Wilkinson. (2006). *Social Determinants of Health.* New York: Oxford University Press.
This book provides an overview of the social and economic factors that are now known to be the most powerful determinants of population health in modern nations.

Raphael, D. (2004). *Social Determinants of Health: Canadian Perspectives.* Toronto: Canadian Scholars' Press.
This book summarizes how socio-economic factors affect the health of Canadians, surveys the current state of 11 social determinants of health across Canada, and provides an analysis of how these determinants affect Canadians' health.

Relevant Web Sites

Canadian Centre for Policy Alternatives (CCPA)
www.policyalternatives.ca
   The centre monitors developments and promotes research on economic and social issues facing Canada and provides alternatives to the views of business research institutes and many government agencies.

Canadian Council on Social Development (CCSD)
www.ccsd.ca
   The CCSD focuses on social welfare issues of poverty, social inclusion, disability, cultural diversity, child well-being, employment, and housing. It provides statistics and reports on these issues.

Centre for Social Justice (CSJ)
www.socialjustice.org
   The CSJ works on narrowing the gap between rich and poor, challenging corporate domination of Canadian politics, and pressing for economic and social justice. It provides information, statistics, and reports.

Health Canada Population Health Approach
www.phac-aspc.gc.ca/ph-sp/phdd/
   This Web site provides details about how the population health aims to improve the health of the entire population by acting upon the broad range of factors and conditions that influence health.

National Council on Welfare (NCW)
www.ncwcnbes.net
   The NCW advises the Canadian government on matters related to social welfare and the needs of low-income Canadians. NCW publishes reports on poverty and social policy issues.

Glossary

Equity in health: Is an ethical value grounded in the ethical principle of distributive justice and consonant with human rights principles. Equity in health can be defined as the absence of disparities in health (and in its key social determinants) that are systematically associated with social advantage or disadvantage. Health inequities systematically put populations who are already socially disadvantaged by virtue of being poor, female, or members of a disenfranchised racial, ethnic, or religious group at further disadvantage with respect to their health (Braveman and Gruskin 2003).

Poverty: Is the condition whereby individuals, families, and groups in the population lack the resources to obtain the type of diet, participate in the activities, and have the living conditions and amenities that are customary, or at least widely encouraged or approved, in the societies to which they belong. Poverty can be considered in terms of absolute poverty whereby individual and families do not have enough resources to keep "body and soul together" or relative poverty whereby they do not have the ability to participate in common activities of daily living (Gordon and Townsend 2000).

Public policy: Is a course of action or inaction chosen by public authorities to address a given problem or interrelated set of problems. Policy is a course of action that is anchored in a set of values regarding appropriate public goals and a set of beliefs about the best way of achieving those goals. The idea of public policy assumes that an issue is no longer a private affair (Wolf 2005).

Social determinants of health: Are the economic and social conditions that influence the health of individuals, communities, and jurisdictions. Social determinants of health determine whether individuals stay healthy or become ill and the extent to which a person or community possesses the physical, social, and personal resources to identify and achieve personal aspirations, satisfy needs, and cope with the environment. Social determinants of health include conditions of childhood, availability and quality of income, food, housing, employment, and health and social services (Raphael 2004a).

Welfare state: Is a state in which organized power is deliberately used to modify the play of market forces in at least three directions: (1) by guaranteeing individuals and families a minimum income irrespective of the market value of their work or property; (2) by narrowing the extent of security by enabling individuals and families to meet certain social contingencies (for example, sickness, old age, and unemployment) that lead otherwise to individual and family crises; (3) by ensuring that all citizens without distinction of status or class are offered the best standards available in relation to a certain agreed range of social services (Briggs 1961).

CHAPTER SIX

SOCIAL CLASS INEQUALITIES IN HEALTH

Does Welfare State Regime Matter?

Carles Muntaner, Carme Borrell, Anton Kunst, Haejoo Chung, Joan Benach, and Selahadin Ibrahim

---

Learning Objectives

At the conclusion of this chapter, the reader will be able to
- define social class and its meaning in nations such as Canada
- define and provide examples of social class inequalities in health
- provide evidence of the relationship between social class and health
- provide evidence on the relationship between social class and health under different forms of welfare state regimes
- identify gaps in the research on welfare state and class inequalities in health

---

Introduction

One of the most consistent findings in health research is that "social class" is strongly related to health status however measured (see Townsend, Davidson, and Whitehead 1992 and Raphael 2001 for reviews). Most research on macro (system-level) political determinants of population health does not consider their relation to social class inequalities in health (Coburn 2004; Macincko and Starfield 2001; Muntaner et al. 2002; Navarro and Shi 2001). Nevertheless, macro political structures such as the type of welfare state regime should have an effect on health differences between social classes (e.g., workers, managers, employers) via processes such as the provision of social and health services and taxation policies and distribution of income (Muntaner and Lynch 1999; Navarro and Muntaner, 2004). In this chapter we examine the relationship between a welfare state regime (i.e., social democratic, Christian democratic, liberal) and class inequalities in health within a comparative framework. We begin by showing the complexity of the relationship between class and health by moving beyond the common use of social stratification measures (e.g., income, education) and looking at Spain, a European post-fascist country with a welfare state that is less developed than the E.U. average. Next we explore mortality differentials by occupational social class in three countries representing the social democratic, the liberal, and the Christian democratic welfare regime types. We end by issuing some recommendations for future research on the role of welfare state regimes in shaping class inequalities in health.

Does Class Matter? The Difference between Social Class and Social Stratification in Population Health Studies

The two major indicators used to assess socio-economic position in studies of social inequalities in health are social stratification and social class. Social stratification usually refers to the ranking of individuals along a continuum of economic attributes such as income or years of education. These rankings are known as "simple gradational measures" (Muntaner et al. 2004). Most social epidemiologists use several measures of social stratification simultaneously because single measures have been insufficient in explaining social inequalities in the health of populations. Measures of social stratification are important predictors of patterns of mortality and morbidity (Lynch and Kaplan 2000). However, despite their usefulness in predicting health outcomes, these measures do not reveal the social mechanisms that explain how individuals come to accumulate different levels of economic, political, and cultural resources (Muntaner and Lynch 1999). This is so because they have generally been selected for pragmatic considerations, i.e., availability of data, rather than for theoretical reasons.

We define social class as representing relations of ownership or control over productive resources (i.e., physical, financial, and organizational). Social class has important consequences for the lives of individuals. The extent of an individual's legal rights and power to control productive assets determines an individual's abilities to acquire income. And income determines in large part the individual's standard of living—(see Chapter 5 in this volume for a discussion of pathways by which income and material conditions of life influence health). Thus, the class position of "business owner" compels its members to hire "workers" and extract labour from them, while the "worker"class position compels its members to find employment and perform labour. Although there have been few empirical studies

---

Box 6.1: Social Class Exploitation

Although there are several definitions of exploitation (e.g., Saint-Simonian, liberal), exploitation is a key concept in the Marxian tradition. In the Marxian view, exploitation refers to the social mechanism underlying social class inequality. Exploitation is a characteristic of employment systems where unpaid labour is systematically forced out of one class and put at the disposal of another. According to a traditional view of exploitation, workers are exploited if they work longer hours than the number of labour hours employed in the goods they consume. Recent definitions incorporate authority in the workplace into the process of exploitation. Capitalist production always involves an apparatus of domination involving surveillance, positive and negative sanctions, and varying forms of hierarchy. Managers and supervisors exercise delegated capitalist class powers as they practise domination within production. The higher an employee rises in the authority hierarchy, the greater the weight of capitalist interests within this class location. The strategic position of managers within the organization of production enables them to make significant claims on a portion of the social surplus—the part of production left over after all inputs have been paid for—in the form of relatively high earnings.

Several studies in the last decade have shown associations between exploitation, in particular its domination aspects, and health outcomes in general population samples.

---

of social class and health, the need to study social class has been noted by social epidemiologists (Krieger et al. 1997; Muntaner and O'Campo 1993).

Social class provides an explicit relational mechanism (property, management) that explains how economic inequalities are generated and how they may affect health. For example, in a recent study, a team of U.S. epidemiologists found that low-level supervisors, who could hire and fire front-line personnel but did not have policy or decision-making authority in the firm, showed higher rates of depression and anxiety disorders than both upper management (who had authority and decision-making attributes) and non-management workers (who had neither) (Muntaner et al. 1998). This finding was predicted by the contradictory class location hypothesis (i.e., supervisors are in conflict with both workers and upper management and do not have control over policy), but was not predicted or explained by indicators of years of education or income gradients. Moreover, the income health hypothesis would have led to the expectation that supervisors, because of their higher incomes, would present *lower* rates of anxiety and depression than workers. Therefore, in a recent study we examined the relationships between measures of social class

(Wright's social class indicators, i.e., relationship to productive assets) and indicators of general health and mental health (Borrell et al. 2004).

The measures of social class we used in our investigation originate from a social class model that has been accumulating empirical support over the last 20 years. Wright's social class indicators assess ownership of productive assets, and control and authority relations in the workplace (control over organizational assets). Property rights over the financial or physical assets used in the production of goods and services generate three class positions: employers, who are self-employed and hire labour; the traditional petit bourgeoisie, who are self-employed, but do not hire labour; and workers who sell their labour. These social class positions reflect relations that underlie economic inequality since productive asset ownership generates economic inequality (i.e., deriving income from owning property).

Control over organizational assets (power and control in the workplace) is determined by two kinds of relations at work: (a) influence over company policy (e.g., making decisions over a number of people employed, the products or services delivered, the amount of work performed, the size and distribution of budgets); and (b) sanctioning authority (granting or preventing pay raises or promotions, hiring, firing, or temporally suspending a subordinate). The supervisory and policy-making functions of managers allow them to enjoy greater wealth than workers, for example, through income derived from shares of stock, incentives, bonuses, and hierarchical pay scales. To complete the social class scheme, Wright includes skills/credentials relations as part of his map of class positions (the expert, semi-skilled, and "unskilled" class positions). Experts are defined as those holding jobs that require skills, particularly credentialed skills, which are scarce relative to their demand by the market. Experts enjoy a credential rent: their wages are usually above the cost of the reproduction of their training. Semi-skilled and "unskilled" class positions are defined as jobs requiring skills that are in large supply, particularly uncredentialed skills. Because credentials provide access to labour markets with higher pay and less hazardous working conditions, experts would be expected to have better health status than "semi-skilled" and "unskilled" workers.

We tested this scheme using the Barcelona Health Interview Survey, a cross-sectional survey of 10,000 residents of the city's non-institutionalized working population of 16–64 years in the year 2000. Only the employed population was included in the analyses (2,345 men and 1,874 women). Health-related variables included self-perceived health, health behaviours, injuries, chronic functional impairment, and a number of chronic disorders. (See Table 6.1.) Findings reveal that, contrary to conventional wisdom, health indicators are often worse for employers than for managers, and that supervisors often fare more poorly than workers. Our findings highlight the potential health consequences of social class positions defined by relations of control over productive assets. They also confirm that social class taps into parts of the social variation in health that are not captured by conventional measures of social stratification (See Glossary).

Table 6.1: Relationship between Social Class, Self-Rated Health, Overweight, Chronic Functional Impairment, Injuries, and Number of Chronic Conditions. Working Population, 16–64 years, Barcelona, 2000

Health Outcomes	Poor Self-Rated Health		Smoking		Overweight		Chronic Limitations of Activity		Injuries		4 or More Chronic Conditions	
Social Class	Male	Female	Male	Female	Male	Female	Male	Female	Male	Female	Male	Female
Capitalists	4.3	12.5	40.6	26.7	13	8.3	3.6	14.7	13.5	7.3	23.6	55.8
Small employer	13.4	15	37.3	37.4	21.8	14.4	10.7	7.5	15.9	9.5	6.5	21.3
Petit bourgeoisie	12.4	13.5	36.8	43.7	20.2	14.6	6.8	10.5	20.5	21.1	10.7	12
Expert												
Managers	3.4	0	44.6	43.5	17.2	4.2	5.1	6.5	9.3	11.9	4.1	5
Supervisor	2.7	10	23.3	33.6	17.6	13.1	4.1	7	20.2	6.5	8.3	31.8
Worker	4.4	3.8	30.7	29.1	14.8	6.8	6.8	7.4	8.5	14.8	4.6	12.4
Semi-skilled												
Managers	0	0	36.1	32.8	36.6	0	14.8	0	8.2	24.4	4.5	0
Supervisor	13.4	7.8	45.5	40.5	28.5	7.7	11.8	13.6	14.6	10.3	9.3	3.5
Worker	9.3	10.1	42.6	29.5	18.5	11.6	5.9	14.4	16.5	16.6	8.9	21.2
Unskilled												
Supervisor	12.8	15.4	47.6	47.7	22.2	15.4	10.5	18.3	23.7	22.4	11.4	19
Worker	14	19	46	37.3	22.6	18.1	11.8	13.5	16.2	14.7	11.9	22.3

What about Canada?

Social class inequalities are pervasive in Canada (Baer et al. 1987). There have been few studies on social class and health inequalities in Canada due to lack of data on social class (see Raphael et al. 2004). Occupational social class, however, is a common measure of social stratification that is available in several large surveys. For example, an analysis of the Canadian Community Health Survey (CCHS) cycle 1.2 (n = 36,984) from which we analyzed the subsample of 18–64 year olds for which occupation and health questions were available (n = 19,907) yields evidence of occupational class inequalities in health (expressed as percents). The rate of poor or fair self-rated mental health is 6.3 percent among workers and 4.5 percent among professionals and managers (the residual category). Similarly, the rate of poor or fair self-rated overall health is 6.8 percent among workers and 3.9 percent among professionals and managers. With regard to the rate of substance use disorders, it is 12.5 percent among workers and 9 percent among professionals and managers. These associations were statistically significant using a Chi-squared test.

Thus, although we do not have much data on social class proper in Canada, we are confident that such analyses would provide evidence of inequalities in health.

Welfare State, Occupational Social Class, and Mortality Differentials

As stated above, welfare state regime types are expected to vary in ways that affect population health. Welfare states regimes with strong working-class power (e.g., social democratic regimes with high union density and social democratic parties in government) will be more likely to implement redistributive policies such as universal health care, poverty reduction, or generous unemployment benefits than Christian democratic (which rely on the family for the provision of social services) or liberal regimes (which rely on the market). In this section we draw on the E.U. comparative study by Kunst et al. (2001), which will allow us to illustrate the relationship between welfare state and class inequalities in health. Mortality differences between men from the working (manual) class and the non-working (non-manual) class have been demonstrated for about 15 European countries with a variety of welfare state regimes (social democratic, liberal, Christian democratic) in the 1980s (Kunst et al. 2001). Canada is considered a liberal welfare state regime (see Chapters 5 and 8 in this volume for a further description of these welfare states and the public policies associated with each state). Studies from some of these countries have shown that class differences in mortality have increased since then. However, changes in inequalities in mortality have not yet been documented for many countries and none of this research has identified countries in terms of their welfare state regimes. A comparative overview of trends by welfare state regime is needed in order to determine whether the widening of health inequalities—often referred to in both scientific and policy documents—is a phenomenon that is influenced by political factors (Kunst et al. 2001).

For individual countries, a reassessment of the data is needed for several reasons. First, in many studies, the potential effect of all possible data problems has not been evaluated systematically, so that the strength of the evidence on widening health inequalities is as yet uncertain. Second, most studies have not taken into account the fact that occupational classes with the largest excess mortality have become smaller over time, i.e., there are fewer and fewer unskilled labourers over time. When increasingly fewer people belong to the groups with high mortality, the total impact of inequalities on mortality in the population at large might diminish (Kunst et al. 2001).

The purpose of this section is to determine whether occupational class differences in all-cause mortality have increased for European countries between the 1980s and 1990s and whether these differences vary by welfare state regime type (social democratic, liberal, Christian democratic). These class differences are expressed both in terms of the magnitude of the mortality difference between two or more classes, and in terms of the public health impact of these differences. We look at the three countries with data from nationally (or regionally) representative longitudinal studies. One country is social democratic (Sweden); one country is liberal (U.K.), and the last piece of data originates from a region in a Christian democratic country (Torino, Italy) (Kunst et al. 2001).

Overview of Data Sources

The number of deaths by five-year age group and occupational class was obtained from longitudinal mortality follow-up of the population censuses carried out in about 1980 and about 1990 respectively (Kunst et al. 2001). People enumerated in the 1990 census were followed from 1990 to 1995. Those enumerated in the 1980 census were followed from 1980 to 1985 and from 1985 to 1989. In this way, three five-year periods between about 1980 and 1995 were distinguished. Most studies covered the entire national population. The data for England and Wales apply to a 1 percent sample of private households. The Italian study is restricted to the city of Turin and its surroundings. Age was measured as the age at the start of each sub-period. Data are analyzed for men in the age group 35–59 years. Men older than 60 years were excluded because of lack of detailed occupational information of retired men in most studies. Women were excluded from analysis because it was impossible for many countries to assign women to occupational classes (on the basis of their own occupation or their partner's occupation) in a way that was both valid and comparable over time.

Four broad occupational classes were distinguished: non-manual workers, manual workers, farmers and farm labourers, and self-employed men. The Erikson-Goldthorpe-Portocarero (EGP) scheme was used as a reference. This scheme can be used as an alternative to the Wright's social class scheme previously described. They both emphasize employment relations as the basis for the assessment of class positions. In Sweden, England, and Wales, EGP algorithms were available for the

1980s, and similar algorithms were applied to data for the 1990s. In Italy, a national social class scheme was used, allowing analyses among the four main social classes. In the Turin study, farmers and farm labourers were not distinguished because they formed a negligible part of the Turin city population.

Table 6.2 presents the distribution of men by occupational class in the three periods. In all countries, the non-manual and manual classes are the largest two classes. The share of self-employed men is modest and stable in our social democratic welfare state, and less so in England and Wales and Turin (liberal and Christian democratic countries, respectively). In nearly all countries, the share of manual and agricultural classes decreases over time, while the share of non-manual classes increases (Kunst et al. 2001).

Table 6.2: Population Distribution by Occupational Class: Men 30–59 Years

Country	Occupational Class	Proportion (%) of the Total Population		
		1980–1984	1985–1989	1990–1994
Sweden	Non-manual	43.6	44.3	46.3
	Self-employed	8.9	9.0	7.5
	Agricultural	5.9	5.4	4.3
	Manual	41.5	41.3	41.9
England/Wales	Non-manual	32.9	33.6	38.3
	Self-employed	10.8	11.2	17.3
	Agricultural	3.0	2.9	2.7
	Manual	53.4	52.2	41.6
Turin	Non-manual	34.1	34.4	42.0
	Self-employed	15.7	15.9	17.5
	Manual	50.1	49.7	40.4

The mortality level per occupational class was measured by means of age-adjusted mortality rates. Standardization by five-year age group was done by means of the direct method, with the European standard population of 1987 as the standard. Thanks to this standardization procedure, control was made for differences in age structure between occupational classes and, in addition, between countries and periods (Kunst et al. 2001).

The magnitude of mortality differences by occupational class was measured by means of two complementary inequality indices (Mackenbach and Kunst 1997).

1. *Rate differences*: These were calculated simply as the absolute difference
    between the age-standardized mortality rates that were observed for
    non-manual and manual classes.
2. *Rate ratios*: These can be calculated simply as the ratio of the two mortality
    rates mentioned above.

In addition, two indices were calculated that explicitly take into account the
distribution of the population over occupational classes (Mackenbach and Kunst
1997):

1. The population attributable risk (PAR), in which the class of non-manual
    workers was the reference group, was calculated on the basis of the
    age-standardized mortality rates according to standard formulae (see
    definition in Mackenbach and Kunst 1997).
2. The index of dissimilarity (ID), based on a distinction between the
    four broad occupational classes, was calculated on the basis of the age-
    standardized mortality rates (see definition in Mackenbach and Kunst
    1997).

Age-Standardized Death Rates

Death rates according to occupational class are presented in Figure 6.1 for Sweden,
Italy (Turin), and England and Wales (Kunst et al. 2001). Each country represents a
major welfare state type (i.e., social democratic, Christian democratic, and liberal).
In each country and period, manual classes have higher mortality rates than non-
manual classes. The mortality rates of the two other classes (self- employed and
agricultural men) are generally in between.

Mortality trends between the 1980s and 1990s are presented in Figure 6.1. National
mortality rates have declined considerably between 1982 and 1992 in most countries,
and this is the case for each occupational class. In absolute terms, the mortality
decline was about the same for manual and non-manual workers in most countries.
In relative terms, mortality declined faster in non-manual classes than in manual
classes in all countries (social democratic, liberal, and Christian democratic alike).
This class difference was relatively large in England and Wales (liberal).

Figure 6.2 shows how these similarities and dissimilarities in mortality declines
influenced the magnitude of class differentials in mortality. For each country, this
magnitude is given in both absolute terms (as rate differences) and in relative terms
(as rate ratios). In absolute terms, the advantage of non-manual classes over manual
classes has remained more or less stable in most countries. In England and Wales,
however, the larger absolute decline in non-manual classes resulted in a widening
of absolute mortality differences. In relative terms, the advantage of non-manual
classes over manual classes increased everywhere.

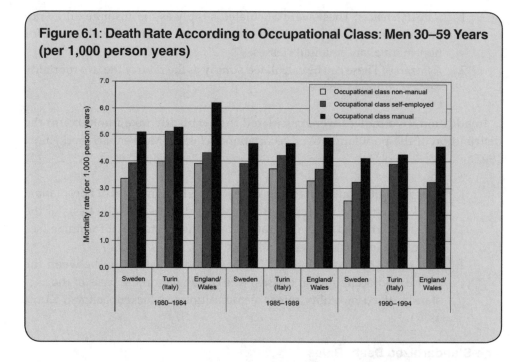

Figure 6.1: Death Rate According to Occupational Class: Men 30–59 Years (per 1,000 person years)

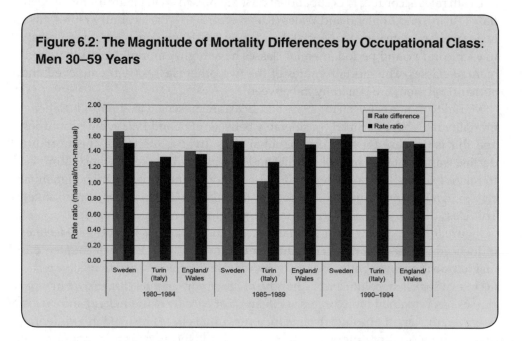

Figure 6.2: The Magnitude of Mortality Differences by Occupational Class: Men 30–59 Years

Until now, we looked mainly at changes by comparing the first to the last period. Some more detailed information can be obtained by looking at the middle period as well. Inequality estimates for the middle period are usually between the estimates for the first and last period. In some countries, however, the trends are less regular. An acceleration of trends (larger increases at the end of the study period) is observed for Sweden and Italy (Turin), whereas a deceleration (smaller increases at the end) seems to have occurred in England and Wales.

Taking into Account Population Distributions

The rate ratios and rate differences do not take into account changes in the occupational composition of the male working population, which changed considerably in a few countries (Kunst et al. 2001). Even though the relative mortality excess of manual classes increased over time, in some countries ever fewer men belonged to manual classes. This population change is taken into account by the population attributable risk (PAR), which is presented in Figure 6.3. The PAR shows essentially the same trends as the rate ratios. The PAR did not decrease in any of the countries, despite the decrease in the share of manual classes. Inspection of Figure 6.3 reveals why: in most countries this decrease is relatively small. Only in England and Wales and Italy (Turin), where the proportion of manual classes declined substantially, did the PAR remain stable despite increasing rate ratios.

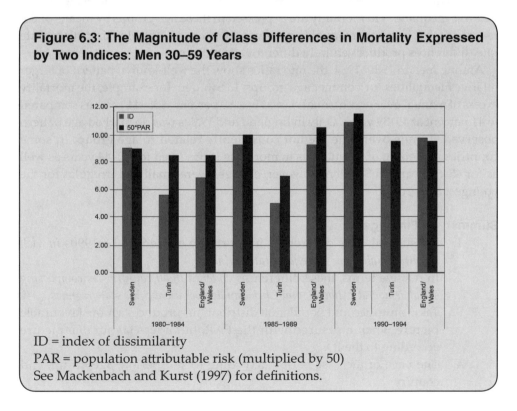

Figure 6.3: The Magnitude of Class Differences in Mortality Expressed by Two Indices: Men 30–59 Years

ID = index of dissimilarity
PAR = population attributable risk (multiplied by 50)
See Mackenbach and Kurst (1997) for definitions.

Figure 6.3 includes another summary index, the index of dissimilarity (ID). The value of about nine for Sweden in the first period can be interpreted to mean that 9 percent of all deaths would have to be redistributed to obtain the same mortality rates for all occupational classes. This value takes into account the population share and mortality level of all classes separately, and it is larger if the classes with, respectively, the highest and lowest mortality rates are larger. The ID shows about the same trends as the PAR. Large increases are observed for some countries, most notably for England and Wales. The increase in England and Wales is related to the mortality trends of farmers and self-employed men. While these classes had an already lower-than-average mortality level in the 1980s, they experienced the largest relative declines in the subsequent decade (Figure 6.1). Thus, these classes approached the non-manual groups (which is a favourable development from the PAR perspective), but moved away from the overall average (which is unfavourable from the ID perspective). The increase in the ID for England and Wales, as well for some countries, thus reflects a general divergence of class-specific mortality rates.

Age-Specific Patterns

The results presented until now collapses the mortality experiences of different ages, and might perhaps conceal divergent trends for more specific age groups (Kunst et al. 2001). For that reason, a distinction by age group is made in Figure 6.4. Relative inequalities in mortality are expressed in these age groups by means of the rate ratios that compare manual to non-manual classes. (Note: looking at absolute rate differences produces entirely different age patterns.)

Among men in 1980–1984, the rate ratios show the well-known pattern of larger relative inequalities for younger age groups. In Sweden, for example, the mortality excess of manual over non-manual classes was 80 percent at 35–44 years as compared to 41 percent at 45–59 years. Only in England and Wales was no marked age pattern observed. Trends over time are not consistently related to age group. In some countries, widening of inequalities in mortality is observed for 30–44 years as well as for 45–59 years. In Sweden, however, changes were small and irregular for the youngest age group.

Summary of Findings

1. Substantial class differences in mortality existed in the 1990s *in each country, in all types of welfare state regimes.*
2. In relative terms, these differences *widened in all countries, encompassing social democratic, liberal, and Christian democratic welfare state regimes.*
3. Taking into account population distributions produces a more favourable picture when measured with the PAR, but a less favourable picture according to the ID.
4. The pace of increase varied according to sub-period, age group, and country.

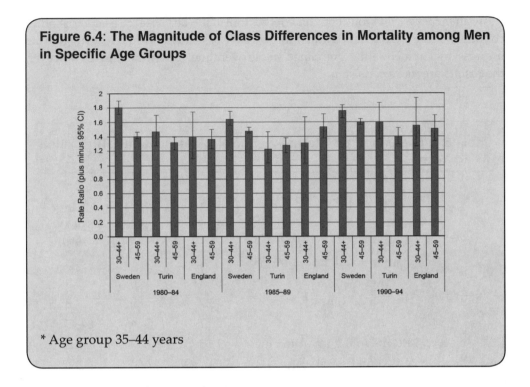

Figure 6.4: The Magnitude of Class Differences in Mortality among Men in Specific Age Groups

* Age group 35–44 years

Alternative Social Class Measures

Even though the Erikson-Goldthorpe-Portocarero social class scheme (which shows a substantial overlap with Wright's scheme presented in the first section of the chapter) was used as a general reference, there was inevitably some variation among countries in the social class schemes used and in the occupational information that was available to construct these schemes (Kunst et al. 2001). This variability raises the question as to what extent the choice for a specific class scheme would influence the observed magnitude and trends in class differences in mortality. One evaluation is presented in Table 6.3. In the Italian study (Turin), two data sets were created based on two different class schemes. For 1982–1986, the two class schemes produced nearly identical results, both in terms of population distribution and in terms of class differences in mortality. For example, the rate ratios that compare manual to non-manual classes were 1.33 and 1.36 for the two class schemes. (Another study found a rate ratio of 1.35 when using the Erikson-Goldthorpe-Portocarero scheme). For 1991–1996, however, the two class schemes produced less consistent results. Population distributions differed mainly because of different ways of defining the class of self-employed men in the 1992 census. Although estimates of class differences in mortality are roughly similar, the two schemes produce different estimates of trends over time. Rate ratios calculated under the first class scheme show an increase that would be considered "normal" (i.e., as large as in most other countries) while the rate ratios under the second class scheme would instead give the impression that inequalities remained stable over time. In terms of the ID, however, the results are more consistent.

Table 6.3: Evaluation of Alternative Social Classifications: Turin, Men 35–59 Years

		1982–1986	1992–1996	Change (1980–1990)
National class scheme	Population distribution (%)			
	- non-manual	34.1	42.0	7.9
	- self-employed	15.7	17.5	1.8
	- manual	50.1	40.4	–9.7
	RR manual vs. non-manual	1.33	1.43	0.10
	Index of dissimilarity	5.67	7.94	2.27
Esping-Andersen scheme	Population distribution (%)			
	- non-manual	32.2	30.4	–1.8
	- self-employed	17.5	25.4	7.9
	- manual	50.2	44.2	–6.0
	RR manual vs. non-manual	1.36	1.39	0.03
	Index of dissimilarity	5.65	6.92	1.27

This example from Italy (Turin) illustrates the more general experience that different social class schemes can produce different impressions of the magnitude and trends of class differences in mortality. However, the example also illustrates that inequality estimates are fairly robust if a classification into a few broad and clearly defined social classes is used.

Differences within Manual and Non-manual Classes

In the analyses up to now, no distinctions were made within the broad classes of manual and non-manual workers respectively (Kunst et al. 2001). The main reasons to do so were that (a) in some countries this distinction could not be made with the available data and (b) in the other countries there may be large problems with the comparability of data over time. Nonetheless, the question arises whether similar trends would be observed when a finer distinction would have been made. Perhaps the broad classes of manual and non-manual workers combine sub-classes with widely different mortality trends. Table 6.4 presents an example of the information that would be gained with a more detailed distinction of social classes. In the longitudinal study for England and Wales, mortality differences are given according to the British registrar-general's class scheme. For each period, the mortality level of each class is expressed as a ratio to the mortality level of the upper non-manual class. In order to secure comparability over time with this more detailed social classification, all estimates are based on a 15-year follow-up to the 1981 cohort. The results for 1981–1985 show the well-known pattern of increasing mortality rates when moving from class I to class V. With this finer classification, larger mortality differences are observed than with the simple contrast between manual and non-manual classes. Between 1981–1985 and 1991–1995, the class differences generally increased, with the larger increases in the lower occupational classes. The mortality trend of the lower non-manual class is somewhat irregular, perhaps due to the relatively small number of deaths in this class (about 200 per sub-period).

Table 6.4: Taking into Account Mortality Differences within the Manual and Non-manual in England and Wales, Men 35–59 Years

Social Class	Relative Mortality Risk (change since 1981–1985)				
	1981–1985	1986–1990		1991–1995	
Class I, II (upper non-manual = reference)	1.00	1.00		1.00	
Class III N (lower non-manual)	1.26	1.20	(–0.06)	1.32	(0.11)
Class III M (skilled worker)	1.32	1.37	(0.05)	1.44	(0.12)
Class IV, V (unskilled/ semi-skilled worker)	1.61	1.72	(0.11)	1.80	(0.19)
Manual as compared to non-manual	1.35	1.43	(0.08)	1.46	(0.11)

Source: ONS data on mortality by social class, according to the registrar-general's scheme, in the 1981 cohort, including men who were "unclassified" at the census.

This example from England and Wales illustrates the more general point that inequality measures based on the simple manual versus non-manual distinction are usually able to represent the general trend in class differences in mortality. However, a further distinction may reveal unexpected patterns, and it can help to identify more precisely those groups in which mortality trends are least favourable (Kunst et al. 2001).

Conclusions

Longitudinal, census-based data on mortality by occupational class can be used to monitor class differences in mortality among middle-aged men to compare trends across welfare state regime types. However, in both the analysis and interpretation of the results, we need to deal with (inactive) men for whom the social class cannot be determined. The trends presented here apply to middle-aged men. Given the scarcity of data and problems with unknown class, it is unlikely that trends in class differences in mortality can be assessed in many countries either for women or for elderly men at this point. Class differences in mortality are still substantial in European welfare states. The similarity of trends across welfare state types underlies that the common economic experience of countries in a given period (i.e., larger reductions in mortality among non-working-class, middle-aged men during the post-Second World War boom) might dwarf the effect of welfare state type on class inequalities in health in developed market economies. In other words, the joint evolution of capitalist economies would seem a stronger determinant of social class inequalities in health than the type of welfare state regime that manages this economy (e.g., social democratic, Christian democratic, liberal) in a particular country. Future research needs to improve the measurement of social class, obtain better data for women and unemployed people, and determine the specific welfare state policies that might reduce class inequalities in health. In that sense the Eurothyne project, financed by the E.U., might help elucidate some of these issues.

Acknowledgments

The authors would like to thank Seeromanie Harding, Orjan Hemstron, and Guiseppe Costa for generously sharing the data from U.K., Sweden, and Italy, respectively.

References

Baer, D., E. Grabb, and W.A. Johnston. (1987). "Class, Crisis and Political Ideology." *Canadian Review of Sociology and Anthropology* 42: 1–22.

Borrell, C., C. Muntaner, J. Benach, and L. Artazcoz. (2004). "Social Class and Self-Reported Health Status among Men and Women: What Is the Role of Work Organisation, Household Material Standards and Household Labour?" *Social Science and Medicine* 58(10): 1869–1887.

Coburn, D. (2004). "Beyond the Income Inequality Hypothesis: Class, Neo-liberalism, and Health Inequalities." *Social Science and Medicine* 58(1): 41–56.

Krieger, N., D.R. Williams, and N.E. Moss. (1997). "Measuring Social Class in U.S. Public Health Research: Concepts, Methodologies, and Guidelines." *Annual Review of Public Health* 18: 341–378.

Kunst, A.E., V. Bos, J.P. Mackenbach, and E.U. Working Group on Inequalities in Health. (2001). *Monitoring Socioeconomic Inequalities in Health in the European Union: Guidelines and Illustrations*. Rotterdam: Erasmus University.

Lynch, J.W., and G.A. Kaplan. (2000). "Socioeconomic Position." In *Social Epidemiology*, edited by L.F. Berkman and I. Kawachi, 76–94. New York: Oxford University Press.

Macinko, J., and B. Starfield. (2001). "The Utility of Social Capital in Research on Health Determinants." *Milbank Quarterly* 79(3): 387–427.

Mackenbach, J., and A. Kunst. (1997). "Measuring the Magnitude of Socio-economic Inequalities in Health: An Overview of Available Measures Illustrated with Two Examples from Europe." *Social Science and Medicine* 44(6): 757–771.

Marshall, S.W., I. Kawachi, N. Pearce, and B. Borman. (1993). "Social-Class Differences in Mortality from Diseases Amenable to Medical Intervention in New Zealand." *International Journal of Epidemiology* 22(2): 255–261.

Muntaner, C., and P. Ocampo. (1993). "A Critical-Appraisal of the Demand Control Model of the Psychosocial Work-Environment—Epistemological, Social, Behavioral and Class Considerations." *Social Science and Medicine* 36(11): 1509–1517.

Muntaner, C., W. Eaton, C. Diala, R. Kessler, and P. Sorlie. (1998). "Social Class, Assets, Organizational Control and the Prevalence of Common Groups of Psychiatric Disorders." *Social Science and Medicine* 47(12): 2043–2053.

Muntaner, C., and J. Lynch. (1999). "Income Inequality, Social Cohesion, and Class Relations: A Critique of Wilkinson's Neo-Durkheimian Research Program." *International Journal of Health Services* 29(1): 59–81.

Muntaner, C., J.W. Lynch, M. Hillemeier, J.H. Lee, D.R. Benach, and C. Borrell. (2002). "Economic Inequality, Working-Class Power, Social Capital and Cause-Specific Mortality in Wealthy Countries." *International Journal of Health Services* 32(4): 629–656.

Muntaner, C., W.W. Eaton, R. Miech, and P. O'Campo. (2004). "Socioeconomic Position and Major Mental Disorders." *Epidemiologic Reviews* 26: 53–62.

Navarro, V., and L. Shi. (2001). "The Political Context of Social Inequalities and Health." *Social Science and Medicine* 52(3): 481–491.

Navarro, V., C. Borrell, J. Benach, C. Muntaner, A. Quiroga, M. Rodriguez, and J. Guma. (2003). "The Importance of the Political and the Social in Explaining Mortality Differentials among the Countries of the OECD." *International Journal Health Services* 33(3): 419–494.

Navarro, V., and C. Muntaner. (2004). *Political and Economic Determinants of Population Health and Well-Being: Controversies and Developments*. Amityville: The Baywood Publishing Company.

Raphael D. (2001). "From Increasing Poverty to Societal Disintegration: How Economic Inequality Affects the Health of Individuals and Communities." In *Unhealthy Times: The Political Economy of Health and Care in Canada*, edited by H. Armstrong and P. Armstrong, 223–246. Toronto: Oxford University Press.

Raphael D., J. Macdonald, R. Labonte, R. Colman, K. Hayward, and R. Torgerson. (2004). "Researching Income and Income Distribution as a Determinant of Health in Canada: Gaps Between Theoretical Knowledge, Research Practice, and Policy Implementation." *Healthy Policy* 72 (2004): 217–232.

Townsend, P. N. Davidson, and M. Whitehead, eds. (1992). *Inequalities in Health: The Black Report and the Health Divide*. New York: Penguin.

• •

Critical Thinking Questions

1. Do social class and social stratification make the same predictions? Give an example from the chapter to illustrate your answer.
2. Do employers always have better health than workers? Give an example from the chapter to support your response.
3. Is there a relationship between welfare state regime type and trends in class inequalities in health from the data?
4. How would you explain the findings on the relationship between welfare state regime type and occupational class inequalities? Are they intuitive or counterintuitive? Justify your response.
5. Identify three needs for improving research on the comparative welfare state regime analysis of class inequalities in health.

Further Readings

Muntaner, C., C. Borrell, J. Benach, M.I. Pasarin, and E. Fernandez. (2003). "The Associations of Social Class and Social Stratification with Patterns of General and Mental Health in a Spanish Population." *International Journal of Epidemiology* 32(6): 950–958.
An empirical demonstration of the differences between social class, occupation strata, and education in health studies.

Navarro, V., and C. Muntaner (2004). *Political and Economic Determinants of Health and Well-Being.* Amityville: Baywood.
A state-of-the-art volume of the pervasive relation between social class and population health.

Wolff, R., and S. Resnick. (1987). *Economics: Marxian vs. Neoclassical.* Baltimore: Johns Hopkins University Press.
This volume provides definitions of class from both the Marxian and neo-classical traditions.

Wright, E.O. (2000). *Class Matters.* New York: Oxford University Press.
Definition and empirical studies of class in the neo-Marxian tradition.

Relevant Web Sites

Department of Epidemiology and Community Medicine, University of Ottawa
http://courseweb.edteched.uottawa.ca/epi6181/Reading_list/SES.htm
   Deals with social aspects of epidemiology.

Centre for the Study of Working Class Life, State University of Stony Brook, New York
http://naples.cc.sunysb.edu/wcm.nsf
   A centre dedicated to exploring the meaning of class in today's world.

Inequality.org
www.inequality.org
   The Inequality Web site includes data and discussion on social inequalities in health (including social class).

Rethinking Marxism: A Journal of Economics, Culture, and Society
www.nd.edu/~remarx/frontmatter/aboutaesa.html
   Devoted to social class as exploitation; mostly social science.

Glossary

Occupation: The meaning of occupation is usually taken for granted, but the significance of occupation varies from place to place. Occupation is a social role, a set of expectations with respect to the knowledge, skills, and experience of workers. Occupations group skills together into sets. These sets become known to employers and workers and serve to organize labour markets; they become, for instance, categories in job-vacancy advertisements. They facilitate the training of workers by providing goals and standards for training, and expectations as to employment prospects for employers, teachers, and trainees that motivate long-term commitments to the transmission and acquisition of skills. Countries differ in the strength of occupational definitions. In the United States, for instance, the boundaries of occupations are generally much more flexible and the significance of occupation in employment systems much less than in Germany. Survey respondents' occupation may be coded and the codes used to classify respondents according to occupational characteristics or exposures. A century ago, Durkheim suggested that, as the division of labour advanced, occupational associations could become a significant force in maintaining social solidarity. Recently this idea has been revisited; some have speculated that strengthening occupational definitions and institutions might be one response to the insecurity created by trends toward flexible and contingent work.

Occupational social class: Many commonly used measures labelled as "occupational class" are really measures of occupational stratification; they roughly rank workers on a hierarchical dimension. Such measures of occupational class are frequently grouped with other measures of stratification as alternative measure of social class. However, the concept of occupational class has developed within a theoretical tradition generally characterized as "Marxian." In this tradition, occupational class is defined by relations of ownership or control over productive resources (i.e., physical, financial, or organizational resources). Occupational class has important systematic consequences for the lives of individuals: the extent of an individual's legal right and power to control productive assets determines the strategies and practices devoted to acquire income and, as a result, determines an individual's standard of living. The composition and importance of occupational class systems vary internationally, but in developed economies, the most important classes are capitalists, the self-employed and small-business owners, workers, and those with contradictory positions (e.g., managers and supervisors who are workers, but who represent the interests of owners in their work).

Unions: Unions are organizations that represent the interests of workers with employers. The size of unions and the scope of union activities vary widely across countries and have also evolved over time. High rates of union membership and strong unions are associated with stronger social safety nets, active state labour-market policies, and greater employment protections for workers. Yet even in countries such as the U.S. where union membership is relatively low, unions make a positive contribution to the welfare of workers by raising wages, improving benefits, giving workers a public or political voice, educating workers, and monitoring work safety and labour relations.

Welfare state: A welfare state is a social system whereby the state assumes primary responsibility for the welfare of its citizens, as in matters of health care, education, employment, and social security or a nation in which such a system operates.

Working-class power: Power is the ability to make happen what one wants, even over the resistance or opposition of others. There are numerous sources of working-class power under capitalist production relations, but they often involve having collective control over generalized resources such as money, organizations, political parties, and communications media. Some sources of working-class power are situation-specific—for example, having access to information networks, having a particular position in an organization, or possessing collective control over particular natural resources. Other sources of power, such as ideological charisma, are personal, although they are expressed via working-class organizations (social democratic parties or unions). Social-class power is manifested through the political processes in government policy, in the actions of labour and working-class parties, and in the definition of agendas and issues whenever working-class material and social conditions are contested.

CHAPTER SEVEN

GENDER, RACE, AND HEALTH INEQUALITIES

Ann Pederson and Dennis Raphael

Learning Objectives

At the conclusion of this chapter, the reader will be able to

- examine how sex and gender influence health status, health care utilization, and experiences of health and illness
- examine why Canadian immigrants of colour might appear to have better health status than people born in Canada
- understand the reasons that the health of non-European immigrants to Canada appears to deteriorate over time
- consider why the living conditions of new Canadians appear to be of poorer quality than those born in Canada
- consider why an examination of gender and diversity should be integrated into health research and health policy

Introduction

Whether one is a man or a woman affects one's health status, use of health services, experience of illness, and engagement in health-related activities such as caring for others or participating in sports. Health is grounded in the context of men's and women's lives: it arises from the roles we play, the expectations we encounter, and the opportunities available to us based upon whether we are women or men, girls or boys. However, while all societies are divided along the "fault lines" of sex and gender (Papanek 1984), there are other social processes and dimensions of social location that also contribute to health. Many people in Canada are disadvantaged as a result of differences in income, power, age, sexual orientation, geographic location, disability, and/or race or as a result of experiences of violence, trauma, migration, or colonization. Racialized discrimination of visible minority groups and Aboriginal peoples has contributed to serious inequalities in health. When the combined effects of gender and race are considered, Aboriginal women are among the most vulnerable members of Canadian society.

This chapter delves briefly into issues of gender, race, and health. In the first section, we consider women's and men's health comparatively but also independently, with particular emphasis on women's health given the continued need to argue for its inclusion as a separate area of study, research, and practice. We argue that gender is a marker of social and economic vulnerability that manifests itself in inequalities in access to health and health care (Standing 1997). For women, income inadequacy and caregiving responsibilities are major contributors to health. The second part of the chapter looks more closely at how race and ethnicity contribute to health in Canada. We consider how the analysis of race and health—with the exception of Aboriginal health—is in its infancy. Recent evidence suggests that while the health of recent immigrants to Canada is excellent, over time health status deteriorates, especially among immigrants of non-European descent. This may be due to the poor living conditions to which these immigrants are subjected. Gender-based and race-related diversity analysis should be incorporated into health research and policy development to both understand and improve health.

Gender and Health

Key Concepts

It can be useful to distinguish between "sex" and "gender" in discussing men's and women's health. "Sex" refers to biological aspects of being male or female. While sex is perhaps most visible in terms of reproduction, there are underlying physiological processes and anatomical features that are typically different in males and females. "Gender," on the other hand, refers to the social attributes commonly ascribed to people who are male or female. All societies are organized in ways that reflect constructions of women and men as different kinds of people, with respective roles, responsibilities, and opportunities, including access to resources and benefits. As a social construct, the particular expressions and understandings of gender can vary over time and place and among communities. Behaviours, customs, roles, and practices are flexible and more variable across societies than the sex-related hormonal, anatomical, or physiological processes that typically characterize male and female bodies.[1]

Gender is a relational concept and involves not only the ascribed attributes that are systematically assigned to each sex but also relations between women and men (Health Canada 2000), including gender power. For example, the legal codes that frame social relationships—such as marriage, divorce, and child custody—have important implications for relations between women and men (as well as for relations between partners of the same sex) by the ways that they shape access to or responsibility for employment, income, housing, child care, and social benefits. Such practices enshrine social norms and values and contribute to individual expectations and personal as well as social identities. These social processes, in turn, contribute to physical and mental well-being through access to resources, opportunities, and power. Thus, sex and gender interact to create health conditions, situations, and problems that are unique to one sex or which vary in terms of prevalence, severity, risk factors, or interventions for women or men (see Greaves et al. 1999). Sex and gender also interact with the other determinants of health discussed in this volume such as socio-economic status, paid and unpaid work, and disability (Janzen 1998).

Standing (1997: 2) describes gender as a marker of vulnerability in two senses in the global context:

> First, women are found disproportionately among the most vulnerable population groups. They tend to be poorer than men on average, to have less access to income earning opportunities and other resources, including health care, and to be more dependent on others for their longer term security .... Second, access to and utilization of health services are importantly influenced by cultural and ideological factors, such as the embargoes on consulting male practitioners, lack of freedom to act without permission from husbands or senior kin and low valuation of the health needs of women and girls compared to that of men and boys.

In Canada, women's health and men's health similarly reflect important sex- and gender-related opportunities and vulnerabilities.

Health Status

According to Statistics Canada, average life expectancy at birth in 1999 was 79.0 years. Broken down by sex, however, women had an average life expectancy of 81.7 years while men had an average life expectancy of 76.3 (Health Canada 2002). This breakdown illustrates the value of even basic sex-disaggregation of data, as the overall figure masks the differences in life expectancy between women and men. However, as noted earlier, differences among women or men are also important to understanding the health of Canadians. Average life expectancy at birth in 1999 for First Nations people living on and off reserve was estimated to be 76.6 years for women and 68.9 years for men, sobering evidence of inequalities in Canada (Health Canada 2002).

The main causes of death among women and men in Canada are similar: coronary heart disease, cancer, and chronic lung disease; however, an analysis of potential years of life lost (PYLL) indicates that a larger number of PYLL are attributable to accidents for men as opposed to cancer for women (DesMeules, Manuel, and Cho 2003). Further, the size of the difference in PYLL between women and men in Canada varies across the lifespan, "with the largest discrepancy between men and women emerging in early and middle adulthood, where death from external causes (e.g., motor vehicle accidents) occurs at a much greater rate for men" (Janzen 1998: 21).

Women's apparent health advantage is reduced when morbidity and health care utilization are examined. For example, women report more frequent long-term disability and more chronic conditions than men (DesMeules, Turner, and Cho 2003). Ruiz and Verbrugge (1997), among others, suggest that the higher mortality rate and lower life expectancy of men compared to women have been misinterpreted to mean that women enjoy superior health, completely ignoring, they contend, the higher prevalence of chronic conditions in women, particularly in later life. Moreover, women's health status may be converging with that of men's: data suggest a narrowing of the gender gap in longevity in industrialized countries, most of it due to improvements in men's life expectancy (Trovato and Lalu 1996). Just as women's life expectancy increased dramatically in the middle of the 20th century as a result of reductions in maternal mortality, the current pattern of life expectancy observed between women and men may not hold in the future.

"Women are sicker, men die quicker" used to be an adage that supposedly summarized sex differences in health in Western industrialized countries such as Canada. Janzen (1998: ii) warns, however, that recent evidence of the complexity and variability of gender differences in health suggests that "broad generalizations about health-related gender differences are inappropriate." Let's consider at least six ways that sex and gender are important in shaping health and health care needs (Donner and Pederson 2004; Greaves et al. 1999).

First, there are sex-specific conditions, including the full spectrum of reproductive issues. These include birth control for women, pregnancy, childbirth, menstruation, menopause, and female infertility, as well as cervical cancer screening. For men, sex-specific conditions include prostate and testicular cancer and other diseases of the reproductive system, as well as male infertility and related problems. Second, there are conditions more prevalent among women or men, such as breast cancer, eating disorders, depression, and self-inflicted injuries in women and substance use, schizophrenia, and HIV/AIDS in men. Third, there are conditions that appear to be sex-neutral, such as heart disease, but where the signs, symptoms, and appropriate treatment may be different in women and men (Grace 2003). Fourth, there are the ways in which women's gendered roles in our society influence their health, including: women's caregiving responsibilities; the sex-segregation of the labour force, both in general and within health care in particular; the demands of women's caregiving responsibilities; women's average lower incomes; and women's greater responsibilities for combining paid work with child care or caring for other family members.

Fifth, gender stereotypes within the health care system itself may negatively affect women's health. These include both stereotypes about women's use of care and stereotypes about women's caregiving roles. For example, women are often assumed to use health care services more than men, but there is good evidence that this is related to sex-specific care and not to male stoicism or to women's predisposition to seek help. For example, in Manitoba in 1994–1995, the per capita cost of providing females with health care services funded by the Medicare system was approximately 30 percent higher than for men. However, after the costs of sex-specific conditions were removed, and considering costs for both physicians' services and acute hospital care, the costs of insured health care services for women were about the same as for men (Mustard et al. 1998). It has also been suggested that negative stereotypes about women lead to women receiving negatively differential treatment in everything from the use of life-saving drugs during heart attacks (Grace 2003) and the secondary prevention of ischemic heart disease (Hippisley-Cox et al. 2001), to physicians being more likely to assume women's physical symptoms are psychological in origin (McKie 2000).

Finally, there is the overmedicalization of normal aspects of women's lives, including pregnancy, childbirth, and menopause. This practice of framing normal life events as medical problems has been challenged by the women's health movement for over 40 years, with some successes (for example, the reintroduction of midwifery into Canada and its organization as a licensed profession, and challenges to the view of menopause as an estrogen-deficiency disease). Recent marketing campaigns for products to manage erectile dysfunction and male-patterned hair loss suggest that men are not immune to this trend to overmedicalization either.

Some Issues Affecting Men's and Women's Health in Canada

While overall tobacco use has declined in Canada, the decline in smoking prevalence among men has been more pronounced than the decline in smoking prevalence among women, with men's prevalence having declined from 61 percent to 25 percent between 1965 and 2001, while women's smoking prevalence declined from 38 percent to 21 percent during the same time period (Kirkland, Greaves, and Devichand 2003). Moreover, smoking rates among teenaged girls are comparable to, or exceed, those of teenaged boys, and there is evidence documenting that girls start to smoke earlier than boys (Kirkland, Greaves, and Devichand 2003). Aboriginal and First Nations peoples have the highest rates of smoking in Canada (62 percent of First Nations peoples and 72 percent of Inuit were smokers in 1997 compared to 29 percent of the general Canadian population) (Reading 1999). Pearce, Schwartz, and Greaves (2005) suggest that there are important gendered patterns within these overall data that link women's tobacco use to poverty, child care responsibilities, few employment opportunities, and poor housing, among other factors.

Poverty is one of the most pressing issues for women in Canada (Boxes 7.1 and 7.2). Women are more likely than men to be poor in Canada, given current patterns of childbearing, child custody following divorce, and women's employment over the lifespan. Families headed by lone mothers are particularly vulnerable to poverty, both in terms of incidence (56 percent were poor in 1997) and depth (incomes for poor lone-mothers families were, on average, $9,046 *less* than the low-income cut-off poverty line in 1997) (Ross, Scott, and Smith 2000).

The availability of child care is an important contributor to women's quality of life as it is essential for the support of their equality (Friendly 2004). It assists

Box 7.1: Canadian Women, Poverty, and the Minimum Wage

Part of the reason the wage gap is as big as it is in Canada is because women make up two-thirds of the minimum-wage earners. In Canada, minimum-wage earnings do not provide people with a fair income. In fact, minimum-wage earnings fall well below the poverty line.

For example, Manitoba's minimum wage of $7.00/hour (as of April 1, 2004) falls well below both the low-income cut-off, a formula determined by Statistics Canada that often acts as Canada's unofficial poverty line, and the acceptable living level, a poverty line determined by anti-poverty organizations in Winnipeg.

	Low-Income Cut-off (urban)	*Minimum Wage Earnings	Acceptable Living Level (pre-tax) in Winnipeg
Family of one	$17,409	$14,560	$14,409
Family of two (one adult, one child)	$21,760	$14,560	n/a
Family of three (one adult, two children)	$27,063	$14,560	$30,697
Family of four (two adults, two children)	$32,238	$29,120	$38,550
Family of four (one adult, three children)	$32,238	$14,560	$38,550

* Based on 40 hours/week, 52 weeks/year, no allowance for sick days, holidays, or periodic layoffs.

Source: The UN Platform for Action Committee (2004). Available on-line at http://unpac.ca/economy/wompoverty4.html.

women in their role as primary child rearers and facilitates employment outside the home (Palacio-Quintin 2000). Similarly, home health and supportive care are important to Canadian women because women are the most likely recipients of such care, the most likely to be employed as formal caregivers, and serve as the primary caregivers of family members (National Coordinating Group on Health Care Reform and Women nd). As such they are most likely to be affected when such care is not available or accessible (Morris, Robinson, and Simpson 1999). These two issues typify how governmental policy directions affect the quality of life of women (Fast and Keating 2000; Friendly 2004; Raphael and Bryant 2004).

Box 7.2: Canadian Women and Poverty

Poverty Hurts Women Most—Activist
Geoff McMaster

April 26, 2002—The erosion of social spending in Canada violates the basic rights of women, says a leading human rights activist.

Shelagh Day, co-author of a study called *Women and the Equality Deficit* and a director of the "Poverty and Human Rights Project," argued that "we are shredding the very bottom of Canada's social safety net," and that those who suffer most are women.

"More women than men are poor in Canada and around the world," said Day.

"Women are the poorest of the poor, and poverty of women is one of the central indicators of inequality. It's not an accident women are poor or living in deeper poverty than men. It's a manifestation of long-standing, structural discrimination against women."

According to Day, the safety net that has been an essential part of the Canadian social fabric since the Depression is quickly disappearing. Canada is now obsessed, she said, as are so many other countries in the West, with a neo-liberal agenda that creates "phony fiscal crises" and favours self-reliance, deregulated markets and the privitization of essential services while assuming we can no longer afford social assistance.

"That safety net has been very important in creating a climate of egalitarianism in Canada, and for the social mobility of particular groups of people, such as women. So many of those programs take the care-giving burden women carry disproportionately and move it to the state, creating egalitarian opportunities for women."

Day pointed out that 19 per cent of adult women are below the poverty line, compared to 13 per cent for men. Single mothers comprise 54 per cent of Canada's poor, and Aboriginal single mothers make up 73 per cent. "It tells us that being female, a mother and unattached are significant indicators—add being of non-white race or with a disability, and you're even more likely to be poor."

Poor women are also afflicted with a number of conditions specific to their gender, exacerbating their poverty, said Day. They get pregnant in order to qualify for better assistance, and they resort to prostitution and get involved in unhealthy relationships for food and shelter. Once they are on the street, they become particular targets for sexual abuse.

"Poverty enlarges every dimension of inequality," she said. "Poor women are sexually commodified and subordinated in their daily interactions with men. They accept it because it's a way to survive ... and they have no political voice."

Sharon McIvor, a lawyer, Aboriginal activist and head of Academi/Indigenous Studies at the Nicola Valley Institute of Technology in Merritt, B.C., echoed Day's assessment, arguing that despite the charter's adoption, conditions for aboriginal women have improved little over the past two decades.

She said the United Nations has repeatedly found fault with the federal government's treatment of Aboriginal women and has encouraged compliance with numerous U.N. resolutions. But Canada has failed to act, she said. It has not even studied the condition of young Aboriginal women who are ill-equipped for parenthood, elderly women who suffer from disproportionate ill health, or the treatment of native women by the criminal justice system, all of which have been identified as areas of serious concern by the U.N.

"The oppression of Aboriginal women flourishes today despite efforts by the United Nations to pave the way for women's equality." The only significant change to legislation was an end to a policy denying women native status and band membership if they married non-native men.

Source: Express News (2002). Available on-line at www.expressnews.ualberta.ca/ExpressNews/ articles/printer.cfm?p_ID=2454.

Experiences of violence differ for women and men, although they report similar rates of victimization (Statistics Canada 2001). As detailed by Eichler (1997), a man is more likely to experience violence on the street whereas a woman is more likely to experience violence from a family member in her own home. Men report higher rates of robbery and assault, but sexual assaults are more likely to be perpetrated against women (see Figure 7.1) (Statistics Canada 2001). The meaning of these gender difference for the physical and psychological safety of women and girls is profound because often "home" does not provide them with security. While violence does affect men in the home, it is a tiny proportion of the violence experienced by men (2.3 percent) whereas it is the single largest type of violence experienced by women (27.5 percent) (Health Canada 2003a). Responses to "family" or "domestic violence" must reflect these gendered patterns if they are to be of any value in reducing the incidence of violence against women.

Mental health and illness also offer interesting illustrations of sex and gender differences in Canada. Sex differences have been noted in the prevalence of specific mental health problems. For example, women are nearly twice as likely as men to be diagnosed with depression (Health Statistics Division 1998) and anxiety (Howell et al. 2001), particularly young women (Canadian Council on Social

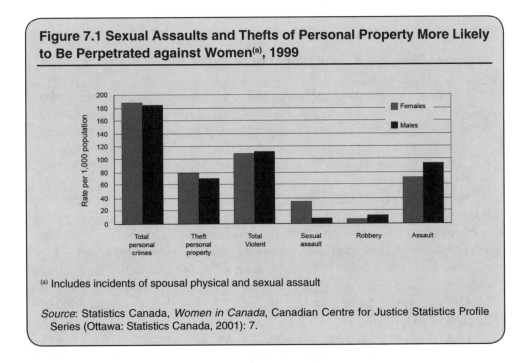

Figure 7.1 Sexual Assaults and Thefts of Personal Property More Likely to Be Perpetrated against Women[a], 1999

[a] Includes incidents of spousal physical and sexual assault

Source: Statistics Canada, *Women in Canada*, Canadian Centre for Justice Statistics Profile Series (Ottawa: Statistics Canada, 2001): 7.

Development 1998). The highest prevalence of depression is found, however, among Aboriginal women, in part as a result of living in impoverished conditions (Health Canada 2003b). Men are more often diagnosed with schizophrenia, certain personality disorders, and substance abuse (Culbertson 1997). Women and men also have different patterns of access to and use of mental health services, with women accessing the system more frequently, receiving treatment more often, and having higher rates of hospitalization for psychiatric problems than men (Federal-Provincial and Territorial Advisory Committee on Population Health 1996; Rhodes and Goering 1994).

Mental illness is associated with experiences of violence and trauma, and being mentally ill puts women at risk for further abuse (Anderson and Chiocchio 1997). Poverty and homelessness are associated with serious mental illness for both men and women in Canada, but less is known about homelessness regarding women than men, in part because the patterns of being without shelter manifest differently for women. Women are more likely, for example, to "couch surf" or stay temporarily with friends and family when they are without shelter, one effect of which is that fewer women appear in homeless shelters and in homelessness research, despite women's higher levels of poverty (see Box 7.3). Differences such as these have led analysts such as Morrow (2003) to call for a comprehensive policy response to women's mental health in Canada.

Box 7.3: **Canadian Women and Homelessness**

Degree of Women's Homelessness Underestimated, Study Finds

The full extent of women's homelessness is severely underestimated, a new study finds. Commissioned by the charitable organization, Sistering, and funded by Health Canada and the Status of Women Canada, *Common Occurrence*: *The Impact of Homelessness on Women's Health* highlights homelessness as a significant women's health issue that seriously impacts women's emotional, mental, spiritual and physical health.

Building on the realization that women's homelessness has not been adequately represented in other studies, and that the continuum of homelessness for women has not been fully understood, researchers sought to incorporate both "hidden" and "visible" homelessness in their report:

Visible homelessness includes women who stay in emergency hostels and shelters and those who sleep rough in places considered unfit for human habitation, such as parks and ravines, doorways, vehicles and abandoned buildings.

Hidden homelessness includes women who are temporarily staying with friends or family or who are staying with a person only in order to obtain shelter, and those living in households where they are the subject of family conflict or violence. Hidden homelessness also includes situations where women are paying so much of their income for housing that they cannot afford the other necessities of life, such as food; those who are at risk of eviction; and those living in illegal or physically unsafe buildings, or in overcrowded households.

"Homelessness has become a women's health issue," says Nancy Blades, the Director of Programming at Sistering. As advocates for the rights of homeless women, Sistering wanted to educate key health care stakeholders about the lived experiences of homeless women in Canada's health care system, and the connection to women's poverty. "We wanted to quantify women's experiences to uncover how women's homelessness is often hidden," says Blades.

Using a gender-based analysis, researchers interviewed more than 125 homeless women in Toronto on their health status, and gathered input from 38 representatives of agencies in Toronto's health, settlement, social services and emergency housing sectors. "We interviewed women in 14 different languages, and of various ages, ethnicities, sexual orientation, disabilities, women with children, street workers, immigrants, women with psychological/emotional/mental illnesses, and more," says Blade. Of the more than 125 women interviewed, 93% of the women reported emotional and mental health issues as a result of their living situations.

In the study, researchers also address women's homeless-specific health concerns, including the barriers homeless women face in the current systems of support. The study finds that social and medical services are not fully responsive to homeless women's health care issues and needs, particularly because there has been little understanding of the continuum of women's homelessness.

Common Occurrence Research Action Report: The Impact of Homelessness on Women's Health is available from Sistering ($20 each, plus $5 shipping). Phone (416) 926-9762 ext. 227 or visit www.sistering.org for details.

Source: Sistering: A Woman's Place. Available on-line at www.cwhn.ca/network-reseau/6-23/6-23pg5.html.

Occupational health research and practice remains largely gender-blind (Messing 1998). The labour force remains largely sex-segregated in some areas, despite the influx of women into many "traditionally" male occupations in the past 40 years. Interestingly, repetitive strain injury is reported equally by both men and women, but there is some evidence suggesting that the percentage of women affected by these problems is rising, particularly women in traditionally male-dominated occupations. Possible explanations include psychosocial aspects of the workplace as well as poorly designed workstations, deadlines, and self-reported stress. In addition, many women's occupational health issues remain hidden in the household because women's labour in this setting is not recognized as work and the health risks associated with unregulated activities in individual households are seldom the target of policy interventions.

Each of these issues illustrates the various ways that sex and gender influence patterns of health and illness among women and men in Canada. Increasing recognition of some of the gender-related differences in health call for action from policy makers, researchers, and clinicians.

Addressing Gender-Based Inequalities in Health

Policy makers in Canada have made numerous commitments to gender equality, as exemplified by being a signatory to international conventions such as the 1981 United Nations *Convention on the Elimination of All Forms of Discrimination against Women* (Waldorf and Bazilli 2000) and the *Platform for Action*, which arose from the 4th World Conference on Women in Beijing in 1995 (Health Canada 2003a). Canada has also taken many steps to support an expanded evidence base on women's health through, for example, supporting a women's health strategy and the Centres of Excellence for Women's Health, establishing a women's health theme within the Canadian Health Network (an electronic resource on health topics), introducing an Institute on Gender and Health as part of the national health research funding infrastructure (Canadian Institutes for Health Research), and developing training in gender-based analysis specific to the health field (see Box 7.4).

Evidence is not always available to facilitate gender-based analysis. For example, Statistics Canada's *Access to Health Care Services in Canada* (Statistics Canada 2001) contains only sex-aggregated data, despite Health Canada's stated commitment to gender-based analysis. The production, analysis, and reporting of sex-disaggregated data are an important step toward understanding gender and health issues; however, it is not sufficient to understand these issues. Gender-based diversity analysis, "which wrestles with issues of women's social location, gender-related power and access to resources, is needed in addition to sex-disaggregated data to fully understand women's lives" (Donner and Pederson 2004: 18). Such analyses rest on an understanding of intersectionality (Weber and Parra-Medina 2003)—that is, an understanding of the multiple social processes underlying social experiences, including gender and race.

Many governments, health authorities, non-governmental organizations, and advocacy groups have developed women's health plans or strategies to address the specific health concerns of women in their communities. However, many of these efforts focus on aspects of care and are consequently addressing health outcomes rather than addressing the underlying social and economic structures that shape women's (and men's) health. Action on these more deeply embedded elements of the social structure may require action far beyond the health sector. Moreover, such strategies need to be developed with an awareness of women's lives so that women are truly able to benefit from the initiative. Financial support for caregiving, for example, is currently part of the Employment Insurance scheme in Canada. Unfortunately, access to this support is limited for the people who need it most—women are the majority of unpaid caregivers—because many women do not qualify for benefits under the scheme because they are not employed full-time.

Race, Ethnicity, and Health

Aside from a long-standing concern with the health status of Canada's Native peoples, analysis of the relationship of race and ethnicity with health is in its infancy in Canada. One reason is the relatively greater historical racial homogeneity of Canadian society as compared, for example, to the U.S. Another reason is that, until recently, health researchers have generally found few health status differences— outside of Aboriginal populations—among racial and ethnic groups in Canada. This is certainly not the case in the U.S. where extensive effort is focused—to the exclusion of social class and income issues—upon identifying racial and ethnic differences in health status.

Increasing attention in Canada is being paid to racial and ethnic issues in health as changing patterns of immigration result in increasing numbers of members of visible minority groups. These Canadian efforts—much of which is being carried out

Box 7.4: Health Canada and Gender Analysis

Health Canada's role is to foster good health by promoting health and protecting Canadians from harmful products, practices, and disease. Gender equality is a broad societal human rights, social justice, and health issue. As such, Health Canada will implement a gender-based analysis to ensure that policies and programs are responsive to sex and gender differences and to women's health needs, which results in remedies to inequality.

Gender-based analysis (GBA) is a method of evaluation and interpretation that takes into account social and economic differences between women and men, whether applied to policy and program development, or general life activities such as work/family roles.

The application of GBA is governed by a number of fundamental principles including:

- gender equality can be achieved only by recognizing the different impact of norms or measures on women and men according to their diverse life situations
- gender-based analysis is an integral part of the substantive analytical process and must be applied at each stage of this process
- gender-based analysis focuses not only on results but also on concepts, arguments, and language used in the work process
- gender-based analysis must lead to remedies to inequality

GBA and Women's Health

When GBA is applied to health policy and program development, gender stereotypes are eliminated and socio-economic factors affecting women's health are acknowledged. When equitable policies are applied to the health system, this sets the stage for the provision of services appropriate to women's needs.

GBA recognizes that the health needs of women and girls, and men and boys are different. It does this by ensuring that an analysis of the determinants of health is undertaken. This accounts for social factors that affect everyone's lives, such as issues of diversity including socio-economic status, ability, ethnicity, and sexual orientation.

Health Canada Initiatives

Health Canada's implementation of a gender-based analysis fully integrates gender into its day-to-day operations. It represents Health Canada's commitment to doing business in a way that is sensitive to women's health needs and concerns.

This federal government commitment is articulated in the Federal Plan for Gender Equality approved by Cabinet in 1995, which states that departments will put forward "A systematic process to inform and guide future legislation and policies at the federal level by assessing any potential differential impact on women and men."

Health Canada will ensure that:

- employees are given professional development seminars to learn the steps involved in GBA
- employees are given a guide on how to apply GBA to the substantive work of the department
- a network of gender equality specialists serve as resource persons for policy/program development and implementation, research, funding, data collection, surveillance, regulatory activities, health promotion, disease prevention, services to First Nations and Inuit, corporate management activities/policies/consultations/communication plans
- managers will dedicate staff time for GBA training, analysis, committee work, etc.
- managers incorporate women's health plans in the development of the annual branch plans and business lines to ensure that gender equality is given priority as an integral part of the strategic planning process

The Women's Health Bureau has prepared a guiding document, *Women's Health Strategy*, which situates gender issues in the context of health, and will be the basis for Health Canada's GBA implementation.

The overall goal is to improve the health of women in Canada by making the health system more responsive to women and women's health.

Sources:

- *Women's Health Strategy*, Women's Health Bureau, Health Canada, 1999.
- *Health Canada's Implementation on Gender-Based Analysis*, Women's Health Bureau, Health Canada, 1999.
- *Exploring Concepts of Gender and Health*, Health Canada, Women's Health Bureau, 2003.
- *Gender-Based Analysis Backgrounder Human Resources Development Canada*, Cat. no. SP-100-01-97E, 1997.
- *Gender-Based Analysis Guide*, Human Resources Development Canada, Cat. no. SP-101-01-97E, 1997.
- *Diversity and Justice: Gender Perspectives, a Guide to Gender Equality Analysis*, Department of Justice Canada, 1998.

> • *Women's Health in the Context of Women's Lives*, Minister of Supply and Services, Cat. no. H39-324/1995E, 1995.
> • *Working Together for Women's Health*: *A Framework for the Development of Policies and Programs*, Federal/Provincial/Territorial Working Group on Women's Health, April 1990.
>
> *Source*: Women's Health Bureau of Health Canada, 2004. Available on-line at www.hc-sc.gc.ca/english/women/.

within an immigration studies focus—are directed at two issues: (a) the relationship of race and ethnicity to health status and (b) analysis of the quality of various social determinants of health experienced by racial and ethnic groups in Canada. A particularly important form this focus is taking is that of examining the health status and economic and social conditions associated with various "racialized groups."

The focus here is upon race with emphasis on the situation of two important groups: Aboriginal peoples and immigrant groups in Canada called "visible minorities" or "racialized groups." "Racialization" is a term that considers how groups of individuals come to be treated in inferior ways compared with the dominant group (Allahar and Cote 1998).

Differences in health status between Aboriginal peoples in Canada and non-Aboriginal peoples are striking. However, differences in traditional indicators of health status between racialized immigrant groups and non-racialized groups were few until recently; frequently the health status of non-White groups is superior to that of Whites. Two recent studies find, however, that the health status of non-European immigrants in Canada appear to deteriorate over time. In addition, recent research finds profound differences in economic and social conditions among racialized—especially recently immigrating—groups. This is important as difficult economic and social conditions are frequently precursors to poor health status and these racialized immigrant groups are a significant proportion of the population in Canadian urban areas.

Race, Ethnicity, and Health

There is a well-developed sociological literature regarding the definition of race, ethnicity, and related issues (McMullin 2004). Clear consensus exists—at least among academics in the social sciences—that race and ethnicity are social constructions representing dominant groups' historical attempts to maintain control and power over those identified as members of "other" races or groups. Many health researchers and health workers do not share this view and for them race and ethnicity are indicators of biological disposition to disease or a convenient marker to identify targets for public health interventions (Cruickshank et al. 2001).

These interventions are frequently focused on modifying behavioural risk factors for disease (such as tobacco use, physical inactivity, or poor diet), or improving access to health care. Less common is a public health concern with addressing the social and economic conditions that members of different racial groups are exposed to and working to modify these risk conditions through public policy (see Chapter 15 in this volume). The concern here is with two issues: (1) How has the race concept been applied to understanding health and its determinants? (2) What is known about health inequalities among members of different racial groups?

Race and Health Status: Concepts

Lee, Mountain, and Koenig (2001: 58) point out that "historically, race, genetics, and disease have been inextricably linked, producing a calculus of risk that implicates race with relative health status." Rather than view the greater incidence of a disease among a group as potentially reflecting social and economic conditions that result from discrimination and prejudice, these associations can be attributed to genetic causes. Duster argues that when the association between race and illness is viewed through a "prism of heritability," environmental and class-related causes of illness among specific racial groups can be ignored or suppressed (Duster 2003). Similarly, Krieger (2003: 195) states: "Myriad epidemiological studies continue to treat 'race' as a purely biological (i.e., genetic) variable or seek to explain racial/ethnic disparities in health absent consideration of the effects of racism on health."

Racial differences in health status can be attributed to exposures to specific material conditions of life that result from both membership in specific social and occupational classes as well as the systematic experience of discrimination and prejudice. Members of racialized groups in Canada are overrepresented in lower-status occupations and experience greater incidence of poverty and low income (Galabuzi 2004, 2006). There is increasing evidence that such overrepresentation is due to discrimination, reflecting the presence of racism in Canadian society.

Jones outlines three forms of racism, all of which will have impacts on health (Jones 2000). *Institutionalized racism* is concerned with the structures of society and may be codified in institutions of practice, law, and governmental inaction in the face of need. *Personally mediated racism* is defined as prejudice and discrimination and can manifest itself as lack of respect, suspicion, devaluation, scapegoating, and dehumanization. *Internalized racism* is when those who are stigmatized accept these messages about their own abilities and intrinsic lack of worth. This can lead to resignation, helplessness, and lack of hope. These concepts are clearly applicable to Canadian society (Galabuzi 2004, 2006).

Race and Health Status: Aboriginal Peoples in Canada

Systematic reviews of health issues facing Canada's Aboriginal peoples are available (Health Canada First Nations and Inuit Health Branch 2003; Shah 2004). Aboriginal peoples overall show significantly greater incidence of a range of afflictions and premature death from a variety of causes. These issues result from the poor state of any number of social determinants of health (e.g., income, housing, food security, employment and working conditions, social exclusion, etc.) and reflect a history of social exclusion from Canadian society.

There is a large gap in mortality between the Aboriginal and the general Canadian population. In 1996–1997, mortality rates among First Nations and Inuit peoples from eastern and western Canada and the prairie provinces were almost 1.5 times higher than the national rate. During this same period, infant mortality rates among First Nations peoples were close to 3.5 times the national infant mortality rates. Neonatal death rates are double the general Canadian rates and post-neonatal mortality rates almost four times higher.

Further, off-reserve Aboriginal peoples rate their health status lower than the overall Canadian population (Tjepkema 2002). For every age group between 25 and 64, the proportion of Aboriginal peoples reporting fair or poor health is double that of the total population. The effect is more pronounced among Aboriginal women. For example, 41 percent of Aboriginal women aged 55–64 reported fair or poor health, compared with 19 percent of women in the same age group in the total Canadian population. Among those aged 65 and over, 45 percent of Aboriginal women reported fair or poor health, compared with 29 percent in the total female population. Poor economic and social conditions are responsible for these differences in health.

Race and Health Status: Non-Aboriginal Peoples in North America

United States

Health disparities among racial and ethnic minorities are the focus of numerous research initiatives, national and state public health agendas, and local public health activity (see Chapter 15 in this volume). Indeed, the focus on racial and ethnic disparities is so great that issues of health differences related to income and wealth, social class, and gender are frequently downplayed or neglected. As a result, a great amount of evidence is available concerning racial and ethnic differences in health status among Americans (U.S. Department of Health and Human Services 2004a). The most recent information on these differences can be succinctly summarized as follows: "There are continuing disparities in the burden of illness and death experienced by African Americans, Hispanic Americans, Asian/Pacific Islanders, and American Indians/Alaska natives, as compared to the US population as a whole" (U.S. Department of Health and Human Services 2004b: 1).

In most cases, these racial/ethnic differences exist in life expectancy, infant mortality, and virtually every other indicator of health status. The predominant focus on the causes of these disparities is unduly focused on access to health care and behavioural risk factors with rather less attention paid to the economic and social conditions of these groups and the public policies that spawn these conditions (see Chapter 15 in this volume). The precarious economic and social conditions under which these minority groups live are well documented, but these issues take a

Box 7.5: **Aboriginal Health in Canada**

Encouraging Signs for Aboriginal People Living off Reserves
Carmelina Prete

Aboriginal people living off reserves are improving their quality of life but still lag behind the average Canadian when it comes to health care, education and housing.

The 2001 Aboriginal Peoples Survey, released yesterday by Statistics Canada, shows health is worse among older female Aboriginals and best among the young. This is encouraging since Aboriginals under 25 are a growing segment of the population and now make up nearly half of the off-reserve Aboriginal population in Canada.

The survey is significant because it updates the statistical portrait of the well-being of Aboriginal people in Canada. The last one was done in 1991. Survey questions were answered by 117,000 Indian, Inuit and Métis people—of mixed native and European descent—including 86,000 living off reserves.

Yesterday's survey dealt solely with Aboriginal people living off reserves, who make up 70 per cent of the total Aboriginal population in Canada.

"Things are getting better but we still have a long way to go," says Bruce Peterkin, executive director of the Aboriginal Health Centre in Hamilton.

Overall, 56 per cent rated their health as good or excellent compared with 65 per cent of all Canadians. The gap was negligible among young natives and widened among elder natives.

For example, four in 10 Aboriginal women aged 55–64 reported fair or poor health, more than double the number of non-native women who said the same.

"I'm not surprised. They're the poorest of the poorest of the poor. They're the bottom rung," says Peterkin.

He says elder natives have greater difficulty gaining access to mainstream medical services, which often means they seek help when they are already quite ill.

Nearly half of Aboriginal adults reported having a chronic illness. Arthritis, rheumatism, high blood pressure and asthma were most common. In every case, Ontario natives reported a higher rate of chronic illness than the national aboriginal average.

For example, 19 per cent of native Canadians reported suffering from arthritis.

The number was 26 per cent in Ontario.

Heather Tait, an author of the report, isn't sure why.

"We're just starting to scratch the surface with these numbers," she said.

The survey also sheds light on why 48 per cent of young Aboriginals off reserves drop out of high school compared with about one-third of non-natives. One-quarter of native girls aged 15 to 19 said they left school because of pregnancy or child-care issues. Twenty-four per cent of boys in the same age group blamed boredom.

Catherine Brooks, an indigenous student counsellor at McMaster University, says roadblocks such as poverty and family responsibilities prevent Aboriginals from completing their education. She said Aboriginals are more likely to start their post-secondary education after they've started a family, which make the pressures more intense. Statistics from the survey also show Aboriginals are more likely to complete their schooling later in life.

Roxanne Miller considers herself privileged.

The 30-year-old Mohawk is finishing an undergraduate degree at McMaster University with plans to start a masters degree in occupational therapy next year. Her goal is to become a doctor and serve the Aboriginal community.

She also works part-time at a native health centre while raising her two children, aged 10 and 3, with the support of her fiancé.

"I know I'm not the norm," she says. "I'm privileged. I had a decent upbringing and a lot of support .... My push is that I want to provide a better life for my children."

Miller is among 100 Aboriginal students at McMaster, which has an enrolment of more than 17,500.

The survey also suggests overcrowding is a serious problem for Aboriginals living off reserves. In 2001, 17 per cent lived with more than one person to a room compared with seven per cent of other Canadians. Crowding was most serious for Aboriginal people in Winnipeg, Regina, Saskatoon and Edmonton where native populations are larger.

The survey didn't offer statistics specific to Hamilton. According to the 2001 census, about 7,300 people living in Hamilton, Burlington and Grimsby identified themselves as Aboriginal—a 33 per cent jump from 1996.

Source: The Hamilton Spectator, News (September 25, 2003): A04.

back seat to traditional health care and public health concerns with behaviour and lifestyle modifications (Raphael 2003).

Canada

Canada's concern with issues of race and health as it relates to immigrant groups has been spurred by changing immigration patterns over the past 20 years. While previously a large proportion of immigrants to Canada were of European descent,

Galabuzi (2004: 239) points out: "There has been a significant change in the source countries with over 75% of new immigrants in the 1980s and 1990s coming from the Global South." Racialized (or visible minority) groups now constitute significant proportions of those living in many urban areas (e.g., Toronto, 36.8 percent; Vancouver, 36.9 percent; Calgary, 17.5 percent; Edmonton, 14.6 percent; Ottawa, 14.1 percent; Montreal, 13.6 percent; Winnipeg, 12.5 percent, etc.). Of particular concern is emerging evidence that the social and economic conditions under which members of racialized groups are living are distinct threats to health.

Unlike the situation in the U.S., there is little evidence—outside of studies of Native peoples—of health differences among racial groups (McMullin 2004). Much of this may be due to what has been termed the healthy immigrant effect whereby immigrants to Canada have superior health status compared to native-born Canadians (Hyman 2001). Since a significant proportion of visible-minority Canadians are recent arrivals in Canada and subject to health screening, it is not surprising that many studies find that non-White status is not associated with poorer health status. Table 7.1 shows data from a very well-quoted study that shows that immigrants—both more recently arrived and those from earlier periods—show evidence of superior health status compared to native-born Canadians.

However, the recent availability of both cross-sectional and longitudinal data from the National Population Health Survey (NPHS) provides compelling evidence that the health of immigrants to Canada, especially non-European immigrants, deteriorates over time as compared to Canadian-born residents and European immigrants. Newbold and Danforth (2003) found that immigrants to Canada were more likely than non-immigrants to rate their health as poor or fair and that this was especially the case for those who have been in Canada longer.

A more nuanced and recent analysis is provided by longitudinal analysis of NPHS data (Ng, Wilkins, Gendron, and Berthelot 2004). They categorized respondents into four groups: recent (10 years or less) European immigrants, recent non-European immigrants, long-term (more than 10 years) European immigrants, and long-term non-European immigrants. They then examined the likelihood that individuals reported a transition from good, very good, or excellent health to either fair or poor health.

They found that, as compared to the Canadian-born population, recent non-European immigrants were twice as likely to report a deterioration in health from 1993–1994 to 2002–2003. Long-term non-European immigrants were also more likely to report such deterioration. There was no effect for either of the two European immigrant groups (Figure 7.2). Of importance was the finding that these differences were reflected in recent non-European immigrants who were 50 percent more likely to become frequent visitors to doctors than the Canadian-born population.

The additional predictors of transition to lower health status included a number of factors best described as social determinants of health. These were low income adequacy, less education, and low support. As the authors commented, "Findings

Table 7.1: Age-Adjusted Prevalence Conditions, by Immigrant Status, Canadian-born and Immigrant, Canada, 1994–1995

	Total[a]	Canadian-Born	All Immigrants[b]	European Immigrants Total[c]	European Immigrants 0–10 Years in Canada	European Immigrants 11+	Non-European Immigrants Total[d]	Non-European Immigrants 0–10 Years in Canada	Non-European Immigrants 11+
Any chronic condition	55.5	56.8	50.3[d]	55.3	46.7	57.7	44.7	37.2[d]	51.2
Sex									
Men	51.7	53.0	46.6[d]	51.1	39.8	54.7	40.8	33.8[d]	46.7
Women	59	260	553.8[d]	59.3	52.3	60.5	48.1	40.1[d]	55.6
Annual household income									
Less than $30,000	57.6	59.7	51.3[d]	57.4	46.3	59.5	45.8[d]	37.4[d]	55.5
#30,000 or more	53.9	54.7	49.8[d]	54.0	46.4	56.8	44.6[d]	39.0[d]	48.7
Education									
Less than secondary graduation	55.5	56.3	52.5	57.7	55.2	58.8	45.7	37.0[d]	58.3
Secondary graduation or more	54.9	56.2	49.6[d]	54.4	45.8	57.0	44.6[d]	35.8[d]	50.1
Specific chronic conditions									
Joints	23.9	24.5	21.7[d]	24.9	28.1	25.7	16.4[d]	10.9[d]	20.0
Allergy	18.9	19.5	16.4[d]	17.3	19.6	16.0	11.2d	20.0	
Hypertension	9.7	9.7	9.6	10.0	—	10.2	8.9	6.8	10.3
Headaches	7.3	7.2	7.4	9.1	—	9.4	5.4	<[d]	7.0
Asthma	5.6	6.0	4.1[d]	4.6	—	5.1	3.6[d]	<[d]	
Heart/stroke	4.9	5.0	4.6	5.2	—	5.4	3.3	<[d]	3.9
Sinusitis	4.3	4.7	3.2[d]	3.5	—	3.9	2.7[d]	—	
Ulcers	3.5	3.5	3.2	3.7	—	4.0	—	—	
Diabetes	3.4	3.5	3.2	2.8	—	2.9	4.2	—	4.3
Bronchitis	3.0	3.5	1.6[d]	2.2[d]	—	2.4	<[d]	<[d]	<[d]
Cancer	1.7	1.7	1.7	2.0	—	2.1	—	—	
Urinary incontinence	1.1	1.2	0.9	1.1	—	1.1	<[d]	—	<[d]

(a) Includes unknown immigrant status
(b) Includes unknown country of birth
(c) Includes unknown years in Canada
(d) Difference compared with Canadian-born significance at 95% confidence level
< or > Value significantly greater or smaller than that of Canadian-born, but not shown because of large sampling error.
Source: National Population Survey, 1994–1995. Reproduced in J. Chen, R. Wilkins, and E. Ng, "Health expectancy by immigrant status, 1986 and 1991," Health Reports (Statistics Canada, Catalogue 82-003-XIE) 1996, 8(3): 29–38.

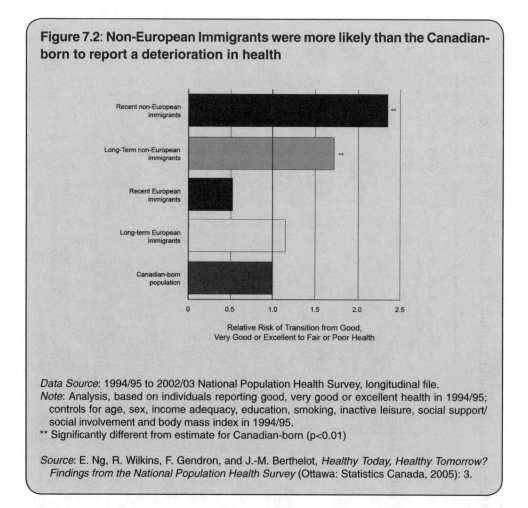

Figure 7.2: Non-European Immigrants were more likely than the Canadian-born to report a deterioration in health

Data Source: 1994/95 to 2002/03 National Population Health Survey, longitudinal file.
Note: Analysis, based on individuals reporting good, very good or excellent health in 1994/95; controls for age, sex, income adequacy, education, smoking, inactive leisure, social support/ social involvement and body mass index in 1994/95.
** Significantly different from estimate for Canadian-born (p<0.01)

Source: E. Ng, R. Wilkins, F. Gendron, and J.-M. Berthelot, *Healthy Today, Healthy Tomorrow? Findings from the National Population Health Survey* (Ottawa: Statistics Canada, 2005): 3.

from the literature on immigrants' integration in Canada have shown that those with non-European origins have low-paid jobs that require little education. Because immigrants with European origins share a similar culture with the Canadian born, they may encounter fewer social, economic, and lifestyle barriers than do those from non-European countries" (Ng, Wilkins, Gendron, and Berthelot 2004: 6). We now turn to these issues.

Racial and Ethnic Differences in Social Determinants of Health

Extensive scholarship is identifying profound issues related to the material conditions of life among Aboriginal and visible-minority immigrants, and non-White Canadians. These are clearly related to social determinants of health such as income, employment and working conditions, housing, education, and recreational opportunities. Indeed, these differences are so profound as to require application of the broad concept of social exclusion as both process and outcome of various societal factors driving these differences (Galabuzi 2004).

Shah provides much evidence concerning the economic and social status of Aboriginal peoples in Canada while Galabuzi (2004, 2006) does so for racialized immigrant groups in Canada. Concerning the latter, these include: (a) a 30 percent income gap in 1998 between racialized and non-racialized groups; (b) higher than average unemployment, with unemployment rates two to three times higher than non-racialized groups; (c) deepening levels of poverty; (d) overrepresentation in lower-paying and lower-status jobs; (e) differential access to housing; (f) increasing racial and economic concentration in Canadian urban areas; and (g) disproportionate contact of racialized groups with the criminal justice system (Ornstein 2000; Pendakur 2000; Reitz 2001).

Statistics Canada has documented differences in income and employment status of recent and earlier immigrants to Canada (Picot 2004). There is a consistent finding that the rate of low income among immigrants (particularly recent immigrants) has been rising during the 1990s while falling for the Canadian-born. Picot attempted to identify the factors responsible for the deteriorating economic welfare of immigrants and found that the rise in low-income status affected immigrants in all education and age groups, including the university educated (Picot 2004). The study found that the economic returns to recent immigrants for their work experience and education were diminished as compared to that seen for earlier immigrants. Considering that 75 percent of these recent immigrants were members of racialized groups, the hypothesis that racism and discrimination are responsible for these diminishing returns must be considered.

As noted, to date health status differences among racialized and non-racialized groups were not consistent. There is evidence from more in-depth studies of members of racialized groups in Canada that these members are encountering significant threats to physical and mental health that are not easily detected by traditional health status measures or are mediated by the "healthy immigrant" effect (Beiser et al. 2002; Canadian Research Institute for the Advancement of Women 2002; Noh et al. 1999). However, international research indicates that exposure to adverse economic and social conditions are reliable precursors to disease. While in the past immigrants to Canada gradually reached income and employment levels comparable to the Canadian-born, this may not continue to be the case.

The pattern of increasing economic and racial concentration in Canadian urban areas suggests cause for concern (Hatfield 1997; Myles, Picot, and Pyper 2000; United Way of Greater Toronto 2004). Such concentration of visible-minority groups has been associated in the U.S. with poor health and increasing social disintegration (Ross, Nobrega, and Dunn 2001). This process may well be underway in many Canadian urban centres, but to date there is little research on the lived experience of members of racialized groups in Canada.

We also know nothing about the experience of discrimination and racism and their effects upon members of racialized groups in Canada. We would expect that such studies would replicate findings that refugees who reported the experience of racial discrimination had higher depression levels that those who did not (Noh et al. 1999). Research on the effects of discrimination in the U.S. and the U.K. suggest attention to this area is needed (Karlsen and Nazroo 2002; Krieger 2003).

Conclusions

This chapter describes evidence of the relationships between gender, race, and health in Canada. Discussions of gender and health, and race and health, share the same challenge of competing explanations. To what extent are gender and race biological and/or social constructs? We believe that these concepts represent the effects of economic and social forces that then determine how these issues are construed by governments, academic researchers, and the public. To the extent that alternative views are held, the dominance of particular understandings will shape research agendas and practical approaches for dealing with these issues.

Gender and Health

Regardless of the issue, it is apparent that probing for the possibility of sex differences is an important first step in analyzing health status, health service utilization, and health policies. Further analysis that considers the potential contribution of sex, gender, and their interaction in accounting for differences in health conditions, outcomes, experiences, and needs for services is useful and can help direct policy makers, program developers, health care providers, and researchers.

A focus on the issue of gender and health can result in a tendency to treat "sex" and "gender" only in comparative terms and to reify the distinctions between men and women at the risk of understanding similarities and of recognizing that facets of the human experience, such as sexuality, are more diverse than is sometimes implied by the focus on "women" and "men." As work on gay, lesbian, bisexual, transgendered, and queer health grows, we learn more about not only the specific health problems of these people but also how issues such as sexual orientation interact with constructs of gender in everyday life, affecting access to opportunities for health as well as health care (OPHA 2000; Ross, Scott, and Wexler 2003).

While it is important to study health comparatively, as we have seen throughout this chapter, the study of women's or men's health independently remains important and necessary. Moreover, the differences among women and among men, as exemplified by the discussion that follows on racialization and health, are critically important because, as this book has illustrated, the determinants of health interact in the lives of individual men and women. Social structures and processes such as heterosexism, racism, ageism, and class call for critical diversity analyses in addition to gender-based analysis, as illustrated by the discussion that follows on race, ethnicity, and health (Jackson et al. 2004). Finally, sex and gender are linked to health inequalities in profound ways worldwide, which has implications for

Canada's role as a global actor as well as for people from all over the world who come to Canada as immigrants and refugees. Indeed, women's health status is a central factor in measuring progress toward gender equity globally. As Doyal (2004) argues, much remains to be done:

> Currently, less than 10% of current global funding for research is spent on diseases that afflict more than 90% of the population. This is referred to as the 10/90 gap in health research, and efforts to close it are mounting as part of the wider equity agenda in health. Increasingly, it is being recognized that gender issues must be central to these efforts, since women comprise the majority of the world's poor. The health of these women is affected not just by their poverty and by failures to meet many of their sex-related (i.e., biological) and reproductive health needs, but also by the wider gender (i.e., social) inqualities that continue to shape their lives. Men's health can also be negatively affected by their masculinity, with the poorest often at the greatest risk. Health researchers will need to take these factors just as seriously as more widely accepted determinants of health such as race, class, and ethnicity. (Doyal 2004: 162)

Research into race and health is a growing area of study. The Canadian Institutes of Health Research support sex- and gender-sensitive health research, though methodological issues remain. There is still much to learn about the effects of sex, gender, and their interaction in order to understand the health of Canadian women, men, girls, and boys.

Race and Health

The literature on the health effects of economic and social conditions suggests cause for concern regarding the health of members of racialized groups in Canada, many of whom are recent immigrants.

The economic situation of these individuals—many of whom are concentrated in urban areas—is clearly inferior to the situation of earlier arrived immigrants and the Canadian-born. Findings that these increased levels of poverty, unemployment, and social and economic exclusion are more persistent than that seen for earlier arrived immigrants is disturbing. The sources of these differences appears to reside in a general deterioration of Canadian social and economic environments (see Chapter 8 in this volume) that interacts with processes of racial discrimination directed toward newly arrived members of racialized groups (Krieger 2000; Williams, Neighbors, and Jackson 2003). As argued by Galabuzi:

> At a time when Canada's population growth and stability are increasingly dependent on immigration, with racialized group members now forming 13.5% of the population and growing and immigrants now 18.4% and projected to account for 25% of the population by 2015, these issues represent an important area of health policy and research. (Galabuzi 2004: 236)

Any attempts to improve the health of Canadians must seriously address the key issues faced by women, recent immigrants, and people of colour in Canada. These issues include economic vulnerability, ingrained attitudes that prejudice the life chances of these groups, and public policy decisions that increase conditions of risk. Research must consider how increased economic and social insecurity interacts with gender and racial and immigrant status to influence health and well-being. At the same times concrete actions need to be taken to address these conditions of risk and promote actions that will promote the health of Canadians in general and members of these groups in particular.

References

Allahar, A., and J. Cote. (1998). *Richer and Poorer: The Structure of Inequality in Canada.* Toronto: Lorimer.

Anderson, C., and K. Chiocchio. (1997). "The Interface of Homelessness, Addictions and Mental Illness in the Lives of Trauma Survivors." In *Sexual Abuse in the Lives of Women Diagnosed with Serious Mental Illness,* edited by M. Harris and C. Landis, 21–38. Amsterdam: Oversees Publisher's Association.

Beiser, M., F. Hou, I. Hyman, M. Tousignant. (2002). "Poverty, Family Process, and the Mental Health of Immigrant Children in Canada." *American Journal of Public Health* 92(2): 220–227.

Canadian Council on Social Development. (1998). *The Progress of Canada's Children, Focus on Youth.* Ottawa: Canadian Council on Social Development.

Canadian Research Institute for the Advancement of Women. (2002). *Women's Experience of Racism: How Race and Gender Interact.* Ottawa: CRIAW.

Chen, J., Wilkins, R., Ng, E. (1996). "Health Expectancy by Immigrant Status, 1986 and 1991." *Health Reports* 8(3). Ottawa: Statistics Canada, Catalogue 82-003-XIE: 29-38.

Cruickshank, J., J.C. Mbanya, R. Wilks, B. Balkas,N. McFarlane-Anderson, and T. Forrester. (2001). "Sick Genes, Sick Individuals or Sick Populations with Chronic Disease? The Emergence of Diabetes and High Blood Pressure in African-Origin Populations." *International Journal of Epidemiology* 30(1): 111–117.

Culbertson, F.M. (1997). "Depression and Gender: An International Review." *American Psychologist* 52(1): 25–31.

DesMeules, M., D. Manuel, and R. Cho. (2003). "Health Status of Canadian Women." *Women's Health Surveillance Report: A Multi-dimensional Look at the Health of Canadian Women.* Ottawa: Health Canada, Canadian Population Health Initiative.

DesMeules, M., L. Turner, and R. Cho. (2003). "Morbidity Experiences and Disability among Canadian Women." In *Women's Health Surveillance Report: A Multi-dimensional Look at the Health of Canadian Women,* edited by M. DesMueles, D. Stewart, A. Kazanjian, H. McLean, J. Poyne, B. Vissandjée, 19-20. Ottawa: Health Canada, Canadian Population Health Initiative.

Donner, L., and A. Pederson. (2004). "Beyond Vectors and Vessels: Women and Primary Health Care Reform in Canada," prepared for the National Workshop on Primary Care and Women, February 6–7, 2004, Winnipeg, Sponsored by the National Coordinating Group on Health Care Reform and Women and the Prairie Women's Health Centre of Excellence.

Doyal, L. (2004). "Gender and the 10/90 Gap in Health Research." *Bulletin of the World Health Organization* 82: 162.

Duster, T. (2003). *Backdoor to Eugenics.* New York: Routledge.

Eichler, M. (1997). *Family Shifts: Families, Policies, and Gender Equality.* Toronto: Oxford University Press.

Fast J., and N. Keating. (2000). *Family Caregiving and Consequences for Careers: Towards a Policy Research Agenda.* Ottawa: Canadian Policy Research Networks.

Federal-Provincial and Territorial Advisory Committee on Population Health. (1996). *Report on the Health of Canadians: Technical Appendix.* Toronto: Federal Provincial and Territorial Advisory Committee on Population Health.

Friendly, M. (2004). "Early Childhood Education and Care." In *Social Determinants of Health: Canadian Perspectives,* edited by D. Raphael, 109–124. Toronto: Canadian Scholars' Press.

Galabuzi, G.E. (2005). "Social Exclusion." In *Social Determinants of Health: Canadian Perspectives,* edited by D. Raphael, 235–252. Toronto: Canadian Scholars' Press.

_____. (2006). *Canada's Economic Apartheid: The Social Exclusion of Racialized Groups in the New Century.* Toronto: Canadian Scholars' Press.

Grace, S. (2003). "Presentation, Delay, and Contraindication to Thrombolytic Treatment in Females and Males with Myocardial Infarction." *Women's Health Issues* 13(6): 214–221.

Greaves, L., et al. (1999). *CIHR 2000: Sex, Gender and Women's Health.* Vancouver: British Columbia Centre of Excellence for Women's Health.

Hatfield, M. (1997). *Concentrations of Poverty and Distressed Neighbourhoods in Canada.* Ottawa: Applied Research Branch, Human Resources Development Canada (HRDC).

Health Canada. (2000). *Health Canada's Gender-Based Analysis Policy.* Ottawa: Minister of Public Works and Government Services Canada.

_____. (2002). *Healthy Canadians: A Federal Report on Comparable Health Indicators 2002.* Ottawa: Health Canada.

_____. (2003a). *Exploring Concepts of Gender and Health.* Ottawa: Women's Health Bureau, Health Canada.

_____. (2003b). *The Health of Aboriginal Women.* Ottawa: Health Canada.

Health Canada First Nations and Inuit Health Branch. (2003). *A Statistical Profile on the Health of First Nations in Canada.* Ottawa: Health Canada, First Nations and Inuit Health Branch.

Health Statistics Division. (1998). *National Population Health Survey Overview, 1996/97.* Ottawa: Statistics Canada.

Hippisley-Cox, J., M. Pringle, N. Crown, A. Beal, and A. Wynn. (2001). "Sex Inequalities in Ischaemic Heart Disease in General Practice: Cross-sectional Survey." *British Medical Journal* 322: 832.

Howell, H.B., Brawman-Mintzer, J. Monier, K.A. Yonkers. (2001). "Generalized Anxiety Disorders in Women." *Psychiatric Clinics of North America* 24(1): 165–178.

Hyman, I. (2001). *Immigration and Health.* Working Paper Series. Ottawa: Applied Research and Analysis Directorate, Health Canada.

Jackson, B., A. Pederson, P. Armstrong, M. Boscoe, B. Chow, K.R. Grant, N. Gubermann, and K. Wilson. (2004). "'Quality Care Is Like a Carton of Eggs': Using a Gender-Based Diversity Analysis to Assess Quality of Health Care." *Canadian Woman Studies* 24:1 (Fall 2004): 15–22.

Janzen, B.L. (1998). *Women, Gender and Health: A Review of the Recent Literature*. Winnipeg: Prairie Women's Health Centre of Excellence.

Jones, C. (2000). "Levels of Racism: A Theoretic Framework and a Gardener's Tale." *American Journal of Public Health* 90(8): 1212–1215.

Karlsen, S., and J.Y. Nazroo. (2002). "Relation between Racial Discrimination, Social Class, and Health among Ethnic Minority Groups." *American Journal of Public Health* 92(4): 624–632.

Kirkland, S., L. Greaves, and P. Devichand. (2003). "Gender Differences in Smoking and Self-Reported Indicators of Health." In *Women's Health Surveillance Report: A Multi-dimensional Look at the Health of Canadian Women*, edited by M. DesMueles, D. Stewart, A. Kazanjian, H. McLean, J. Poyne, and B. Vissandjée, 11–12. Ottawa: Health Canada, Canadian Population Health Initiative.

Krieger, N.A. (2003). "Does Racism Harm Health? Did Child Abuse Exist before 1962? On Explicit Questions, Critical Science, and Current Controversies: An Ecosocial Perspective." *American Journal of Public Health* 93(2): 194–199.

Krieger, N.A. (2000). "Refiguring 'Race': Epidemiology, Racialized Biology, and Biological Expressions of Race Relations." *International Journal of Health Services* 30: 211–216.

Lee, S.S., J. Mountain, and B.A. Koenig. (2001). "The Meanings of Race in the New Genomics: Implications for Health Disparities Research." *Yale Journal of Health Policy, Law and Ethics* 1: 33–75.

McKie, R. (2000). "Moaning Men Push Women to Back of Health Queue." *U.K. Observer* (May 7).

McMullin, J. (2004). *Understanding Social Inequality: Intersections of Class, Age, Gender, Ethnicity and Race in Canada*. Toronto: Oxford University Press.

Messing, K. (1998). *One-Eyed Science: Occupational Health and Women Workers*. Philadelphia: Temple University Press.

Morris, M., J. Robinson, and J. Simpson. (1999). *The Changing Nature of Home Care and Its Impact on Women's Vulnerability to Poverty*. Ottawa: Status of Women Canada.

Morrow, M. (2003). *Mainstreaming Women's Mental Health: Building a Canadian Strategy*. Vancouver: British Columbia Centre of Excellence for Women's Health.

Mustard, C., et al. (1998). "Sex Differences in the Use of Health Services." *New England Journal of Medicine* 338: 1678.

Myles, J., G. Picot, and W. Pyper. (2000). *Neighbourhood Inequality in Canadian Cities*. Ottawa: Statistics Canada, Business and Labour Market Analysis Division.

National Coordinating Group on Health Care Reform and Women. (nd). *Women and Home Care: Why Does Home Care Matter to Women?* Winnipeg: National Coordinating Group on Health Care Reform and Women.

Newbold, K.B., and J. Danforth. (2003). "Health Status and Canada's Immigrant Population." *Social Science and Medicine* 57: 1981-1995.

Ng, E., R. Wilkins, F. Gendron, and J.-M. Berthelot. (2004). *Dynamics of Immigrants' Health in Canada: Evidence from the National Population Health Survey*. Ottawa: Statistics Canada.

Ng, E., R. Wilkins, F.Gendron, and J.-M. Berthelot. (2005). *Healthy Today, Healthy Tomorrow? Findings from the National Population Health Survey*. Ottawa: Statistics Canada.

Noh, S., M. Beiser, V. Kaspar, F. Hou, and A. Rummens. (1999). "Perceived Racial Discrimination, Depression, and Coping: A Study of Southeast Asian Refugees in Canada." *Journal of Health and Social Behavior* 40: 193–207.

Ontario Public Health Association. (2000). *Improving the Access to and Quality of Public Health Services for Lesbians and Gay Men*. Toronto: OPHA.

Ornstein, M. (2000). *Ethno-Racial Inequality in the City of Toronto: An Analysis of the 1996 Census*. Toronto: Access and Equity Unit, Strategic and Corporate Policy Division, Chief Administrator's Office.

Palacio-Quintin, E. (2000). "The Impact of Day Care on Child Development." *Isuma* 1(2): 17–22.

Papanek, H. (1984). *Women in Development and Women's Studies: Agenda for the Future*. East Lansing: Office of Women in International Development, Michigan State University.

Pearce, D., D. Schwartz, and L. Greaves. (2005). *No Gift: Tobacco Policy and Aboriginal People in Canada*. Vancouver: British Columbia Centre of Excellence for Women's Health.

Pendakur, R. (2000). *Immigrants and the Labour Force: Policy, Regulation and Impact*. Montreal: McGill-Queen's University Press.

Picot, G. (2004). *The Deteriorating Economic Welfare of Immigrants and Possible Causes*. Ottawa: Statistics Canada.

Raphael, D. (2003). "A Society in Decline: The Social, Economic, and Political Determinants of Health Inequalities in the U.S.A." In *Health and Social Justice: A Reader on Politics, Ideology, and Inequity in the Distribution of Disease*, edited by R. Hofrichter, 59–88. San Francisco: Jossey Bass.

Raphael, D., and T. Bryant. (2004). "The Welfare State as a Determinant of Women's Health: Support for Women's Quality of Life in Canada and Four Comparison Nations." *Health Policy* 68: 63–79.

Reading, J. (1999). *The Tobacco Report: First Nations and Inuit Regional Health Surveys*. Winnipeg: Northern Health Research Unit, University of Manitoba.

Reitz, J.G. (2001). "Immigrant Skill Utilization in the Canadian Labour Market: Implications of Human Capital Research." *Journal of International Migration and Integration* 2: 347–378.

Rhodes, A., and P. Goering. (1994). "Gender Differences in the Use of Outpatient Mental Health Services." *Journal of Mental Health Administration* 21(4): 338–347.

Ross, D., K. Scott, and P. Smith. (2000). *The Canadian Fact Book on Poverty, 2000*. Ottawa: Canadian Council on Social Development.

Ross, N., K. Nobrega, and J.R. Dunn. (2001). "Income Segregation, Income Inequality and Mortality in North American Metropolitan Areas." *GeoJournal* 53(2): 117–124.

Ross, E., M. Scott, and E. Wexler. (2003). *Environmental Scan on the Health and Housing Nees of Aging Lesbians*. Toronto: Older Lesbians in Valued Environments (OLIVE) and Sherbourne Health Centre.

Ruiz, M.T., and L.M. Verbrugge. (1997). "A Two-Way View of Gender Bias in Medicine." *Journal of Epidemiology and Community Health* 51: 106–109.

Shah, C. (2004). "Aboriginal Health." *Social Determinants of Health: Canadian Perspectives*, edited by D. Raphael, 267–280. Toronto: Canadian Scholars' Press.

Standing, H. (1997). "Gender and Equity in Health Sector Reform Programmes: A Review." *Health Policy and Planning* 12(1): 1–18.

Statistics Canada. (2001). *Women in Canada*. Canadian Centre for Justice Statistics Profile Series. Ottawa: Statistics Canada.

Tjepkema, M. (2002). "The Health of the Off-reserve Aboriginal Population." *Health Reports Supplement* 13: 1–17.

Trovato, F., and N.M. Lalu. (1996). "Narrowing Sex Differentials in Life Expectancy in the Industrialized World: Early 1970s to Early 1990s." *Social Biology* 43(1–2): 20–37.

U.S. Department of Health and Human Services. (2004a). *Health, United States 2004.* Washington: U.S. Department of Health and Human Services.

U.S. Department of Health and Human Services. (2004b). *HHS Fact Sheet.* Washington: U.S. Department of Health and Human Services.

United Way of Greater Toronto. (2004). *Poverty by Postal Code: The Geography of Neighbourhood Poverty, 1981–2001.* Toronto: United Way of Greater Toronto.

Waldorf, L., and S. Bazilli. (2000). *The CEDAW Impact Study.* Toronto: York University Centre for Feminist Studies.

Weber, L., and D. Parra-Medina. (2003). "Intersectionality and Women's Health: Charting a Path to Eliminating Health Disparities. In *Advances in Gender Research*, edited by M. Texler Segal, V. Demos, and J. Kronenfeld, 181–230. Oxford: Elsevier.

Williams, D.R., H.W. Neighbors, and J.S. Jackson. (2003). "Racial/Ethnic Discrimination and Health: Findings from Community Studies." *American Journal of Public Health* 93(2): 200–208.

Note

1. On the other hand, research continues to grow indicating the vast variability in the human body, including its structures and functioning. Despite our customary belief in two sexes, there is wide variability among individuals with respect to the presentation of sex-based physical characteristics, and research has demonstrated the complicated nature of sexual classification systems. One in 2000 infants are born with so-called ambiguous genitalia, with sometimes dramatic results. Parents in North America, for example, are typically encouraged to decided upon the sex of their child very quickly and then to raise the child according to sex-appropriate norms. Such practices illustrate the tremendous significance of sex and gender in everyday life. People often want to know how to identify and label other individuals, and sex-based criteria are a major element of such practices.

• •

Critical Thinking Questions

1. What are the likely consequences of ignoring gender issues in health policy making and research?
2. How are women's health and men's health portrayed in the media? What are the implications of these portraits?
3. What is it about Canadian society that makes women so susceptible to economic and social public policies?

4. What are the health and social implications of racial discrimination in employment and educational opportunities continuing for (a) members of racialized groups? and (b) Canadian society in general? To what extent and in what ways is racial discrimination a current topic of discussion among policy makers, the media, and the public at large?

5. What are some of the political, economic, and social barriers to health and well-being that women of colour experience in Canada? What can be done to help remove these barriers?

Further Readings

Colman, R. (2003). *A Profile of Women's Health Indicators in Canada.* Halifax: GPI Atlantic.
This report offers a statistical analysis of economic, social-psychological, health behaviours, lifestyle, and environmental determinants of health; healthy child development; reproductive health; health outcomes; and health system performance in Canada and the Atlantic provinces. The report was prepared for the Women's Health Bureau, Health Canada by GPI Atlantic. Available on-line at www.gpiatlantic.org/pdf/health/womens/whbreport.pdf.

Doyal, L. (2004). "Gender and the 10/90 Gap in Health Research." *Bulletin of the World Health Organization* 82(3): 126.
This brief editorial summarizes gender and its worldwide relationship to health for women and men, persuasively arguing that ignoring issues of sex and gender is detrimental to improving health globally.

Galabuzi, G.E. (2006). *Canada's Economic Apartheid: The Social Exclusion of Racialized Groups in the New Century.* Toronto: Canadian Scholars' Press.
This book calls attention to the growing racialization of the gap between rich and poor, which, despite the dire implications for Canadian society, is proceeding with minimal public and policy attention. Dr. Galabuzi points to the role of historical patterns of systemic racial discrimination as essential in understanding the persistent overrepresentation of racialized groups in low-paying occupations.

Statistics Canada. (2002). *Women in Canada 2000: A Gender-Based Statistical Report.* Ottawa: Statistics Canada.
Statistics Canada has produced an updated and expanded version of the original publication, first released in March 1985. This report analyzes the situation of Canadian women by exploring their demographic and cultural characteristics, living arrangements, income, labour force activity, health, and criminal and victimization characteristics. Supported by more than 65 key colour charts and 190 tables, this report presents this wealth of information in a clear and concise form.

Relevant Web Sites

Canadian Research Institute for the Advancement of Women (CRIAW)
www.criaw-icref.ca/indexFrame_e.htm
    CRIAW is a research institute that provides tools to facilitate organizations taking action to advance social justice and equality for all women. CRIAW recognizes women's diverse experiences and perspectives; creates spaces for developing women's knowledge; bridges regional isolation; and provides communication links between/among researchers and organizations actively working to promote social justice and equality for all women.

Centres of Excellence for Women's Health
www.cewh-cesf.ca/en/index.shtml
    The Women's Health Contribution Program supports policy research and education on women's health issues. Managed by the Bureau of Women's Health and Gender Analysis, Health Canada, the program is a partnership between multiple stakeholders interested in women's health, including academics, community organizations, policy makers, and clinicians.

Joint Centre of Excellence for Research on Immigration and Settlement (CERIS)
http://ceris.metropolis.net/frameset_e.html
    CERIS is a consortium of Toronto-area universities and community partners. CERIS goals include: promoting research about the impact of immigration on the Greater Toronto Area and on the integration of immigrants into Canadian society; providing training opportunities; and disseminating policy and program-relevant research information.

Women and the Economy, a Project of UNPAC
http://unpac.ca/economy/ecorace.html
    The Women and Economy Web site makes clear that women's experiences of the economy are very different from men's. However, gender is not the only factor that plays a major part in one's place in the economy. Race and racism are other important determinants.

Women's Health Surveillance Report
http://secure.cihi.ca/cihiweb/dispPage.jsp?cw_page=PG_29_Eandcw_topic=29andcw_rel=AR_342_E#full
    The *Women's Health Surveillance Report* provides information and descriptive statistics on determinants of health, health status, and health outcomes for Canadian women. Each chapter presents new, gender-relevant information on a health condition or issue identified as important to women's health during national expert and stakeholder consultations in 1999.

World Health Organization Department on Gender, Women, and Health
www.who.int/gender/en/

The World Health Organization has adopted a policy of gender mainstreaming in order to support equity for women and improve women's health. This site introduces all aspects of the WHO program and provides links to key documents, policy initiatives, and contacts.

Glossary

Gender: Refers to the socially constructed roles, rights, responsibilities, possibilities, and limitations that, in a given society, are assigned to men and women—in other words, to what is considered "masculine" and "feminine" in a given time and place.

Racism: A set of beliefs that asserts the natural superiority of one racial group over another at the individual but also the institutional level. In one sense, racism refers to the belief that biology rather than culture is the primary determinant of group attitudes and actions. Racism goes beyond ideology; it involves discriminatory practices that protect and maintain the position of certain groups and sustain the inferior position of others. (Canada Immigrant Job Issues available on-line at www.canadaimmigrants.com/glossary.asp#R).

Sex: The biological and physiological characteristics of male and female animals: genitalia, reproductive organs, chromosomal complement, hormonal environment, etc.

Sexism: A form of discrimination. It is a set of beliefs that asserts the superiority of one sex over another and can be expressed individually or institutionally. That is, individual people may express beliefs that one sex or the other is more suited for certain tasks or societal roles than the other. Sexism may also be expressed through procedures and assumptions that permeate organizations, legislation, and the law and which again assume that one sex or the other is naturally suited or capable or likely to perform certain roles and hold certain responsibilities as opposed to seeing people of either sex as possessing a diverse range of abilities. Sexism may reflect a limited appreciation of the extent to which differences between the sexes have been socially constructed and are often arbitrarily exaggerated through social codes, custom, and historical practices.

Acknowledgment/Disclaimer

The British Columbia Centre of Excellence for Women's Health and its activities and products have been made possible through a financial contribution from Health Canada. The views expressed herein do not necessarily represent the views of Health Canada.

CHAPTER EIGHT

POLITICS, PUBLIC POLICY, AND POPULATION HEALTH

Toba Bryant

> ### Learning Objectives
>
> At the conclusion of this chapter, the reader will be able to
> - define public policy and its impact on the quality of the social determinants of health
> - identify the political and economic forces that influence public policy
> - explore specific examples of public policy and their impacts on health and well-being
> - consider the Canadian situation in an international context
> - outline policy directions for Canadian society

Introduction

Social determinants of health such as income and its distribution; availability and affordability of housing and food; stability and quality of employment; and the provision of health and social services profoundly influence health. Governments' public policy decisions influence the quality of these social determinants of health. These public policy decisions are themselves shaped by political, economic, and social forces within jurisdictions that allow some approaches and exclude others. This chapter explores why some jurisdictions implement public policies that support the social determinants of health and others do not. To do so it examines the political, economic, and social forces that shape Canadian public policy and nations with similar traditions such as the U.S. and the U.K. Sweden is used as a comparison nation since it has a very well-developed welfare state. A main argument of this chapter is that government actions in public policy domains not usually considered as health-related have strong influence upon population health and citizen well-being. Canadian policy making is compared to other nations on the basis of its potential to create health-enhancing environments.

What Is Public Policy?

At a minimum, public policy is decisions made by governments. The following definition of public policy considers what governments do to address problems and the values that guide problem definition and solution:

> Public policy is a course of action or inaction chosen by public authorities to address a given problem or interrelated set of problems. Policy is a course of action that is anchored in a set of values regarding appropriate public goals and a set of beliefs about the best way of achieving those goals. The idea of public policy assumes that an issue is no longer a private affair. (Wolf 2005: 1)

Esping-Andersen argues that a primary concern of modern welfare states such as Canada is to provide sufficient economic resources to support citizens across the lifespan (Esping-Andersen 2002). Changes in the occupational structure of post-industrial societies require the accumulation of "cognitive and social capital" among citizens. It is especially important to provide children with these assets: "Since it is well established that the ability and motivation to learn in the first place depends on the economic and social conditions of childhood, policies aimed to safeguard child welfare must be regarded as an investment on par with and, perhaps, more urgent than educational investments" (Esping-Anderson 2002: 9). These assets provide intellectual and social flexibility that supports learning new skills and adaptation to changing work environments. Economies also benefit by having women in the workplace and providing training opportunities to assist workers in coping with changing employment situations.

These key public policy issues show similarities with population health formulations that emphasize the accumulation of health assets across the lifespan. In particular Shaw and colleagues emphasize the importance of societal supports for significant transitions across the lifespan such as entering and leaving school, gaining and possibly losing employment, and entering retirement (Shaw, Dorling, Gordon, and Smith 1999). These supports include provision of income and employment security, equitable distribution of resources, and educational and training opportunities across the lifespan. How can we evaluate whether nations are committed to such goals? What indicators of healthy public policy are available? What do these indicators tell us about governmental ideology and public policy?

Political economy conceives politics and economics as both related to each other and to societal functioning (Armstrong, Armstrong, and Coburn 2001). Political economists examine a variety of indicators that reflect government commitments to achieving a well-functioning economy and a vibrant and healthy society. These measures include government's transfer of resources from revenues to citizens in the forms of cash benefits, provision of health and social services, and employment, educational, and family supports. A number of indicators of such commitments are explored in the following sections.

There are a variety of explanations as to how such commitments come about. Some argue these commitments reflect the capacity of progressive political forces such as "left political parties" and working-class power to influence the policy change process. Others look at the influence of civil society and the extent to which political and cultural traditions support equitable approaches to governance. The elements outlined above — the role of the state, the balance between the market and political forces, and civil society — all contribute to understanding how public policy is made. One important indicator of the general shape of public policy is the extent to which nations distribute resources among the population.

Overall Spending on Transfers

The Organisation for Economic Co-operation and Development (OECD) regularly provides indicators of government operations, including provision of supports and services. An especially important indicator is that of government transfers. Transfers refer to governments taking fiscal resources that are generated by the economy and distributing them to the population as services, monetary supports, or investments in social infrastructure. Such infrastructure includes education, employment training, social assistance or welfare payments, family supports, pensions, health and social services, and other benefits.

Among the developed nations of the OECD, the average public social expenditure is 21 percent of gross domestic product (GDP). There is rather large variation among countries with Sweden among the highest public social spender at 31 percent of GDP.

Table 8.1: Social Spending as a Percentage of Gross Domestic Product, 1998

Country	Total	Income Support	Health	Pensions	Social Services
Canada	18.8	3.0	6.3	5.5	4.0
United States	14.6	1.8	5.9	6.1	.8
United Kingdom	20.8	4.3	5.0	6.5	4.0
Sweden	31.0	7.0	6.5	8.0	9.0

Source: Organisation for Economic Co-operation and Development, Society at a Glance: OECD Social Indicators (Paris: OECD, 2003).

Canada ranks among the bottom countries, spending just 18 percent of its GDP on programs. The U.S. spends 14.6 percent and the U.K. 20 percent (Organisation for Economic Co-operation and Development 2003).

The OECD identifies three main domains of social transfers: pensions (about 8 percent of GDP); health (5.5 percent); and income transfers to the working-age population (4.7 percent). Spending in support of families and children averages almost 2 percent of GDP. Table 8.1 shows expenditures on health, income support, pensions, and social services in Canada, the U.S., the U.K., and Sweden as a percentage of GDP in 1998.

Health refers to public spending on health services for the population. The U.S. does not provide universal health care coverage, so the spending presented is for two publicly funded health programs that cover low-income Americans. Canada, the U.K., and Sweden offer government-operated programs for all, though the U.K. also has a separate for-profit health care system.

Income support includes family benefits, wage subsidies, and child support paid by governments to help keep low-income individuals and families out of poverty. Social assistance refers to governments' provision of a basic minimum income for citizens. In all nations, people who lack resources must meet specific criteria—some nations' criteria are more stringent than others—to be eligible for such income programs.

Pension figures refer to government payments to citizens upon retirement from employment. Employers can also provide pensions that employees pay into during employment. The U.S. spends more on public pension programs than Canada does, but there are attempts underway to privatize—and, some argue, subsequently destroy—the U.S. pension program known as Social Security.

Social services include roads, clean water supply, garbage collection, electricity, and telecommunications. In some nations services such as counselling, employment supports, or community health care may be directed to low-income citizens, while in others these services may be universally available.

In these non-health areas, Sweden spends much more than Canada, the U.S., and the U.K. Sweden and other Nordic countries have very different orientations toward social spending than Anglo-Saxon nations. Sweden's welfare state is one of the oldest, having begun building its state programs in the 1920s (Burstrom, Diderichsen, Ostlin, and Ostergren 2002). Many Western countries, including Canada, the U.S., and the U.K., developed their welfare states after the Second World War (Teeple 2000).

Many factors influence the development of public policy orientations. Social spending can be highly contentious in Canada and is especially so in the U.S. Political dynamics such as government ideology and public attitudes toward those in need are significant determinants of the generosity of social spending. Ruling governments' ideologies can be translated into commitment to income redistribution from higher- to lower-income groups and the provision of programs to support citizens in major life activities and transitions.

As an illustration of the role governments play in promoting health and well-being, consider the incidence of poverty before government programs and benefits are applied (Nelson 2004).The pre-transfer poverty rates in the 1990s was 28.8 percent for the U.K.; 28.3 percent for Sweden; 23 percent for the U.S.; and 21 percent for Canada. However, after benefits were applied, Sweden's rate dropped to 3.3 percent, Canada's was reduced to 11.4 percent, but the U.K. remained high at 16.4 percent and the U.S. at 18.6 percent. Clearly, leaving poverty reduction to market forces cannot be an effective approach to poverty reduction.

Sweden has a political ethos of supporting its population and undertaking measures to improve and maintain population health (Swedish National Institute for Public Health 2003). Although it reduced social spending in some areas during the 1990s, Sweden has maintained the highest social spending compared to most Western nations (Figure 8.1). The Swedish Parliament and most political parties are committed to improving and maintaining public welfare. As a result, Sweden has the lowest poverty rates among developed countries and one of the best population health profiles (Innocenti Research Centre 2000, 2001).

The U.S. and Canada have what is called a residualist approach to social welfare and service provision. This is a situation where responsibility for well-being falls largely to individuals. When the individual encounters difficulties, it is expected that

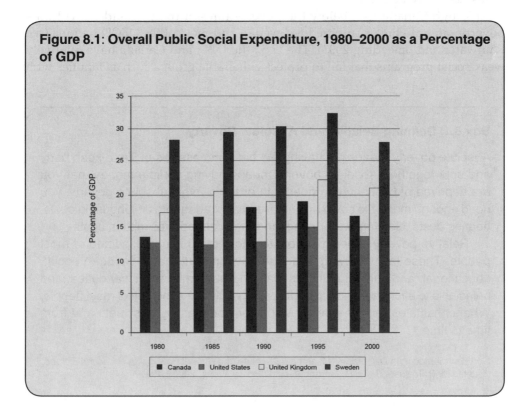

Figure 8.1: **Overall Public Social Expenditure, 1980–2000 as a Percentage of GDP**

families and, if necessary, community-based agencies will provide support (Esping-Andersen 1990, 1999). This approach has been found to result in considerably higher poverty rates than where there is commitment to public service provision.

Poverty Rates as an Indicator of Progressive Public Policy

An essential indicator of the general approach to public policy is the extent to which nations are committed to reducing the incidence of poverty. Poverty profoundly affects health and well-being, and, at the very least, sets individuals upon disadvantageous health and educational trajectories (Auger, Raynault, Lessard, and Choinière 2004). Poverty reduction is essential for the accumulation of cognitive and social capital, essential for an informed and productive workforce (Esping-Andersen 2002). Where does Canada stand on this indicator of commitment to its citizenry?

The Luxembourg Income Study (LIS) provides income and demographic information on households in over 25 nations from 1967 to the present. Table 8.2 shows that using the commonly accepted international indicator of poverty as receiving income less than half the median population income—an indicator of ability to participate in a normal way in society—Canada has lower rates than the U.S. and the U.K. The U.S. measure of poverty, which is set very low, serves as a measure of unambiguous material deprivation that makes daily living very difficult (Rank 2004) (see Box 8.1).

Although Canada falls below the poverty rates of the U.S. and the U.K., its poverty rates are high compared to Sweden and most other OECD nations (see Rainwater and Smeeding 2003). The U.S., the U.K., and Canada have relatively weak social programs that fail to protect vulnerable groups such as families with

---

Box 8.1: Defining Relative and Absolute Poverty

Absolute poverty means not having the basic necessities of life to keep body and soul together. Absolute poverty means having so little money that you are deprived of basic human needs. In order to avoid absolute poverty, you need enough money to cover all of these things: adequate diet, housing costs, heating costs, clothing, water rates, and medical and prescription costs.

Relative poverty is being unable to afford to do things expected of most people. These include living in a safe environment; participating in social, educational, and cultural activities; carrying out family and local duties; and being able to afford transport to participate in activities expected of most people. What constitutes relative poverty will differ from society to society and from time to time.

Source: Adapted from D. Gordon, "Measuring Absolute and Overall Poverty," in Breadline Europe, edited by P. Townsend and D. Gordon (Bristol: Policy Press, 2000): 49–77.

Table 8.2: Rates of Poverty Using Relative and Absolute Rates for Various Groups in Canada, the U.S., the U.K., and Sweden during the 1990s

Country	Percentage of Population below 50% of Median Income			Percentage of Population below U.S. Poverty Line
	Overall	Children	Elderly	Overall
Canada	11.4	15.3	4.7	7.4
United States	17.8	22.3	20.7	13.6
United Kingdom	13.2	20.1	13.9	15.7
Sweden	6.5	2.6	2.6	6.3

Source: M.R. Rank, One Nation, Underprivileged: Why American Poverty Affects Us All (New York: Oxford University Press, 2004): 34.

children from poverty. Poverty rates for elderly families in Canada are, however, very low, a result of public policy initiatives on pensions and benefits carried out over the past two decades.

The different poverty rates of these countries reflect different orientations to social provision. In a sense, these nations represent profoundly different manifestations of what is normally termed the welfare state. All developed nations have some form of welfare state.

In capitalist economies, the welfare state is defined as one that uses government or state power to modify the influence of market forces in at least three ways:

- guarantees individuals and families a minimum income irrespective of the market value of their work or property
- narrows the extent of insecurity by enabling individuals and families to meet certain social contingencies such as sickness, old age, and unemployment, which lead otherwise to individual and family crises
- ensures that all citizens—without distinction of status or class—are offered the best standards available in relation to a certain agreed range of social services. (Briggs 1961)

What kind of welfare state does Canada have? Is it well developed or underdeveloped as compared to other modern industrialized nations? Work on the form that welfare states can take reveals that Canada is seen—consistent with our findings presented above—as having a relatively weak welfare state, showing more similarities with the U.S. than with many European nations.

Box 8.2: **Canada's Total Social Spending Compared to Other Western Nations**

Canada's net social spending has been falling dramatically. In its most recent comparative assessment of social spending in 15 countries, Canada ranks near the bottom. In addition, Canada's 1997 spending level, 18.9 percent of GDP, is a sharp decline from the 1995 level of 20.4 percent of GDP. No other country in the OECD survey had such a sharp cut in net social spending.

"Total social expenditure" is defined in the OECD research as the provision by public and private institutions of benefits to, and financial contributions targeted at, households and individuals in order to provide support during circumstances that adversely affect their welfare.

These benefits can be cash transfers, or can be the direct (in-kind) provision of goods and services. Tax system benefits are included. It is "net," meaning after tax (the benefits an individual or household receives minus any tax they pay on the benefits).

The aim is to provide a comparable measure for that part of an economy's domestic production that is allocated to people in need of social benefits. It is an indicator of the share of resources a nation devoted to meeting social need in 1997 (the latest available data). Data limitations currently preclude analysis of all OECD countries.

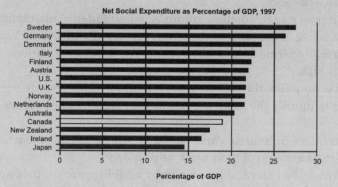

Net Social Expenditure as Percentage of GDP, 1997

Source: Willem Adema, *Net Social Expenditure*, 2nd ed., Labour Market and Social Policy, Occasional Papers no. 52 (Paris: OECD, 2001).

Canada, therefore, can do better. The problem is not one of Canada doing too much for its citizens and thereby potentially affecting the country's competitive situation. Too much has been stripped from one group of Canadians—lower-income households. The burden of fighting the deficit was not equally shared.

Source: D. Hulchanski, *Can Canada Afford to Help Cities, Provide Social Housing, and End Homelessness? Why Are Provincial Governments Doing So Little?* (Toronto: Centre for Urban and Community Studies, University of Toronto, 2002). www.tdrc.net/Report-02-07-DH.htm.

Welfare States and Public Policy

A variety of theoretical frameworks have been devised to understand how public policy components fit together to define a specific type of welfare state. Esping-Andersen devised a typology of capitalist welfare states that has generated much attention and research (Esping-Andersen 1990, 1999). Social democratic, liberal, and conservative welfare states form a continuum of government support to citizens ranging from high government intervention welfare systems in the social democratic (SD) countries to residual welfare systems as seen in liberal nations (LN). Conservative (CN) nations fall midway between these others in service provision and citizen supports.

Sweden is representative of SD welfare states, while the U.S., U.K., and Canada are LN welfare states. The level of welfare-oriented policies in Canada represents both its similarities to the other LN nations as well as its placement within the LN cluster. While Canada frequently appears to be very different from the U.S. in its policies, in comparison, it is closer to the U.S. in its welfare provisions than it is to other SD and CN nations such as France and Germany.

Conservative welfare states (CW) such as France, Germany, and Italy tie benefits to one's occupation and earnings, and tend to stratify citizens rather than promote equality. There is less attempt to support families or women. The vast majority of benefits are earnings-related and contributory rather than universal entitlements as is the case with SD nations.

Esping-Andersen defines the LN welfare state as involving means-tested assistance, modest universal transfers, and modest social-insurance plans. Means testing refers to benefits in the LN welfare state being primarily geared to low-income groups. Social assistance is limited by traditional, liberal work-ethic attitudes that stigmatize the needy and attribute failure to the individual rather than to society. LN nations limit welfare benefits since it is believed that generous benefits lead to a preference for welfare dependency rather than gainful employment.

The nature of benefits in LN nations result from an implicit—and frequently explicit—view that low-income or poor people are poor due to moral failings. This individualistic view fails to acknowledge the structural causes of low income such as high unemployment rates, which have plagued all OECD countries since the 1980s. They also fail to acknowledge the role that poor material conditions of life play in contributing to poor educational and social development in deprived communities. Differences in the form the welfare state takes should be related to overall population health, and indeed there is evidence to this effect.

Welfare States and Population Health Profiles

Navarro and Shi drew upon Esping-Andersen's insights to identify nations governed predominantly from 1945–1980 by social democratic (Sweden, Finland, Norway, Denmark, and Austria), Christian democratic (Belgium, Netherlands, Germany, France, Italy, and Switzerland), or Anglo-Saxon liberal political parties (Canada,

Ireland, the U.K., and the U.S.) (Navarro and Shi 2002). They then compared these nations on a range of political, economic, and population health indicators.

The social democratic regimes presented higher levels of union density—that is, a greater proportion of workers belong to organized labour unions. SD regimes also had higher levels of social security and public employment expenditures. Between 1960 and 1990, these regimes had the highest public health care expenditures, and the most extensive health care coverage of citizens. These nations implemented full employment strategies, attained high rates of female employment, and showed the lowest levels of income inequality and poverty rates. Social democratic nations also had the lowest percentage of national income derived from capital investment and the largest from wages, indicating less wealth accumulation by those already wealthy. On a key indicator of population health—infant mortality—these countries had the lowest rates from 1960 to 1996.

The Christian democratic regimes were second to the social democratic regimes in public health care expenditures. These countries had lower public health care coverage of citizens, but levels higher than the liberal regimes. A smaller proportion of the working-age population was employed by governments and a lower proportion of women were employed overall compared to the social democratic regimes. Christian democratic countries had high income inequalities compared to social democratic countries. This is due to more favourable treatment of wealth and investments and lower redistributive effect of the state.

Anglo-Saxon liberal political economies had the lowest health care expenditures and the lowest coverage by public medical care. They had greater incidence of low-wage earnings, higher income inequalities, and the highest poverty rates. These economies derived the greatest proportion of income from capital investment rather than wages. These liberal countries have the lowest improvement rates in infant mortality rates from 1960 to 1996.

More recently, Navarro and colleagues examined how the political orientation of the governments operates through labour market and welfare policies to influence social inequalities and health status among citizens of 18 OECD nations between 1970 and 1996 (Navarro et al. 2004). Power relations (electoral behaviour and trade union solidarity) interact with civic behaviour (trust in government, corruption, and cynicism) to produce labour market and welfare state policies. When these policies ameliorate social and economic inequalities, population health as measured by infant mortality, cause-specific mortality, and life expectancy should improve.

Indeed, they found that characteristics found in well-developed welfare states— especially social democratic political regimes—were reliably associated with declines in infant mortality and increases in both male and female life expectancy over the study period. These declines in infant mortality and increases in life expectancy were related to:

- increasing support for social democratic parties
- increases in the proportion of the population voting

- increases in public health care coverage
- increases in the proportion of the population employed
- increases in female labour force participation
- increasing income equality
- increases in national wealth

Clearly, then, politics influences public policy and population health. What are the specific forces that determine the trajectory that a nation takes in its establishment of a welfare state? Esping-Andersen (1999) argues that unique historical and cultural forces set a nation on a general path. For the Nordic nations, the advanced welfare state developed as a result of alliances established between workers and farmers supported by the presence of electoral democracy that applied proportional representation (Esping-Andersen 1985). In Canada such alliances have rarely existed. Failure to develop these political alliances in Canada is responsible in part for Canada's relatively weak welfare state. In addition, Canada's welfare state appears to be under even further threat. We now turn to these threats.

Political, Economic, and Social Forces That Shape Public Policy in Liberal Economies

Within the typology of welfare states, there is room for national variation. Both global and national political, economic, and social forces influence public policy and the shape of the welfare state in Canada. Within the Canadian system, these dynamics include political ideologies of the government of the day and competing interests. The rise of neo-liberalism has influenced welfare state policies in Canada.

Coburn (2000) defines neo-liberalism as a political ideology that is committed to a market economy as the best allocator of resources and wealth in a society. It perceives individuals as motivated by material and economic concerns. Competition is considered the primary market instrument for innovations. An unfettered market ensures economic development and a fair distribution of resources.

Lynch agrees that income and health inequalities result from a combination of political ideology interacting with national and region-specific historical factors (Lynch 2000). Neo-liberal public policy helps explain the increases in income and wealth inequalities of the past 20 years. Welfare-state policies that developed after the Second World War reduced the influence of market forces and limited income inequality.

Considering that Canada is already identified as a liberal political economy within Esping-Andersen's typology, it may be especially susceptible to neo-liberal ideology (see Vandenbroucke 2002 for a discussion of European Union resistance to neo-liberal influences). And, indeed many have argued that this has been the case. The growth of the welfare state in Canada levelled off in the early 1980s, and since 1990 there has been a drastic decline in public expenditures in support of a variety of welfare state policies (Stanford 2004).

Teeple (2000) provides a well-developed analysis of the role neo-liberalism has played in the decline of Canada's welfare state. Neo-liberalism serves as a justification for increasing economic globalization and concentrating wealth and power to increase corporate profits. For Teeple, the unrestrained economic power of private property has eroded the post-Second World War welfare state that supported redistribution of wealth and the provision of strong health and social services.

Coburn and Teeple describe a state and a process of economic globalization in which the market determines political, social, and economic activity. The rise of neo-liberalism in liberal political economies (e.g., Thatcherism in the United Kingdom; Reaganism in the United States; and Mulroneyism in Canada) has created increased income inequalities and the weakening of social provision. Certainly, policies followed by Finance Minister Paul Martin during the 1990s reflect both a neo-liberal approach and a distinct threat to the Canadian welfare state (Scarth 2004).

Toward the Future

Canada has a relatively weak welfare state as compared to other nations, and even this state is under threat. What do we know about the determinants of a strong welfare state that can assist those wishing to resist these threats and strengthen public policy in the service of health?

The influence of "left political parties" is important to the development of the welfare state and its maintenance in the post-industrial capitalist era. These parties support redistribution of wealth and advocate for universal social and health programs. Both Esping-Andersen and Navarro, as shown above, have demonstrated how political power influences public policy processes. Additional research supports this view. Rainwater and Smeeding used data from the Luxembourg Income Study to consider the role that left representation played in reducing child poverty (Rainwater and Smeeding 2003).

Among 14 nations between 1946 and 1990, the presence of left parties in government was strongly related to the probability that a child would not experience poverty. The correlation was a very strong .84. Sweden had a 32 percent left Cabinet share with 42-1 odds of escaping child poverty. The U.K. had a 15 percent Cabinet share and 5.5-1 odds of escaping child poverty. Canada has zero percent left Cabinet share and 7-1 odds of escaping child poverty. And the U.S. has the lowest of the 14 countries at zero percent left Cabinet share and 4-1 odds of escaping child poverty.

Brady studies 16 Western democracies for the period from 1967 to 1997 and looked at the impact of left political institutions on a nation's poverty rate (Brady 2003). The findings showed that left political institutions have a powerful effect on poverty reduction through high voter turnout and support of left parties that support the welfare state. In addition, coordination of wage negotiation, a result of strong union density, combine with welfare state policy to reduce poverty. While the welfare state is an essential determinant of poverty, left political institutions are critical to understanding comparative historical variation in both the strength of welfare states and level of poverty among the population.

One important process that has assisted left political parties in having influence is proportional representation in elections. Esping-Andersen identifies proportional representation as essential to the development of the Nordic welfare state (Esping-Andersen 1985). Alesina and Glaeser (2004) provide an extended examination of how proportional representation enhanced the growth and influence of left political parties, thereby strengthening the welfare state. Such political systems enable more parties—particularly political parties that are pro-redistribution—to gain representation that contributes to the formation of more fragmented legislatures or minority governments. Proportional representation systems buffer welfare programs from spending cuts. The relative position of the four nations discussed here, reflecting the strength of left parties, can be easily discerned along a left-right continuum:

LEFT—Sweden—United Kingdom—Canada—United States—RIGHT

Importantly, proportional representation is on the public policy agenda of both the federal and provincial governments. In British Columbia, New Brunswick, and Ontario governments have initiated processes of electoral reform. If proportional representation were to be implemented in Canada, this would provide strong support for strengthening the welfare state and bring in health-supportive public policies. In a sense, governments would be in a permanent minority government situation, a situation that has been associated with progressive public policy in Canada at both the federal and provincial levels.

Politics and Perceptions of Poverty

Another important issue for the future of Canada's welfare state is the politics of poverty, which is concerned with how political institutions and civil society organizations address issues of poverty in a country. In other words, are there pro-redistribution forces within the political realm? To what extent are anti-poverty organizations and the trade union movement able to influence national social policies?

In Canada, such influences appear weak. In 1989, the House of Commons unanimously approved a motion to abolish child poverty by the year 2000. This has not come close to being accomplished. Instead, it has been argued that increasing poverty seems to be an important government agenda item! Public attitudes and values influence the extent to which poverty alleviation will take place. Alesina and Glaeser (2004) found that Americans' beliefs about the presumed laziness of the poor correlates highly with views on whether nations should increase welfare spending. They found that 88 percent of Americans who consider welfare spending to be too high attribute poverty to the laziness of the poor.

At a national level, they also found that high welfare spending correlates strongly with the belief that poverty is society's fault. Among developed nations whose citizens are more likely to attribute poverty to societal causes rather than individual flaws, welfare spending is higher. Educating the public about the societal causes of poverty would go a long way in strengthening support for the welfare state in Canada and elsewhere.

Arts and Gelissen (2001) looked at national differences in citizen beliefs on issues involving social solidarity and justice. These tapped issues of whether governments should provide a job for everyone; provide health care for the sick; provide a decent standard of living for the elderly; reduce income differences; help students from low-income families; and provide decent housing for those who cannot afford it. Britons and Swedes scored the highest and Americans scored the lowest. Canada's score was closer to the U.S. than to the U.K. and Sweden.

It is also important to consider the public's self-perceived political position. In the *1999–2002 World Values Survey and European Values Study*, Canada, the U.S., the U.K., and Sweden reflected different configurations of the political right, political left, and the political centre (Inglehart, Basanez, Diez-Medrano, Halman, and Luijkx 2004). Table 8.3 shows how respondents in each of the four countries located themselves on the political spectrum in 1990 and 2000.

Table 8.3: Self-Positioning on Political Scale by Country, 1990 and 2000

Country	Political Right		Political Centre		Political Left	
	1990	2000	1990	2000	1990	2000
Canada	26	25	58	54	16	21
United States	29	32	54	51	17	18
United Kingdom	27	16	50	58	24	26
Sweden	35	32	37	34	28	34

The distribution of the different political leanings reflect the general orientation toward social spending in each country. The U.S. has the largest increase in those who position themselves on the right between 1990 and 2000. Canada, the U.S., and the U.K. all have a significant proportion of their populations in the political centre. Canada and Sweden increased their left proportion between 1990 and 2000. Canada, the U.S., and the U.K. do not have proportional representation. If this were the case, then the voices of this increasing significant minority in Canada would not be ignored.

Labour Union and Labour Density

The strength of labour is an important determinant of the strength of the welfare state. In particular, class structure and union density are important. The proportion of the workforce that belongs to unions in Sweden is 79 percent, the U.K. 29 percent; Canada 38 percent; and the U.S. 13 percent (Navarro et al. 2004). Zweig (2000) contends that the more than 60 percent of Americans who make up the working class in the U.S. have interests fundamentally at odds with the 200,000 who serve on the governing boards of national corporations. Despite these corporations using their power and influence to undermine the institutions and services that support working-class Americans, working-class Americans have little comprehension of their class-related interests. This may also be the case, though to a lesser extent, in Canada.

Navarro and colleagues (Navarro et al. 2004) found that left party governance correlates strongly with unionization rates and that both are associated with strong welfare states and numerous indicators of health. In the U.S., unionization and the ability to organize is weakly supported and actively opposed (Zweig 2004). Union power is somewhat greater in Canada, but also has been under some attack. These findings beg the question as to whose interests are served by discouraging unionization and the development of institutions that serve the interests of the working class. Research into population health seldom considers the implications of such forces on population health and well-being, particularly of the groups that are least well off as a result. The diverse social conditions of Canada, the U.S., the U.K., and Sweden reflect differing political dynamics that influence social spending.

Application to Specific Canadian Public Policy Domains

Canada is placed within the liberal type of welfare state. Although Canadian governments tend to play to the political centre, they have implemented many neo-liberal policies in recent years. This became particularly apparent during the 1990s in housing, early childhood education and care, social assistance, and labour policy as the federal and provincial governments reduced social spending in all of these areas (Figure 8.2).

Housing: Hulchanski (2003) reviews how both federal and provincial governments—with the exception of Quebec—have stopped providing affordable housing. In Ontario, Canada's largest province, social housing starts declined from 15,000 social housing starts in 1970 to 1998 when there were none. Not surprisingly, there is a crisis in homelessness across Canada. Comprehensive overviews of housing policy and its effects upon health are available (Bryant 2004; Shapcott 2004).

Early childhood education and care: Early childhood education and care is a patchwork of for-profit and non-profit programs across Canada (Friendly 2004). In October 2004, an international review team assembled by the OECD released its report on the range of programs and services available. The report identified limited availability and uneven quality of early childhood education and care services across

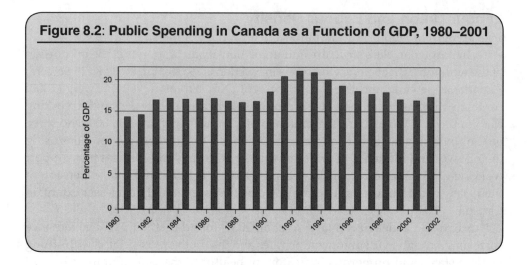

Figure 8.2: Public Spending in Canada as a Function of GDP, 1980–2001

the country and recommended action to ensure a child development and learning focus for early childhood education and care services in Canada (Doherty and Friendly 2004). Numerous studies confirm the value of early childhood education and care in preparation for school and lifelong learning.

There is pressure to establish a national child care program and the federal government has committed to work with the provincial and territorial governments to establish the foundations for a national system of early learning and child care. Canada lags behind many countries in this area, although the U.S. appears to be an exceptionally poor provider of family supports (see Box 8.3).

Social assistance: Social assistance or welfare programs are administered by the provincial and territorial governments in Canada. Canada falls behind most other OECD countries such as Sweden in this area. Canadian governments have been slower than western European governments to upgrade or improve spending on social assistance. In a study of welfare incomes in 2002, the National Council on Welfare (2004) gathered the basic social assistance incomes available for different family types in each province and territory. The evidence shows that these programs generally fail to come close to meeting the basic needs of those on social assistance.

Labour policy: Active labour policy consists of formal classroom training, on-the-job training programs, subsidies to private-sector employers, job-search assistance (i.e., job clubs, individual counselling, etc.), special training programs for youth (i.e., training, employment subsidies, direct job-creation measures), and direct job creation for adult workers. Nations use such programs to eradicate high and persistent unemployment and reduce low pay and poverty among the working-age population. Canada's active labour market policies comprised .53 percent of its GDP from 1980–1996, compared to Sweden's 1.69 percent, the U.K.'s .58 percent,

Box 8.3: **U.S. Family Policy in International Perspective**

Research Finds U.S. Lags Far behind Scores of Countries Globally in Guaranteeing Working Conditions That Support Working Families for immediate release: Wednesday, June 16, 2004

Boston, MA—A new report of research on 168 countries led by Jody Heymann, Associate Professor of Society, Health and Human Development at the Harvard School of Public Health (HSPH), finds that working conditions in the United States that support working families, lag far behind scores of other countries. The report, *The Work, Family and Equity Index: Where Does the United States Stand Globally?* is being released today in Washington DC.

Among the report's findings:

- More than 160 countries offer guaranteed paid leave to women in connection with childbirth. The U.S. does not.
- The only other industrialized country which does not have paid maternity or parental leave for women, Australia, guarantees a full year of unpaid leave to all women in the country. The Family Medical Leave Act in the U.S. provides only 12 weeks of unpaid leave to approximately half of mothers and nothing for the remainder.
- 45 countries ensure that fathers either receive paid paternity leave or have a right to paid paternity leave. The U.S. does not guarantee either.
- At least 96 countries around the world in all geographic regions and at all economic levels provide for paid annual leave. The U.S. does not ensure paid annual leave.
- 76 countries guarantee working mothers the right to breastfeed. The U.S. does not protect the ability of working mothers to breastfeed, despite its importance to the health of baby and mother alike.
- 139 countries mandate paid sick leave. 117 of these countries ensure at least one week. The U.S. does not guarantee even one day leave for illness.

"The United States trails enormously far behind the rest of the world when it comes to legislation to protect the health and welfare of working families. Scores of countries guarantee paid leave for new mothers and fathers, the opportunity to breastfeed, sick leave, and some minimum annual leave that can be spent with children, elderly parents or other family members. The United States guarantees none of these to working Americans or their families." Jody Heymann explained, "This is only the beginning of the list. Protections against extreme work hours or weeks with no breaks are among the other areas where the U.S. lags. Moreover, we have fallen behind when it comes to services for pre-school and school age children, as well as in working conditions. The costs are enormous to the health and welfare of children, the disabled and elderly, and the working adults who care for them."

Source: Press release, Harvard School of Public Health. Available on-line at www.hsph.harvard. edu/press/releases/press06162004.html.

and the U.S.'s .22 percent (Ross 2004). Sweden's more generous labour market policy provides more extensive job training and retraining for older workers. These are key areas for promoting the cognitive and social skills necessary for Canada and other welfare states to provide healthy economic and social conditions.

These policy issues are important to Canadians' health and well-being and should be debated and acted upon. The increasing focus on what is called the Social Union Framework Agreement provides an opportunity for such action. In February 1999, the federal, provincial, and territorial governments, except Quebec, signed an agreement to establish more constructive and co-operative relationships between the two levels of government in social policy (Fortin, Noel, and St-Hilaire 2003). The agreement was to meet the needs of Canadians by ensuring access to essential social programs and services, including welfare and health care of "reasonably comparable" quality. To date, this has not occurred. A minority government situation—that is, no one party can govern without the consent of one or other parties in Parliament—may increase sensitivity to these issues. The issues discussed in this chapter section should be included in any national debate about the future of Canadian public policy.

Conclusions

There is little consideration given to public policy in the population health literature. Political economy approaches focus on how the market and economics, political ideology, and other dynamics are integrally related and influence the nature of public policy. These are not preordained or natural processes, but socially determined by politics and the power of groups that strive to influence government decisions to achieve policy objectives.

Spending on health and social spending can be politically contentious yet in the end determine citizens' health and well-being. Moreover, political economy approaches can identify interests that benefit from low social spending and how these interests operate through the political system to influence public decision making on these issues. Political ideology profoundly influences income redistribution and the policies that affect income, social, and health inequalities.

However, there has been little, if any, consideration of these concepts in population health research and discussion. There is a need to move away from biomedical and epidemiological models to consider the influence of political ideology, social organization, and economic infrastructure to understand how economic and social inequalities lead to health inequalities. Directing the health sector's gaze to broader political and economic factors may be the most effective means of improving population health and reducing inequalities in health.

References

Alesina, A., and E.L. Glaeser. (2004). *Fighting Poverty in the U.S. and Europe: A World of Difference*. Toronto: Oxford University Press.

Armstrong, P., H. Armstrong, and D. Coburn, eds. (2001). *Unhealthy Times: The Political Economy of Health and Care in Canada*. Toronto: Oxford University Press.

Arts, W., and J. Gelissen. (2001). "Welfare States, Solidarity and Justice Principles: Does the Type Really Matter?" *ACTA Sociologica* 44: 283–299.

Auger, N., M. Raynault, R. Lessard, and R. Choinière. (2004). "Income and Health in Canada." In *Social Determinants of Health: Canadian Perspectives*, edited by D. Raphael, 39–52. Toronto: Canadian Scholars' Press.

Brady, D. (2003). "The Politics of Poverty: Left Political Institutions, the Welfare State, and Poverty." *Social Forces* 82: 557–588.

Briggs, A. (1961). "The Welfare State in Historical Perspective." *European Journal of Sociology* 2: 251–259.

Bryant, T. (2004). "Housing and Health." In *Social Determinants of Health: Canadian Perspectives*, edited by D. Raphael, 217–232. Toronto: Canadian Scholars' Press.

Burstrom, B., F. Diderichsen, P. Ostlin, and P.O. Ostergren. (2002). "Sweden." In *Reducing Inequalities in Health: A European Perspective*, edited by M. Bakker, 274–283. London: Routledge.

Coburn, D. (2000). "Income Inequality, Social Cohesion and the Health Status of Populations: The Role of Neo-liberalism." *Social Science and Medicine* 51(1): 135–146.

Doherty, G., and M. Friendly. (2004). *OECD Thematic Review of Early Childhood Education and Care*. Ottawa: Government of Canada.

Esping-Andersen, G. (1985). *Politics against Markets: The Social Democratic Road to Power*. Princeton: Princeton University Press.

_____. (1990). *The Three Worlds of Welfare Capitalism*. Princeton: Princeton University Press.

_____. (1999). *Social Foundations of Post-industrial Economies*. New York: Oxford University Press.

_____, ed. (2002). *Why We Need a New Welfare State*. Oxford: Oxford University Press.

Fortin, S., A. Noel, and F. St-Hilaire, eds. (2003). *Forging the Canadian Social Union: SUFA and Beyond*. Montreal: Institute for Research on Public Policy.

Friendly, M. (2004). "Early Childhood Education and Care." In *Social Determinants of Health Canadian Perspectives*, edited by D. Raphael, 109–123. Toronto: Canadian Scholars' Press.

Hulchanski, D. (2003). *Housing Policy for Tomorrow's Cities*. Ottawa: Canadian Policy Research Networks.

Inglehart, R., M. Basanez, J. Diez-Medrano, L. Halman, and R. Luijkx, eds. (2004). *Human Beliefs and Values: A Cross-cultural Sourcebook Based on the 1999–2002 Values Survey*. Delegacion Coyoacan: Siglo XXI Editores.

Innocenti Research Centre. (2000). *A League Table of Child Poverty in Rich Nations*. Florence: Innocenti Research Centre.

_____. (2001). *A League Table of Child Deaths by Injury in Rich Nations*. Florence: Innocenti Research Centre.

Lynch, J. (2000). "Income Inequality and Health: Expanding the Debate." *Social Science and Medicine* 51: 1001–1005.

National Council of Welfare. (2004). *Poverty Profile 2001*. Ottawa: National Council of Welfare.

Navarro, V., and L. Shi. (2002). "The Political Context of Social Inequalities and Health." In *The Political Economy of Social Inequalities: Consequences for Health and Quality of Life*, edited by V. Navarro. Amityville: Baywood Press.

Navarro, V., C. Borrell, J. Benach, C. Muntaner, A. Quiroga, M. Rodrigues-Sanz, N. Verges, J. Guma, and M.I. Pasarin. (2004). "The Importance of the Political and the Social in Explaining Mortality Differentials among the Countries of the OECD, 1950–1998." In *The Political and Social Contexts of Health*, edited by V. Navarro, 11–86. Amityville: Baywood Press.

Nelson, K. (2004). "Mechanisms of Poverty Alleviation: Anti-poverty Effects of Non-means and Means-Tested Benefits in Five Welfare States." *Journal of European Public Policy* 14: 371–390.

Organisation for Economic Co-operation and Development. (2003). *Society at a Glance: OECD Social Indicators 2002 Edition*. Paris: OECD.

Rainwater, L., and T.M. Smeeding. (2003). *Poor Kids in a Rich Country: America's Children in Comparative Perspective*. New York: Russell Sage Foundation.

Rank, M.R. (2004). *One Nation, Underprivileged: Why American Poverty Affects Us All*. New York: Oxford University Press.

Ross, N. (2004). *What Have We Learned Studying Income Inequality and Population Health?* Ottawa: Canadian Population Health Initiative.

Scarth, T., ed. (2004). *Hell and High Water: An Assessment of Paul Martin's Record and Implications for the Future*. Ottawa: Canadian Centre for Policy Alternatives.

Shapcott, M. (2004). "Housing." In *Social Determinants of Health: Canadian Perspectives*, edited by D. Raphael, 201–215. Toronto: Canadian Scholars' Press.

Shaw, M., D. Dorling, D. Gordon, and G.D. Smith. (1999). *The Widening Gap: Health Inequalities and Policy in Britain*. Bristol: The Policy Press.

Stanford, J. (2004). "Paul Martin, the Deficit, and the Debt: Taking Another Look." In *Hell and High Water: An Assessment of Paul Martin's Record and Implications for the Future*, edited by T. Scarth, 31–54. Ottawa: Canadian Centre for Policy Alternatives.

Swedish National Institute for Public Health. (2003). *Sweden's New Public Health Policy*. Stockholm: Swedish National Institute for Public Health.

Teeple, G. (2000). *Globalization and the Decline of Social Reform: Into the Twenty-First Century*. Aurora: Garamond Press.

Vandenbroucke, F. (2002). "Foreword." In *Why We Need a New Welfare State*, edited by G. Esping-Andersen, viii–xxvi. New York: Oxford University Press.

Wolf, R. (2005). "What Is Public Policy?" Queen's University. Retrieved January 31, 2005. Available on-line at www.ginsler.com/html/toolbox.htp.

Zweig, M. (2000). *The Working-Class Majority: America's Best Kept Secret*. Ithaca: Cornell University Press.

_____, ed. (2004). *What's Class Got to Do with It?: American Society in the Twenty-First Century*. Ithaca: Cornell University Press.

• •

Critical Thinking Questions

1. Prior to reading this chapter, what were your views concerning the extent of poverty in Canada? Did you feel that Canada was doing a good or poor job in addressing the issue? What is the effect on public perceptions and public policy making of having the U.S., with its very high poverty rates, as a neighbour?

2. What are some political, social, and economic barriers to having progressive social policies such those seen in Sweden implemented in Canada?

3. Why are Canadian families not lobbying for family-friendly policies? Why aren't Canadian workers pressuring governments for active labour market policies, such as increased job training for youth and retraining for older workers?

4. To what extent is proportional representation an issue in Canada? What are the barriers to implementing it in Canada? How can proportional representation be placed on the public policy agenda in Canada?

5. How much influence does the labour movement have in making Canadian public policy? What are your views concerning the role that organized labour should play in making public policy? Would you personally benefit from increased labour influence? Why or why not?

Further Readings

Alesina, A., and E.L. Glaeser. (2004). *Fighting Poverty in the U.S. and Europe: A World of Difference*. Oxford: Oxford University Press.
The authors provide an analysis of how differing historical traditions and political and social structures explain differences between American and European approaches to fighting poverty. Their presentations include data from Canada in addition to the U.S. and Europe.

Esping-Andersen, G. (1990). *The Three Worlds of Welfare Capitalism*. Princeton: Princeton University Press.
_____. (1999). *Social Foundations of Postindustrial Economies*. Toronto: Oxford University Press.
These books provide a typology of Western welfare states that takes into account a range of social policies and links these with variations in the historical development of Western countries. The author describes how profound differences among liberal (e.g., the U.S., Canada, and the U.K.), conservative (e.g., Germany, France, and Italy), and social democratic (e.g., Sweden, Norway, and Denmark) political economies translate into widely differing lived experiences among citizens of these nations.

Esping-Andersen, G., ed. (2002). *Why We Need a New Welfare State*. Oxford: Oxford University Press.
Contributors argue that welfare states need to consider issues of social inclusion and justice. The volume focuses on four social domains: the aged and transition to retirement; welfare issues related to changes in working life; risks and needs that arise in households, especially in families with young children; and the challenges of creating gender equality.

Rainwater, L., and T.M. Smeeding. (2003). *Poor Kids in a Rich Country: America's Children in Comparative Perspective*. New York: Russell Sage Foundation.
The authors consider why poverty rates are so high in the U.S. By comparing the situation of American children in low-income families with their counterparts in western Europe, Australia, and Canada, they provide a detailed perspective on the dynamics of child poverty in developed nations.

Teeple, G. (2000). *Globalization and the Decline of Social Reform: Into the Twenty-First Century*. Aurora: Garamond Press.
Teeple sees the welfare state as being threatened by the rise of economic and political forces associated with global capitalism. He warns that the consequences of weakened welfare states include declining national sovereignty, increasing economic inequality, and increasing insecurity for citizens.

Relevant Web Sites

Economic and Social National Data Rates and Rankings
http://dataranking.com/default.htm
   Kenji Suzuki, of the European Institute of Japanese Studies at the Stockholm School of Economics, maintains a current repository of a wide range of national data. The site provides rates and rankings for each nation compared to the world, developed nations, continents, etc.

Human Development Reports
http://hdr.undp.org/
   The Human Development Report was first launched in 1990 with the goal of placing people at the centre of the development process in terms of economic debate, policy, and advocacy. The Human Development Reports provide current information on a range of development topics.

Institute for Research on Public Policy
www.irpp.org/
   IRPP's mission is to assist Canadians in making more effective policy choices. Their research aims to enhance the quality of the debate on the issues

related to economic performance, social progress, and sound democratic governance.

Luxembourg Income Studies
www.lisproject.org/publications/wpapers.htm
   The Luxembourg Income Studies provide working papers on a range of issues related to income and other indicators. The working papers can be downloaded from this site.

Organisation for Economic Co-operation and Development
www.oecd.org/home/
   This site provides a wealth of reports, publications, and statistics about every aspect of society in modern industrialized states. Many of its contents are free or available electronically through your local university's library.

Glossary

Active labour policy: A government's policies and programs developed to create or maintain jobs. These range from sheltered workshops and other job-creation measures for workers with disabilities to employment in regular public service and public works projects (i.e., building and highway construction). It also covers subsidies to private business to hire new employees or extend seasonal work throughout the year; apprenticeship training, on-the-job training and retraining, work-study programs to ease transition from school to employment; and job-transition training for workers facing layoffs.

Family policy: Policies and programs designed to provide a secure growing environment for children and to ensure that parents have the material and psychological supports for rearing children. Through these policies, usually involving various forms of financial support and the system of child care, society compensates citizens for some of the costs borne by families with children.

Gross domestic product (GDP): The total market value of all goods and services produced in a country in a given year. It is equal to total consumer, investment, and government spending, plus the value of exports, minus the value of imports.

Left political parties: Political parties that support the redistribution of wealth by way of income support, and publicly funded programs for individuals with disabilities, and families and individuals with low income. Strongly aligned with the labour movement, they also advocate for policies to support workers and other policy initiatives that reduce social and health inequalities in a population. The New Democrats in Canada, the Social

Democrats in Sweden, and the Labour Party in the U.K. are considered left parties. The U.S. does not have a politically relevant left party.

Proportional representation: A variety of systems used for electing a legislature in which the number of seats a party wins is more or less proportional to the percentage of popular votes cast. This is in contrast to the first-past-the-post approach where the party candidate with the most votes in each constituency wins the seat. Proportional representation is the norm in most European nations. It is seen as contributing to the influence of left parties on progressive legislation in many modern welfare states.

PART III

CANADA'S HEALTH CARE SYSTEM

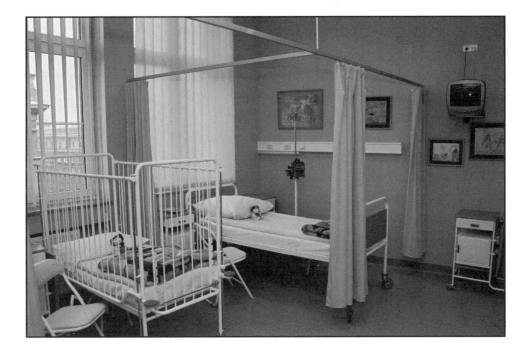

One of the most commented upon differences between Canada and the U.S. is that every Canadian is entitled to doctor and hospital care while many Americans are subject to bankruptcy and destitution if they become ill. Indeed, the health care system in Canada is typically considered the "crown jewel" of Canada's welfare state. These differences in approaches to health care between Canada and the U.S. are of relatively recent origin, however, and reflect different political dynamics in these two nations.

Not surprisingly, health care policy is a dominant feature of ongoing public debate and governmental concern in both Canada and the U.S. And the recent decade has seen ongoing attempts to reform and modernize both health care systems to meet changing needs and priorities. Central to these attempts at reform are issues of public versus private financing and public versus for-profit health care services.

Any understanding of the evolution and future of health care in Canada must consider issues of power and influence. What political and economic forces led to the development of the Canadian health care system? How are these forces influencing the current attempts at reform? How do political, economic, and other forces influence the organization and delivery of health care and the responsibilities of various health care professionals within this system?

This section considers the history of health care in Canada and how Canada's health care system came about. It explores its similarities with—and differences from—the U.S. health care system and the forces that led to these differences. Current trends in reform are examined and issues that will determine its future direction are outlined. Running through all of these issues are questions about public versus private financing and public versus private health care services.

In Chapter 9, Georgina Feldberg and Robert Vipond review the history of health care in Canada. They identify the key populations, patterns of illness, institutions, and funding mechanisms that have shaped the evolution of Canadian health care. They show how, until relatively recently, the health care systems of Canada and the U.S. were similar, as were the health profiles of the two nations. They then examine the divergence of health care approaches in Canada and the U.S. and the health consequences of those differences. Included in this examination are the political developments that led to universal access to health care in Canada and the population-based Medicare and Medicaid program in the U.S. Some of the powerful economic and political forces that continue to influence these developments such as recent fiscal crises are outlined.

In Chapter 10, Mary Wiktorowicz outlines some of the key aspects of health care systems in Canada and the U.S. She traces very recent developments in health care reform in both nations and identifies the political, economic, and social forces driving such developments. She also considers lessons that can be learned from other nations and the unique features of change that have occurred in Canada and the U.S. Political structures of Canada and the U.S. are seen as key determinants of whether legislation to reform health care systems is successful or not. Some of the key dimensions considered in examination of these health care systems are public versus private financing of health care and public versus private delivery of health care. In Canada, concerns with regionalization or jurisdictional organization of health care and integration of services are emerging as key planning issues.

In Chapter 11, Ivy Bourgeault reviews the development and division of responsibilities in the health care system. She highlights the gendered nature of the division of labour and how this has led to the devaluing of the health care professions dominated by women with a particular focus on nursing. Bourgeault is also concerned with how the health care division of labour has been differentially affected by recent reforms such as managed care and the privatization of some health care services. She describes the development of managed care and raises critical questions about this approach. She also examines how increasing privatization of the health care system is affecting those in various health care professions.

·······································

CHAPTER NINE

CRACKS IN THE FOUNDATION

The Origins and Development of the Canadian and American Health Care Systems

Georgina Feldberg and Robert Vipond

·······································

Learning Objectives

At the conclusion of this chapter, the reader will be able to
- understand the historical development of health and healing in Canada and the U.S.
- identify key populations, patterns of illness, institutions, and funding mechanisms that have shaped the evolution of Canadian health care
- recognize similarities and differences in the evolution of Medicare
- develop awareness of the cracks in the historical foundations of Canada's health care system that create vulnerabilities

---

Introduction

In a CBC on-line poll, conducted in the fall of 2004, Canadians registered their pride in Canada's health care system by naming Tommy Douglas, the father of Medicare, the "greatest Canadian" of all time. Almost simultaneously, the Supreme Court of Canada ruled that "[t]he Canada Health Act and the relevant [provincial] legislation do not promise that any Canadian will receive funding for all medically required treatments." The court's language, part of its decision on payment for autism treatments, startled many Canadians. The decision shook Canadians' pride in a universal, publicly funded system that we believe is comprehensive, serves the needs of all, and distinguishes us from our American neighbours. It seemed to undermine what former Minister of Health Monique Begin (1988) called "Canada's right to health." Faced with change, we have come to expect that services will expand to meet new needs, whether through the inclusion of ever-expanding medical and surgical interventions or, as in the case of autism treatments, with an acknowledgment of the social determinants of health that extends health care funding into non-traditional domains.

As Canadians confront unwelcome challenges to health care, they regularly invoke "history"—the Canadian tradition—to provide a clear set of standards or ideals by which change can be judged. History is used to justify our expectations and, most regularly, to distinguish what is truly Canadian from "American" ways and practices that do not measure up to our social commitments. However, what is called history is often actually nostalgia, a constructed memory of better ways and better times that glosses over problems, conflicts, and inconsistencies. Despite affirmations of difference, Canada and the U.S. share markedly similar health care pasts. Until late in the 20th century, the evolution of healing methods, the design of health care institutions and funding systems, and patterns of illness closely paralleled one another. Those similarities suggest that some of the disturbing changes in the Canadian health care system do not represent new "Americanization" but, rather, cracks in the historical foundation of Canada's health care system. In this chapter, we expose those cracks so that history can be used to outline a path for change rather than to lament a paradise lost.

The Demographic and Social Origins of North American Health and Health Care (1700–1900)

The marked similarities in the evolution of health care in English Canada[1] and the United States reflect other shared traditions that shape and intersect with health, disease, and healing. Because the two young, industrialized nations were both originally colonies of England, they have common political, cultural, and economic heritages. Both operate under a federal system in which responsibility for health care is split between national and local levels of government, and in which the welfare state reflects the dominance of a liberal political tradition. Both nations were built by immigrants; their populations are a mix of Native, European, Asian, and African descendants. Their populations are sparse and spread over similar geographies, large expanses of land that cover diverse climates and terrains. Both built capitalist economies whose growth centred on the creation of transcontinental markets, and that are now deeply integrated with each other.

The history of health care in North America begins with the informal healing traditions that emerged in the pre-colonial and colonial periods and predominated until the late 19th century. Prior to the 20th century, few Canadians would have visited a doctor or a hospital. McGill College granted "Canada's" first medical degree in 1833, and both European and locally trained physicians practised in

Upper and Lower Canada (now Ontario and Quebec), but their practices were limited and located primarily in cities. Hospitals, which had strong ties to religious orders, were institutions for the destitute and dying (Connor 2000). Most Canadians, especially those living outside of cities, relied on informal healing traditions—such as herbalism and midwifery—that had both indigenous (or local) and European origins. Prior to the arrival of British and French settlers, a range of First Nations practised herbalism. Teas, smoke, and tinctures (made from the fruit, leaves, berries, or bark of local grasses, plants, or trees) provided remedies for the respiratory, digestive, and skin conditions most common during this period. European colonists similarly relied on herbal and botanical remedies. Though the European preparations were initially distinct, with time the imported and local traditions mixed (Crellin 1994; Kelm 1998).

Box 9.1: Canadian Timeline

1400–1850	Contact between European and indigenous populations creates new diseases and patterns of spread
1867	BNA Act
1882	Robert Koch identifies the tubercle bacillus
1912	Lloyd George introduces the Insurance Act in Great Britain
1939–1945	Second World War
1945	Early attempts at health insurance in Canada and the U.S.
1957	Hospital and Diagnostic Services Act (Canada)
1962	Saskatchewan doctors' strike
1965	U.S. Medicare/Medicaid
1967	Medical Care Act (Canada)
1984	Canada Health Act

Science, licensing, and regulation were not part of the early healing traditions. Herbalists, midwives, and other healers learned through apprenticeship. Lore, tradition, and reputation ensured the integrity of their healing practices, but there were few formal rules for education or accreditation. The lack of formal regulation allowed for diverse and widespread participation in healing practices that were often informal or rooted in the domestic economy. There were expert herbalists, but mothers regularly taught their daughters how to grow and brew common and essential remedies, recipes for which they included in family cookbooks. Women regularly gave birth at home, assisted by their family, neighbours, or by the local midwife (Biggs 1983; Mitchinson 2002).

The British North America (BNA) Act (1867), which shaped the constitutional framework of the Canadian federation, reflected contemporary experiences with disease and the relative unimportance of what we now call scientific medicine. Prior to Confederation, Canadians regularly confronted infections and epidemic diseases that had huge social and economic costs. Tuberculosis, typhoid, cholera, and smallpox—the most common infections—decimated Native populations. They disrupted trade, killed young productive citizens, and caused disability that shortened working lives. Throughout the 19th century, most American and Canadian physicians ascribed these diseases to filth and decay rather than germs. Building on the "sanitary ideal" that had developed in Britain, they argued the need for city planning and development that would reduce garbage, promote clean water, and ensure the proper design of communities (Cassel, 1994; MacDougall 1990). The structures of Canadian government that the BNA Act created reflected both the immediacy of health hazards posed by infections and the state of health knowledge. The BNA Act split jurisdiction for health care between the federal government and the provinces. Recognizing the economic significance of infections, and their implications for trade and the military, it assigned to the federal government responsibility for quarantines and marine hospitals. Recognizing that most other interventions against infection (e.g., sanitation) took place at the local level, it implicitly assigned the remaining responsibility for health to provinces and cities. The act created a relationship between the control of infections, public health, and the state, but it largely ignored curative medicine.

What is now called modern or allopathic biomedicine came into dominance during the late 19th century and changed the structure and delivery of North American health care. In 1882, the German physician Robert Koch provoked a "bacteriologic, immunologic, and chemotherapeutic" revolution when he isolated the bacterium that caused tuberculosis. Koch's postulates allowed physicians and public health departments to focus their attention on the microbes that caused diseases, rather than on the social and physical conditions in which they bred. While some historians argue that many physicians never lost sight of the social and other factors that made individuals vulnerable to bacteria (Feldberg 1995; Leavitt 1992), North American medicine nonetheless changed dramatically after 1900. Medical education and research became increasingly scientific and institutional. Health care professions became increasingly regulated and stratified by race, class, and gender; male and class dominance emerged in medical practice. Hospitals became centres of care.

By the early decades of the 20th century, North Americans recognized the need to reshape and regulate medical practice. As rigid standards for medical training and licensing emerged, medical schools, which had previously existed informally or independently, sought affiliation with universities. Women, who had played significant roles in informal caregiving, were now excluded from education and practice, and sought access to formal medical education. Some of Canada's earliest

> **Box 9.2: The Bacteriologic Revolution and the Transformation of Health Care**
>
> Prior to the late19th century, physicians and public health authorities understood that diseases could be spread from person to person. However, they attributed infections to filth and dirt, bad air, smells, and unsanitary conditions, and they believed that behavioural and environmental change were most effective.
>
> In 1882, the German physician Robert Koch isolated the bacterium that caused tuberculosis (TB). Using what became known as Koch's postulates, Koch established a causal relationship between bacterial infection and disease. First, Koch isolated bacteria from the blood of a diseased animal. He grew the microbes in a petri dish, injected them back into animals, and observed that these animals developed all the signs and symptoms of the original disease. He then drew blood from the sick animals and showed that he could isolate the same microbes in it.
>
> Koch's work is thought to have inspired a revolution that transformed both the theory and practice of public health. It allowed physicians to focus on controlling bacteria rather than behaviours. It paved the way for the development of antibiotics and vaccines that would treat or prevent infections. By the middle of the 20th century, physicians and pharmaceutical manufacturers had capitalized on the knowledge that bacteria caused infections, and they believed that they had successfully eradicated many infectious diseases.
>
> The bacteriologic revolution was never conceptually or practically complete. Even at its height many physicians continued to recognize that when healthy women and men were exposed to bacteria, they did not always fall ill. Because a healthy host seemed to resist infection, they argued that individuals who ate correctly, slept well, worked and played in moderation, and lived in clean and well-ventilated houses could avoid falling ill. Newly emerging infections, such as SARS and BSE, have also challenged public confidence in the bacteriologic revolution.

women physicians went to the U.S. to study. Others founded independent women's medical colleges. Still others demanded access to existing schools and programs.

It is important to note that these changes in medical training and practice affected Canada and the United States in broadly similar ways. In 1910, Abraham Flexner undertook a review of medical schools in the United States and Canada designed to standardize and improve education and care. Canada was included in Flexner's review because of long-standing medical exchanges between the two nations. Like many others, Emily Stowe, Canada's first woman doctor, travelled to the U.S. to study medicine. Leaders of Canadian medicine and nursing, such as Frank Rattray

Lillie, William Osler, and Isabel Maitland Stewart, left Canada for the U.S., where they played key roles in education, practice, and research. Philanthropic and voluntary associations, such as the National Tuberculosis Association, spanned both countries. The Rockefeller Foundation, a prominent American funding agency, founded and intellectually shaped public health programs at Ontario and Quebec universities.

Throughout the early decades of the 20th century, a market for health care and a basket of medical services that North Americans sought access to emerged. Instead of relying on informal healing traditions and public health interventions, Americans and Canadians sought the expertise and technology of physicians and hospitals. The ability to pay for these services consequently became paramount, as did the relationship of curative medicine to the state.

Insuring Health (1900–1980)

Differences in health insurance coverage represent the great divide between Canada and the U.S., yet Canada and U.S. also share early traditions of health care insurance. Prior to 1900, when hospitals were primarily institutes for the dying and destitute and medicines were compounded locally, health care was limited and cheap. Professionalism and science combined to make health care more necessary and more costly. By the end of the First World War, most European nations, including England, recognized a public need for access to hospital and medical care and established some form of government-administered health insurance. Canada and the United States had not. Between 1912 and 1929, American physicians were "almost persuaded" (Numbers 1978). Despite strong ties with Britain, Canadian doctors avoided and resisted discussions of national health insurance. In 1912, after British Prime Minister Lloyd George introduced his Insurance Act, an entry in the *Canadian Medical Association Journal* warned that government insurance plans would undermine the spirit of charity in medicine, turn physicians into civil servants, and create a culture of private practice. The Depression cast national health insurance in a different light. Physicians' medical practices declined during the 1930s and they struggled to earn a living by bartering services for goods. In this climate of economic crisis, existing insurance plans—offered by benevolent associations, religious orders, or insurance providers—either failed or proved inadequate. Medical associations consequently began to lobby for government health plans that would ensure access to care and payment to care providers. In 1934, the Canadian Medical Association accused provincial and municipal governments of failing to provide necessary medical care for the indigent and unemployed, and it proposed the remedy of "state health insurance." As late as 1943, a strong majority of physicians who belonged to the CMA continued to support this position (Bothwell and English 1976).

Following the Second World War, plans for national health insurance emerged in both Canada and the United States. In 1945, Prime Minister William Lyon Mackenzie King introduced his plan for national health insurance to the Dominion-Provincial

Conference on Reconstruction. Merely months later, President Harry S. Truman presented an ambitious plan for universal health insurance to Congress. Both plans failed. Fears of socialism and government encroachment on individual liberties blocked Truman's efforts (Koojiman 1999). The bickering over provincial-federal jurisdiction that has come to characterize discussions of health reform proved the Canadian obstacle; several Canadian provinces rejected King's plans for a national health insurance scheme on grounds that it encroached on provincial jurisdiction in health (Tuohy 1999).

Early plans for national health insurance failed, but during the 1950s government spending on health care nonetheless increased in both Canada and the U.S. Setting what might be seen as a pattern, Ottawa approved new expenditures for hospital construction throughout the decade. The United States Congress made extensive investments in medical research, medical education, and hospital construction during the same period. In short, both countries invested heavily in medical education, research, and hospitals, but neither moved to ensure broad access to medical services.

The growth of hospitals, their emergence as treatment centres, and the escalating costs of hospital care prompted the need for broader insurance coverage. In 1957, Canada responded to an emerging crisis by implementing the Hospital and Diagnostic Services Act. This plan made coverage of hospital services more readily and widely available, but even then, only half of Canadians had coverage for any other kind of expense. Patterns of coverage were similar in the United States, where employment-based and veterans' plans provided coverage for many families, and Blue Cross emerged as a major hospital insurance provider. In both countries, about 60 percent of services were covered, but disparities were huge. Over 90 percent of those Americans who worked in the highly unionized manufacturing sector had extensive coverage, but only 40 percent of farm workers had any. First Nations communities, women, and immigrants were underserved in both countries. Urban-rural and regional disparities were also great (Starr 1982).

The struggle to instate health insurance as a democratic right of citizenship took real shape in 1961 when Premier Tommy Douglas, a Baptist minister and leader of Saskatchewan's social democratic government, introduced a comprehensive medical insurance plan in the province. By the 1960s, medicine had become lucrative, and the CMA members who had supported national or public health insurance plans no longer needed government funding. They prospered financially, and they commanded considerable respect from their patients and communities. Hence, Saskatchewan's physicians now staunchly opposed Douglas's efforts. The Saskatchewan Medicare plan, which culminated in the historic doctors' strike of 1962, fundamentally shaped the structure and tensions of Canadian health care by institutionalizing the model of private practice/public payment. In introducing Medicare, the Douglas government committed itself to creating a system that was "acceptable both to those providing the service and those receiving it" (Naylor 1986: 182). On the one hand, the Saskatchewan plan promised all citizens, regardless of financial circumstances, a comprehensive system of medical services that was financed through taxes and administered publicly. On the other, the Saskatchewan plan acknowledged the powerful interests of physicians. From the outset, the Douglas plan rejected European models that paid physicians by capitation (the number of patients listed in their practice) or salary in favour of the traditional fee-for-service model of payment. Physicians continued to practise as individuals and to bill by service, but the government, rather than the individual patient or an insurance company, now paid the bill.

Saskatchewan's plan became the inspiration for Canada's national health insurance program, known as Medicare. It put into place the guiding principles of the 1967 Medical Care Act: universality (all citizens are entitled to health coverage), comprehensiveness (all "medically necessary" services are covered), and portability (all Canadian citizens and permanent residents are entitled to care regardless of where in Canada they live or travel). By 1972, when the Yukon introduced its medical services insurance plan, Medicare was in place throughout Canada.

The implementation of national health insurance seemed to distinguish Canada and the U.S. starkly. However, the differences were not initially very great. Throughout the 1960s and 1970s, the U.S. government also implemented programs that made health services available to a broader public. The U.S. focused its efforts on vulnerable populations. The Migrant Health Act of 1962 and President Lyndon B. Johnson's "War on Poverty" provided U.S. federal funding for rural health clinics, maternal and child health programs, community mental health services, and neighbourhood health centres. In 1965, amendments to the Social Security Act established Medicare and Medicaid, which extended coverage to the elderly and the poor. Medicare, a national program with uniform standards for eligibility and benefits, covered all hospital and some physician costs for Americans over 65 and some people with disabilities. Medicaid, a joint federal-state program, provided federal grants to the states to reimburse doctors and hospitals that cared for medical indigents and people on welfare.

Costs, coverage, and health status did not differ significantly north and south of the Canadian border either. In 1971, the U.S. and Canada spent essentially the same percentage of their gross national product on health care—7.6 percent and 7.4 percent respectively—and the vast majority of citizens had access to some medical services. In 1976, nearly 90 percent of Americans had either public or private health insurance, a rate not so very different from Canada. Throughout the first half of the 20th century, mortality and morbidity from the leading causes of death—infectious diseases, like tuberculosis—were similar in Canada and the U.S. Thereafter, key health status indicators, such as infant and maternal mortality, remained comparable. In 1940, maternal mortality, calculated as maternal deaths per 100,000 live births, stood at 400 in Canada and 376 in the U.S. After 1950, infant and maternal mortality rates declined significantly, and by 1960 maternal deaths in both countries had decreased by half, to about 200. During the next two decades, they fell to less than 10 per 100,000 (U.S. Bureau of the Census 1975: 109).

Box 9.3: **Measuring the Impacts of Medical Interventions**

During the 20th century, national and international health agencies regularly used a series of indicators to measure the effectiveness of medical and public health interventions. Because public health interventions originally developed in Europe as part of mercantilist assumptions about the economic benefits of a strong population, many indicators focused on population growth. Life expectancy (the number of years men or women could expect to live to) was one indicator. National rates of maternal and infant mortality also became common measures of the success of health care systems. Maternal mortality is the number of women who die in childbirth; infant mortality is the number of children under one year of age who die. Reducing maternal and infant mortality was a key health goal of the early health care policy reforms. Reductions in maternal and infant mortality were taken as signs that medical and technological interventions into birth had been successful. They were seen as evidence that medical "advances" had reduced infections associated with birth and early childhood and that those medical procedures had been made widely available.

There are two problems with historical mortality indicators. First, national averages hide significant race and class differences. It is important to note that in both Canada and the U.S. the average rates do not expose the significant death rates in Native, African-American, Hispanic, and other minority populations. For example, in Canada, rates of maternal and infant mortality have traditionally been, and continue to be, much higher in northern First Nations communities than in the rest of the country. In the U.S., minority populations similarly have higher rates of maternal and infant mortality. Second, statistics are difficult to keep when births occur outside hospitals. Most important, while reductions in mortality are often attributed to medical intervention, changes may actually reflect social and economic changes.

Changes in Health, Changes in Coverage (1984–2000)

The Canada Health Act of 1984 changed the delivery of health care and marked a point of significant departure between Canada and the U.S. Canada's national health plan insured services. The United States had chosen instead to insure populations. By the 1980s, inequities resulting from both approaches were apparent. Canada's Medical Care Act (1967) had allowed for private billing above the Medicare cap. This included provincial premiums and co-payments for specialist services. In particular, obstetricians and gynecologists could bill patients above the approved government rate, and this "extra billing" reduced access to care. Canadians living in remote areas, women, and minorities were differentially disadvantaged by the premiums and co-payments that national health insurance allowed.

In the U.S., Medicare and Medicaid covered less than half the medical expenses of senior citizens and one-third of health costs for the poor. Like private insurance plans, Medicare limited coverage of hospital stays to a set number of days, and it paid only a part of approved physicians' fees or other forms of out-patient care. Recipients were responsible for the remaining charges, and many purchased supplementary private insurance to help cover the extra costs. Seniors who could not afford the co-payment required by Medicare, either because they were already poor or because a long illness drained their bank accounts, often found themselves on Medicaid. Because Medicaid was funded out of general revenues at both the state and federal level, the base coverage from state to state was uneven. Moreover, Medicaid carried a stigma of welfare or public assistance.

The Canada Health Act of 1984 strengthened Canada's commitment to universal health insurance by prohibiting premiums and extra billing. It ensured that virtually all Canadians had access to medical services. In contrast, public and private commitments to health insurance declined in the U.S. In 1988, 13 percent of Americans under 65 had no private or public health insurance. The number of Americans without health insurance rose dramatically thereafter. Drastic reductions in funding for Medicare and Medicaid provided one source of decreased coverage. The rising costs of health benefits eroded pre-tax corporate profits, so that many companies reduced health insurance coverage. As a result, employees paid greater percentages of premiums and costs. The percentage of Americans with no insurance coverage also increased because of corporate restructuring; full-time staff were replaced by part-time employees who had no entitlement to benefits. By 1992, the number of Americans who were not insured had risen to 38.9 million, or 17.4 percent of the population under 65. Another 40 million were underinsured. Health care even began to seem unaffordable to middle-class Americans, many of whom worried that they might have financial difficulty paying for the costs of a major illness (Tuohy 1999).

Key health status indicators began to reflect these national differences in access to health care. Maternal mortality once again provides an example. Dramatic declines in maternal mortality, often attributed to increased and improved access to medical care, occurred in both the U.S. and Canada between 1900 and 1980. However, between 1982 and 1999, there was no further decline in maternal mortality in the U.S. By 1990, the U.S. rate of 12/100,000 was double the Canadian rate of 6/100,000 (World Health Organization 1996). The difference in rates reflected the ability of young and indigent mothers to access appropriate medical care. It also reflected different levels of access to social and economic resources that are key to health.

The Canada Health Act was passed during a period of broad, global rethinking of health care and the determinants of health. The change in name, from Medical Care to Health, reflected this new approach. Four sources of discontent affected the ways in which this rethinking occurred in Canada and the U.S.: (1) apparent increases in the costs of health care spending; (2) changing patterns of disease that drew attention to the limitation of existing insurance plans; (3) a commitment to alternative forms of service delivery; (4) and populist critiques of scientific medicine that intersected with a consumer rights and activist agenda. This latter stream included critics who saw the value of medical interventions but wanted relief from unnecessary medical procedures and other abuses of medical power; it also included those who questioned the priority given to biomedicine and looked for extra-medical alternatives.

At the end of the 1980s, Canada spent only 8.6 percent of its GNP on health care while in the United States, spending had risen to 11.4 percent. But by the 1990s, some Canadian health economists also sounded the alarm over rising health care expenditures: the portion of GNP spent on health care had jumped by 10 percent. As the North American medical system grew more expensive, escalating costs seemed to present a crisis. Subsequent studies would attribute the apparent rise in Canadian health care spending to a decline in the economy as a whole, rather than an absolute rise in health care expenditures, but physicians, politicians, economists, and the public all worried that costs were spiralling out of control while the quality of care declined (Tuohy 1999).

Some responded to the apparent fiscal crisis by focusing on excesses in "consumer demand." Seeking culprits, American politicians and physicians blamed Medicare and Medicaid, which, having finally made medical services accessible to senior citizens and the poor, achieved their objectives of democratizing use. When Medicare or Medicaid coverage made it possible for Americans to visit physicians, the number of office visits often increased in the covered populations. One study suggested that, in 1964, poor Americans went to the doctor 20 percent *less* often than more affluent Americans; 10 years later, they visited the doctor 18 percent *more often* (Starr 1982). Canadians, like Ontario Premier Mike Harris, also blamed "consumer abuse" of the system. Others focused on the "supply side" of the equation. When the Canada Health and Social Transfer (CHST) reduced federal transfer payments, Manitoba, Ontario, and other provinces imposed caps on the amount physicians could bill in any given year, and hence on the numbers of patients they could see. Doctors and administrators tried to cut spending by restructuring the hospital system in ways that would reduce expenditures on costly hospital services and shift care into the community. Many provinces delisted services they considered non-essential (like in vitro fertilization and cosmetic surgery) from compulsory coverage. Provincial leaders with strained budgets questioned whether new immigrants, especially those with pre-existing chronic illness, should be eligible for health care benefits. These changes intensified regional, economic, and gender-based disparities in access to care. Canadians living in small towns, rural areas, and the North complained about the concentration of new technology in large cities. Increasing numbers of homeless Canadians found themselves without adequate access to care.

Other "reformers" seized the opportunity to develop new options for financing and delivering medical care. They critiqued fee-for-service and other payment schemes that created incentives for the use of costly services, and they proposed alternatives, like the health maintenance organizations (HMO). First introduced in the 1970s, HMOs and their Canadian counterpart, the health service organization (HSO), initially promised to provide integrated care at lower cost. Prepaid a fixed sum per patient, administrators received bonuses for keeping costs low and patients out of hospitals. Many provinces took part in the experiment in group practice. Quebec led the way with local community health centres and English Canada introduced a range of alternative forms of service delivery, community health centres among them.

HMOs, HSOs, and other alternative delivery plans also promised to broaden health coverage. Panic over rising costs hijacked the health care debate, and the intensity of concerns about financing drew attention away from more fundamental questions about the definitions of health and health care. After 1950, infectious diseases declined in North America. Tuberculosis, which had been the "costliest of communicable diseases" and "the leading cause of death," all but disappeared from view. Chronic diseases—heart disease, cancer, diabetes, and depression—replaced infections as the leading causes of North American deaths.

Table 9.1: Changes in Mortality, 1900–1975, Deaths per 100,000

Year	Tuberculosis	Heart Disease	Cancers
1900	194	137	64
1950	30	322	135
1975	3.9	1037	351

Source: United States Bureau of the Census. *Historical Statistics of the United States: Colonial Times to 1970*, (Washington, D.C.: Government Printing Office, 1975).

As Canadians reflected on their health care system, many critics also noted that health care services needed to shift to prevent and accommodate new conditions. They drew attention to the interconnections between poverty, life experience, and disease. They drew distinctions between preventive public health and medical care; they argued for public investment in health rather than health care.

Proposals for new forms of service delivery attempted to address some of these concerns about the limits to modern medicine. HMOs, for example, provided an opportunity to change both the kind of care that was delivered and the way it was delivered. Attractive to those who sought to reduce costs, HMOs also had appeal across the political spectrum because prepaid group practices seemed to provide an opportunity to achieve "equity and access" (Fein 1972). They combatted the focus on physicians and the limitations of solo practice. Early models, such as the Harvard Community Health Plan, appealed to the progressive left because they integrated the services of a range of health care providers. In Canada, HSOs and CLSCs (local community health centres) also found support because they reduced and broadened the scope of care. The Medical Services Act, as reflected in its title, provided payment only for medical services that *physicians* delivered. HSOs and CLSCs finessed these limitations. They encouraged physicians to work in groups with other practitioners (such as massage therapists or psychologists) whose services were not included in the Medicare basket. The HSO paid physicians a salary or capitation fee, rather than the approved fee for service, and any savings could be used to publicly finance non-medical services. The new practices also shifted the site of integrated care from hospital to community.

HMOs became symbols of the chaotic American medical scene, "managed care," and consumer discontent. In the U.S., they shifted the "problem" from overmedicalization to undertreatment. Yet, undertreatment is a problem only if tests and prescriptions are actually necessary. As proponents have noted, HMOs can lack the incentive to overtreat and emphasize and encourage preventive health measures, such as Pap smears. They rely on family physicians or nurse practitioners, who use fewer tests and less invasive procedures than specialists. In many HMOs, for example, nurse-midwives, rather than obstetricians, deliver babies in normal births.

HMOs, HSOs, and other alternative forms of service delivery helped to reduce health care costs, promised to enhance access to care, and broadened the meaning of care. Despite this, they addressed only part of the problem. As the government of Canada renewed its commitment to universal coverage for medical care, increasing numbers of historians, demographers, and epidemiologists challenged the relationship between medicine and health. Thomas McKeown's *The Role of Medicine* questioned whether medicine had improved the health of Europeans and attributed increasing longevity and declining mortality to improvements in the standard of living (McKeown 1979). National governments, led by the World Health Organization, affirmed that health was more than the absence of disease, and at Alma Ata they affirmed the importance of economic and social determinants of health (World Health Organization 1978). The re-emergence of tuberculosis and other infections drew attention to historical patterns of disease and disease control and shaped a challenge to the premises of the bacteriologic revolution. Physicians, they found, had rarely focused narrowly on the bacterial causes of disease; they had regularly argued that these diseases were due in large part to "social misery." Epidemiologic and other analyses consistently showed a correlation between social spending and health status, so that Nordic and northern European countries had the best indicators.

North American health policy did not always heed this new emphasis on health or these new directions in health research. The Canada Health Act changed the parameters of funding and language, but it did not change the emphasis or direction of spending. Rather than integrating social and health spending, when Canadian governments reframed and reviewed health care financing during the 1990s, they repeatedly revised funding formulas to divorce social spending from health care spending. The separation of funding envelopes for health, education, and welfare allowed spending on medical care to increase and investment in health — education, work, and housing that increase health status — to decrease.

Conclusions

Saskatchewan's celebrated public-health insurance plan provided the model for Canadian Medicare. It also set some of the cracks in Canada's health care foundation. It provided the model for private practice/public payment that has challenged the very existence of Canadian Medicare; it reinforced battles over provincial and federal jurisdiction; and it set the framework for an insurance scheme in which medicine and medical care dominated.

Canada's national Medicare plan did much to address who paid for medical services, but it did little to change the delivery of services. Canadian doctors remained in private practice and billed Medicare for a set fee per service. To an important extent, then, the founders of Medicare, first in Saskatchewan then nationally, built a tension into the health care system between the egalitarian ends (universal and accessible medical services) and the market-based means (delivery by physicians in private practice). Defenders of Medicare worry that the establishment of a parallel system of private clinics in provinces like Alberta will create a two-tiered health care system in which wealthier citizens will have preferential access to treatment. It is important to realize that this challenge feeds off the original compromises that created room, within Canada's health care system, for wealth-maximizing private practice.

This fee structure was determined by negotiations between doctors and each province. The national health insurance system was financed partly by the federal government, but since the Canadian constitution assigns responsibility for health care to the provinces, Medicare is administered at the provincial level. From the start, hospitals and physicians were also the backbone of the system. Until 1984, when the Canada Health Act prohibited extra billing, co-payments, in the form of provincial premiums, were allowed, and specialists, including obstetricians and gynecologists, were permitted to bill patients above the government rate. As in the United States, hospitals rather than community clinics remained the site of most health care delivery.

The original Medicare plan, incubated in Saskatchewan and then appropriated nationally, is often used as an example of what is good about federalism. Yet it is also clear that the peculiar division of jurisdiction in the Canadian federation — in which the federal government has the dominant fiscal capacity while the provinces possess most of the constitutional authority to deliver programs—has created a policy environment in which discord and competition is endemic. More than this, the disconnect between payment (Ottawa) and delivery (provinces) of social programs has made it extremely difficult to imagine how the two levels of government would work together to accomplish what the Nordic countries have done—namely, to seriously frame programs that go beyond medical services and address the social determinants of health.

The Supreme Court of Canada's decision regarding autism treatments points to a third crack in the foundation of Canada's health care system. Canadians enjoy a publicly funded health insurance scheme in which eligibility is universal and not predicated on income, marriage, or employment. However, the emphasis on medical care restricts the range of services covered. Ironically, midwifery was not covered under Canada's universal health system. Legalized only within the past decade, coverage for midwifery remains outside the public financing system of many provinces. Similarly, alternative health services—including counselling, chiropractic, naturopathic therapy, homeopathic therapy, and hydrotherapy—available through many private insurers in the United States, are not made publicly available to Canadians.

More critically, a range of health-promoting services fall outside of the domain of both federal and provincial health departments. New patterns of mortality and morbidity have created new needs and expectations, not all of which are or can be met by our current system. The limitations reflect our history. The BNA Act initially made public health interventions the domain of the state; it overlooked private practice and curative medicine. The reforms of the 1960s addressed the new status of biomedicine and brought physicians and treatment into public financing plans. However, as those reforms took place, patterns of disease shifted. The new diseases, often labelled lifestyle diseases, are actually diseases of circumstance. They reflect living conditions, poverty, and access to housing and income. For historical reasons, Canada has not integrated these social and economic domains into the modern organization or financing of health.

References

Begin, Monique. (1988). *Medicare: Canada's Right to Health*. Montreal: Optimum Publishing International.

Biggs, C. Lesley. (1983). "The Case of the Missing Midwives: A History of Midwifery in Ontario from 1795–1900." *Ontario History* 75: 21–36.

Bothwell, R.S., and J. English. (1976). "Pragmatic Physicians: Canadian Medicine and Healthcare Insurance, 1910–1945." *University of Western Ontario Medical Journal* 47(3): 14–17.

Cassel, J. (1994). "Public Health in Canada." In *A History of Public Health and the Modern State*, edited by D. Porter, 276–312. Amsterdam and Atlanta: G.A. Rodopi.

Connor, J.T.H. (2000). *Doing Good: The Life of Toronto's General Hospital*. Toronto: University of Toronto Press.

Crellin, J.K. (1994). *Home Medicine: The Newfoundland Experience*. Montreal: McGill-Queen's University Press.

Fein, R. (1972). "Equity and Access in Healthcare." *Milbank Memorial Quarterly* (4): 157–190.

Feldberg, G. (1995). *Disease and Class: Tuberculosis and the Shaping of Modern North American Society*. New Brunswick: Rutgers University Press.

Kelm, M. (1998). *Colonizing Bodies: Aboriginal Health and Healing in British Columbia, 1900–1950*. Vancouver: UBC Press.

Kooijman, J. (1999). *And the Pursuit of National Health: The Incremental Strategy toward National Health Insurance*. Amsterdam and Atlanta: G.A. Rodopoi.

Leavitt, J. (1992). "Typhoid Mary Strikes Back: Bacteriological Theory and Practice in Early Public Health." *Isis* 83: 608–629.

Lomas, J., J. Abelson, and B.Hutchison. (1995). "Registering Patients and Paying Capitation in Family Practice: Lessons from Canada." *British Medical Journal* 311: 1317–1318.

Lomas, J., C. Fooks, T. Rice, and R.J. Labelle. (1989). "Paying Physicians in Canada: Minding Our Ps and Qus." *Health Affairs* 8: 80–102.

MacDougall, H. (1990). *Activists and Advocates: Toronto's Health Department, 1883–1983*. Toronto and Oxford: Dundurn.

Marmor, T. (1973). *The Politics of Medicare*. New York: Aldine-Atheson.

McKeown, T. (1979). *The Role of Medicine: Dream, Mirage or Nemesis*. Princeton: Princeton University Press.

Mitchinson, W. (2002). *Giving Birth in Canada, 1900–1950*. Toronto: University of Toronto Press.

Naylor, C.D. (1986). *Private Practice, Public Payment: Canadian Medicine and the Politics of Health Insurance, 1911–1966*. Kingston and Montreal: McGill-Queen's University Press.

Numbers, R. (1978). *Almost Persuaded: American Physicians and Compulsory Health Insurance 1912–1920*. Baltimore: Johns Hopkins Press.

Starr, P. (1982). *The Social Transformation of American Medicine*. New York: Basic Books.

Tuohy, C.H. (1999). *Accidental Logics: The Dynamics of Change in the Health Care Arena in the United States, Britain and Canada*. New York and Oxford: Oxford University Press.

United States Bureau of the Census. (1975). *Historical Statistics of the United States: Colonial Times to 1970*. Washington, D.C.: Government Printing Office.

World Health Organization. (1978). *Alma Ata Declaration*. Available on-line at www/who. int.

———. (1996). "Revised 1990 Estimates of Maternal Mortality." Geneva: World Health Organization.

Note

1. The evolution of health care and healing in Quebec has distinctive characteristics that are beyond the scope of this essay.

• •

Critical Thinking Questions

1. What distinguished the delivery of health care in the periods before and after 1900?
2. In what three ways were health care systems in the U.S. and Canada similar before 1980?
3. Saskatchewan's experiment in publicly funded health insurance laid the foundation for Canadian Medicare. What principles did the Saskatchewan model establish?
4. What are three foundational cracks in Canada's national health insurance plan?
5. How did the Medical Care Act enhance health care in Canada, and how did it compromise the achievement of health?

Further Readings

Feldberg, G., M. Ladd-Taylor, A. Li, and K. McPherson. (2003). *Women, Health and Nation: Canada and the U.S. since 1945*. Montreal and Kingston: McGill-Queen's University Press.
Changes in the financing and delivery of health care had special implications for women. The introduction to this collection outlines the diverging and converging histories of health and health care in Canada and the U.S. The essays explore the ways in which women promoted and were affected by changes in the financing and delivery of health care.

McKeown, T. (1976). *The Modern Rise of Population*. New York: Academic Press.
This classic work challenges the received wisdom that European population growth was the result of medical "advances," such as the conquest of infectious disease. McKeown was one of the first to suggest that social and economic factors played a critical role.

National Advisory Committee on SARS and Public Health. (2003). *Learning from SARS: Renewal of Public Health in Canada, a Report of the National Advisory Committee on SARS*. Ottawa: National Advisory Committee on SARS and Public Health.
A report to Health Canada, this document outlines the history of public health initiatives and points to the ways in which historical patterns shape current health responses.

Naylor, C.D. (1986). *Private Practice, Public Payment: Canadian Medicine and the Politics of Health Insurance, 1911–1966*. Kingston and Montreal: McGill-Queen's University Press.
An outline of the development of publicly funded health insurance in Canada, this book describes and explains the tensions built into the Medicare system.

It underscores the ways in which fee-for-service models threaten universal health insurance.

Tuohy, C. Hughes. (1999). *Accidental Logics: The Dynamics of Change in the Health Care Arena in the United States, Britain and Canada*. New York and Oxford: Oxford University Press.
An analysis of the compounded financial crises facing the health care systems in Canada, the United States, and Britain. The book shows how different "accidents" of history have shaped the dilemmas facing the health care systems in the three countries.

Relevant Web Sites

Statistics Canada
www.statscan.ca/english/freepub.
This Statistics Canada Web site contains historical statistics for Canada that can be used to track patterns of health and disease.

Weyburn Review
www.weyburnreview.com/
This Web site chronicles the achievements of Tommy Douglas, the father of Canadian Medicare. It provides sections on his life as a minister, his political career, and his interest in Medicare.

U.S. Census Bureau
www2.census.gov/prod2/statcomp
This U.S. government Web site contains historical statistics for the United States from the 1700s onward. It can be used to track changes in health and disease.

World Health Organization
www.who.int
This Web site for the World Health Organization includes historical disease and health statistics along with declarations about health services and health care interventions.

Glossary

Alternative service delivery: A general term used to refer to the organization and payment of medical services. Includes group practices, such as health maintenance organizations (HMO), health service organizations (HSO), or CLSCs (centres locaux de santé communitaire), designed to reduce health care spending, ensure continuity of care, and extend coverage to a wider range of services. More recently, they have been associated with efforts to contain costs and reduce the quality of care.

Canada Health Act (1984): The CHA supplanted the Medical Care Act as the foundation of the Canadian Medicare system. In particular, the CHA reinforced the principles of Canadian Medicare by penalizing provinces financially if they allowed physicians to extra bill—that is, charge patients over and above the amount paid by the government for their services.

Medicare: In both Canada and the United States, Medicare refers to a government-funded program of health insurance. In Canada, Medicare is defined by the hospital and medical services that are provided. In the United States, Medicare is delimited by the population it serves, specifically the elderly.

Medical Care Act (1967): The act of Parliament that enshrined a national program of hospital and medical insurance on the "Saskatchewan model." The act established joint responsibility for the delivery of health care in Canada, with the federal government providing funding and the provincial governments responsible for delivering health care. By 1972, the Medical Care Act was in place across the country in 10 provinces and two territories.

·······························

CHAPTER TEN

HEALTH CARE SYSTEMS
IN EVOLUTION

Mary E. Wiktorowicz

·······························

Learning Objectives

At the conclusion of this chapter, the reader will be able to
- explore the divergent premises that shaped the health care systems in Canada and the U.S., including ideological perspectives and political institutions
- understand the different organizational designs on which different health care systems are based, including the modes of financing and delivering health care services
- clarify the recent reforms to Medicare and Medicaid in the U.S., and the current challenges managed care is facing
- identify the areas of convergence and divergence between the health care system in Canada and the U.S., including integrated health systems, and access to pharmaceuticals

Introduction

This chapter provides an overview of the status of health care systems in Canada and the U.S. with emphasis upon recent attempts at reform. The focus is on the effect of the political and economic forces on the organization of care. Lessons from developments in other nations are considered and unique aspects of change in Canada and the U.S. are examined for their impact upon the health of citizens. Recent developments in Medicare in Canada and the U.S. are of special interest.

At the close of the 20th century, Canada and the United States reflected diverging patterns in the organization and delivery of their health care systems. Each nation's health care system was founded on different ideological premises and political authority, and these same forces continue to shape their evolution. Canada and the U.S.'s response to the challenges of access to and escalating costs of health care has in turn led them to embrace different approaches with some similarities, for example, with respect to organizational management approaches to achieve "integrated health systems." At the same time, the strategies adopted to address issues of pharmaceutical cost and access demonstrate divergent paths. This chapter explores the most important aspects of the divergent and convergent approaches that Canada and the U.S. have adopted toward their health care sectors. We consider how the different political systems in each state have shaped its recent restructuring efforts, and how international systems of care have informed the directions taken.

Diverging Premises for Health Care Systems

The legislative and political structures that guide democratic reform in Canada and the U.S. shape their approaches to social policy, and the health care sector represents one of the most significant areas of divergence. Several political and historical forces have influenced the design and delivery of health care in Canada and the United States, which we explore through the lenses of ideological perspective, political authority, and modes of financing and delivery.

Ideological Perspective

Most countries have common goals regarding health care that include:

- *Social protection*: Enable those with fewer resources to access health care.
- *Redistribution*: Redistribute health care costs among individuals, employers, and society.
- *Efficiency*: Ensure efficiency in the production and consumption of health services.

At the same time, the development and reform of national health care systems is highly politicized. How health care is organized and funded fuels many debates within each nation. These debates are based on different opinions about the role of government in health care, which arise from different values and national traditions. These in turn shape the insurance systems and administrative processes through which health professionals deliver services.

Health care in the U.S. is based on a system of private health insurance. There are also programs of public health insurance for people on social security (aged 65 and older) referred to as Medicare, and on social assistance referred to as Medicaid. Access to health care for the remainder of the population is through private insurance, which much of the population receives as a benefit of employment, or through other benefit plans such as those for veterans, through the Veterans Administration. At the same time, approximately 45 million people remain uninsured, and several million are underinsured such that their health insurance plan does not cover all the health care services they require. By contrast, Canada has a universal system of public health insurance, in which provincial public insurance plans develop contracts with private non-profit health care institutions such as hospitals and practitioners to deliver care to the population. The differences in the two health care systems have evolved as a result of different ideological conceptions and political institutional processes through which legislation is developed (Maioni 1998; Tuohy 1999).

Box 10.1: Liberalism and Socialism

Liberalism comes from the word *libre*, and emphasizes the following:
- *Personal freedom*: Absence of coercion; individuals can pursue their own interests.
- *Limited government*: Government acts only as an umpire to enforce the rules of society needed to sustain a free market. The limits on government are defined in the constitution, which clarifies the government's jurisdiction in different areas.
- *Equality of right*: Everyone must abide by the same rules. Reform Liberals redefined the notion of equality to equality of opportunity. Reform Liberals consider the positive role of the state in promoting individuals' potential.
- *Consent of the governed*: Elections.

Alternatively, socialism is motivated by a dislike of the consequences of the market economy that are inherent in the liberal vision. Instead, socialism:
- Emphasizes assets are owned by the community, while benefits are distributed to all, not just select private owners.
- Aspires to a higher degree of "equality of result."
- Works toward political gradualism. The goal is to make the state more politically accountable. (MacLean and Wood 2000: 57)

In many ways, national health insurance symbolizes the great divide between: liberalism and socialism; the free market and the planned economy (see Box 10.1). Such principles are deeply rooted within each nation. For example, the Canadian constitution is based on such principles as "peace, order, and good government." By contrast, the American constitution emphasizes "life, liberty, and the pursuit of happiness."

In most industrialized nations, public health insurance has been adopted at least partially to address the market failure in the health sector (see Box 10.2), and societal judgments concerning equitable access to necessary care irrespective of ability to

---

Box 10.2: Market Failure: A Rationale for Government Intervention

Free market:
Liberal economists believe public welfare is promoted by a competitive market through the so-called "invisible hand": People's utility-maximizing behaviour and firms' profit-maximizing behaviour will, through the "invisible hand," lead to an optimal distribution of goods.

But economic reality differs from the assumptions of the competitive model:
Efficient outcomes are not always promoted by the market, leading to market failures, which provide the economic rationale for government intervention.

The market fails for such public goods as:
- primary and secondary education
- health care

Society benefits from an educated population whose health care needs are addressed. The market does not, however, distribute these on a universal basis, which provides the rationale for government involvement (Weimer and Vining 1989).

---

pay and differences in "need." Such a perspective reflects Rawls's (1971) *A Theory of Justice*, which suggests that those who design rules put themselves behind a "veil of ignorance," where their position in the resulting distribution is unknown. Under these circumstances, most individuals would have *social primary goods distributed equally* to preserve the dignity of all individuals, but still allow social and economic inequalities if they worked to everyone's advantage. The driving force of publicly operated health systems is to extend coverage based on social justice. As Stone (1988: 81) suggests, "[t]he pattern of public needs is the signature of a society. In its definition of public needs, a society says what it means to be human and to have dignity in that culture." Such ideologies can be referred to as dominant ideas that prevail within a society at a given time (Doern and Phidd 1988; Dyson 1980; Simeon 1976). While dominant ideas are important, they are only one factor in the constellation of political dynamics that shape health policy in each nation.

Political Institutions and Historical Perspective
There are several political and historical forces that shape the different paths that Canada and the U.S. have taken in developing their health care systems, and that influenced their subsequent reforms. Although health care emerged as a political issue in both nations as early as the 1930s, it was not until the 1960s that the basis of each system was formulated through their respective legislative processes.

In the U.S., policy reforms based on new laws must be passed by a majority of the members in both the Senate and the House of Representatives, in addition to receiving the support of the president. Any new legislative policy proposal thus requires the support of the majority of the members of the two legislative houses, as well as the president, which in turn represents three potential levels of veto.

Since the various regions across the U.S. are well represented in the Senate (each state has two seats) and the House of Representatives (seats are assigned based on population), the result is that there are only two major political parties in the United States: Republicans and Democrats. Health reformers in the Democratic Party who proposed a national system of universal health care were forced to modify and dilute their plans to appeal to a broad coalition of groups (such as the unions and the labour movement) that the Democratic Party represents. This forced the Democrats to abandon many of the tenets on which their proposal for health reform was based, as they would otherwise risk losing the support of key groups. Even if the Democrats succeeded in attaining consensus within their party, an additional hurdle remained. The absence of party discipline in the Senate and House of Representatives—where members of a political party are not required to vote for the measures their party proposes—means there is no assurance that all Democratic members would vote for the legislation.

Moreover, several interest groups—such as the American Medical Association and the private health insurance companies—oppose legislation that would change the conditions under which they practise. Such interest groups and the lobbyists they employ seek to influence elected members of the Senate, the House of Representatives, and the president to oppose the proposed changes. Introducing legislation that would change how health professionals practise and insurance companies conduct their business, and increase the level of taxes citizens pay to support a program of national health care insurance therefore faces enormous challenges (Maioni 1998).

Additional factors that influenced the policy trajectory toward employer-sponsored health insurance in the 1950s include the labour movement's shift to collective bargaining rather than national politics to gain health insurance, the business community's preference for offering fringe benefits instead of supporting government-run health insurance, and tax reform (enshrined in legislation) that excluded employer-paid premiums from employees' taxable income and subsidized employer-sponsored health insurance, which became the primary health insurance system in the U.S. (Hacker 2002). As a result, advocates of national health insurance shifted their focus from the general population to those who were largely excluded from the workforce: the elderly and low-income people. The public health insurance system was thus targeted to people not expected to work and designed around a private, but tax-subsidized insurance system for employees and their families. Employer-sponsored insurance, however, excludes large numbers of low- and modest-income workers (Feder 2004).

In contrast, passing legislation concerning universal public health insurance in the Canadian Parliament faced fewer obstacles for three reasons. First, Canadian political parties adhere to the concept of party discipline, such that members of a party will generally support the legislation proposed by members of their party. Second, when a political party governs the House of Commons, its members comprise the executive: the prime minister and a select group of ministers referred to as the Cabinet. The fusion between the governing party and the executive means that interest groups such as the Canadian Medical Association (CMA), which opposed the legislation enshrining public health insurance, had few alternate avenues through which they could influence the legislative process. Such was the case when the CMA attempted to block the Medical Care Act in 1957.

A third factor that supports the introduction of innovations in Canada is the absence of a system of regional representation, which led to the establishment of a third party. Although representation in Parliament is based on population distribution, the Senate lacks a formal system of regional representation. Regional interests thus have more incentive to develop political parties outside the two major parties (Liberals and Conservatives) as a vehicle to assert their voice in federal policy. Western-based parties such as the Canadian Commonwealth Federation (CCF), which later evolved into the New Democratic Party (NDP), thus played a decisive role in changing the political landscape by introducing policy proposals that would not have otherwise been raised by the two main traditional parties.

The election of the CCF in Saskatchewan and its adoption of Medicare indeed provided the impetus for a legislative proposal for universal health insurance at the national level. The establishment of the CCF thus created a channel through which the populist Western movement could advance its interests and counter the medical lobby, thereby reshaping the debate on public health insurance. The Canada–U.S. comparison therefore reflects important contrasts between the multiple points of both access for influence and veto inherent in the American separation of powers, and the consolidated power of the Canadian parliamentary system in which executive and legislative powers are effectively fused (Maioni 1998).

Once a health system was adopted in Canada and the U.S., a series of interest groups (medical profession, private insurance companies, allied health professionals) and organizational constructs became entrenched within each national system, making the ability to change courses through subsequent reforms much more difficult in each nation. President Clinton's 1993 attempt to achieve universal health insurance coverage through legislative reform, for example, failed to gain support. Instead, reforms in the U.S. and Canadian health care systems reflect logical progressions of the organizational dynamics on which they were founded (Tuohy 1999). In the U.S., private insurance companies, which deliver employee-sponsored health care, resisted further government involvement. Private insurance companies also diminished the autonomy of the medical profession by placing limits on the types of treatments clients' insurance plans covered, which effectively restricted how physicians could practise. Once the elderly and the poor were covered through Medicare and Medicaid, subsidization of health insurance for the economically disadvantaged became a political challenge, as any new measures would financially disrupt the insured population (Feder 2004). Innovations in health care instead occurred through organizational aspects of the private insurance delivery systems.

In Canada, despite considerable "restructuring" and realignment of the hospital sector within each province, the medical profession maintains its clinical autonomy, even though fiscal pressures have led the government to tame the medical profession's entrepreneurial discretion (Tuohy 1999). The new frontier in Canadian health reform has instead occurred through regionalization of provincial health care systems. Individual organizations' and the province of Alberta's attempts to expand private health care delivery have largely been resisted, but continue nevertheless.

Organizational Design: Modes of Financing and Delivery

To better understand the distinctions between the Canadian and U.S. systems, we consider how national health care systems are organized by focusing on three dimensions referred to by economists as:

- *Financing*: How are health care services paid for: publicly or privately?
- *Delivery*: How are health services delivered: publicly or privately?
- *Allocation*: How are the funds allocated to service providers?

Health care services can be *financed* and *delivered* through either public or private means. *Allocation* refers to the way health care professionals are paid, including the kinds of incentives incorporated in different methods of payment. When referring to *financing* and *delivery*, there are strengths and weaknesses in having a publicly or privately financed and delivered health care system. The best way to demonstrate these is by exploring the approaches different nations have adopted, their comparative advantages and disadvantages, and the reforms different nations have used to address their weaknesses (Deber 2004).

Financing: Insuring and Purchasing Health Care Services

Financing health care services includes a system of insurance to protect individuals from the risk and cost of falling ill and requiring costly health care services (diagnosis, treatment, and rehabilitation). In a *publicly financed* health care system, all citizens contribute to and pay for the system of health insurance through their personal income and other taxes. Important advantages include: (1) spreading the risk of illness across the entire population so that insurance is affordable to all citizens, even those with greater risk of falling ill; (2) more effective cost control over health care services; and (3) universal coverage.

Since all citizens face the risk of becoming ill, most would rather pay into a system in which they are protected should they fall ill, even if they are currently healthy. As such, in publicly insured systems, healthy individuals who do not require extensive health care services subsidize those who become ill and require treatment. In contrast, in a privately financed system individuals pay private insurance companies to insure them against the risk of illness and needing costly health care services. To ensure a high profit, private insurance companies are more likely to be selective in choosing those whom they will insure by charging higher premiums to people with pre-existing illnesses. The cost of such high premiums effectively excludes those people who can't afford the premiums. People with a chronic condition such as diabetes, high blood pressure, or even a family history of an illness such as cancer must thus pay a higher charge, which may render the insurance unaffordable and leave them without coverage.

A second advantage of publicly financed systems is relative cost control over health care services. This is achieved because the government is the single purchaser of health care services, endowing it with *monopsony* power. With the *monopsony* power inherent in a single-payer system, the government collects funds from the public, and negotiates with health care providers on the behalf of the public regarding the services to be offered and the remuneration health care providers will receive. If health care professionals are not satisfied with the government's offer, their only recourse is to negotiate better terms or to go on strike by refusing to offer their services. The government is thus in a relatively strong position, as it has the capacity to negotiate more advantageous terms on behalf of the entire population.

Germany and the Netherlands have health care systems that involve *private financing* through private insurance (sickness funds) as shown in Table 10.1. The effect has been that *private financing led to risk shifting among insurers*. Private insurers sought to enrol clients who were healthier, free of chronic conditions, and thus less expensive to care for. They also discouraged clients with chronic conditions from enrolling in their insurance plans by charging them higher fees. The problem then becomes one of affordability. For the elderly and those with chronic conditions, attaining health care insurance became increasingly expensive and many were unable to afford it, leaving them without insurance.

The reforms Germany and the Netherlands have enacted to address this problem included government regulation of the sickness funds. Such insurance funds are prevented from excluding patients with chronic illness by ensuring the range of fees they charge are reasonable, and that the risk is spread throughout the enrolled population. As a result, the sickness funds co-operate by using similar insurance criteria, and thereby operate as a quasi-single payer. A problem associated with privately financed systems is one of *cost control in the absence of monopsony*. If health care providers are not pleased with the remuneration offered by one private insurance company, they can seek higher compensation from another company. As

Table 10.1: International Health Care Systems: Comparing Financing and Delivery

Delivery	Financing	
	Public	Private
Public	Britain, Sweden: National Health Service	___
Private	Canada, France: Public insurance system	Germany,* Netherlands, Switzerland,* U.S.: Private insurance

* Mixture of private insurance and government subsidy: government regulates and subsidizes private mutual aid societies.

companies seek to attract health care professionals through higher remuneration, the cost of providing health care rises. Private insurance thus does not provide an effective cost control, and consumers face higher charges for the same kinds of health care services.

The third advantage of publicly financed systems is universality. Since the entire population contributes to the insurance plan, all citizens have access to it, even those who are least able to contribute. Public financing thus achieves equity across the population.

Critics of publicly financed systems, however, point to the waiting lists for diagnostic and treatment services, suggesting that if private financing were allowed, individuals could purchase private services to reduce their wait for health care services. A parallel private system exists in some publicly financed systems, such as in the United Kingdom and Australia. The problem with allowing a parallel private system is that many of the best health care professionals gravitate to its more lucrative remuneration. As found in Britain, the result is that people who can afford to pay privately move to the front of the queue, while the remainder of the population relying on the public system face an even lengthier wait as health professionals working in the private sector provide fewer services to the public system. As the private system does not provide comprehensive services, however, it still relies on the public national system. When private care expands, support for the public system diminishes, since those who purchase private health care withdraw their support for the public system. Considerable inequities thus result from a parallel private system due to the deterioration in the public system.

France has a different system, where health care is publicly insured up to a certain point depending on the diagnosis (except for low-income people, who are fully insured), and where private insurance supplements the public insurance system.

Public and private insurance thus cover the same health care. Private insurers are also regulated in the same manner as the public insurance system, and the reimbursement rules for health care providers are the same whether they are private not-for-profit, or for-profit (Sandier, Paris, and Polton 2004).

Health Service Delivery: Public or Private

Publicly delivered health care services—where health care providers are considered employees of the state—has been found to result in less than optimal health care as Britain and Sweden demonstrate. The disadvantage of public delivery is that the health care system's responsiveness to clients is questionable. In contrast, with privately delivered health care services, if clients are not pleased with the quality of the service, or if the wait for services is too lengthy, they have the option of seeking health care elsewhere. In the case of a public provider, however, the usual market signal of consumers choosing to purchase care elsewhere is not available. In the case of health care this is further complicated because of what economists refer to as "imperfect information": medical care is complex and consumers cannot easily discern the quality of the services they receive, which is thus another form of market failure. Nor are there obvious ways for the client to signal her or his dissatisfaction with the care received.

A distinction must also be made between *for-profit* and *not-for-profit* private delivery, as *for-profit* delivery is more likely to lead to suboptimal care. The evidence is drawn from a study that compared for-profit and not-for-profit health care firms in the U.S. In comparing dialysis services for patients, for example, not-for-profit companies were more likely to send their patients for kidney transplant to alleviate their renal failure, which eliminated their need for dialysis. In contrast, the for-profit clinics were less likely to send their clients for renal transplant, leading their clients to be dependent on renal dialysis for the remainder of their lives (Devereaux et al. 2002). For-profit delivery is thus acceptable only when outcome standards can be clearly specified and monitored, which is difficult to attain for complex services such as health care (Deber 2004). Private not-for-profit delivery is thus optimal.

Health care systems that include *public financing*, and *public delivery* thus offer good cost control, and good equity, but questionable client responsiveness. Reforms to address the suboptimal client responsiveness have focused on internal markets to realign the incentives to provide quality service delivery, as shown in Box 10.3. These include the purchaser-provider split, where providers are required to compete for service delivery contracts. Under the purchaser-provider split, purchasers are responsible to the budgetary authority for cost control and to patients for the quality and accessibility of care. While the public financing component in these systems has largely remained, a measure of private delivery has been introduced. The role of purchasers has also been enhanced in the U.S.'s managed care plans and selective contracting by insurers. While most countries have used this model for the purchase of hospital services (Australia, Britain, New Zealand, Sweden, Italy,

Box 10.3: **Planned Market Initiatives**

Planned market initiatives reflect a set of conscious choices about how to introduce market-style incentives into existing allocation-based management structures. In other words, to promote efficiency, the government intercedes in a publicly insured health care system by introducing market-based tools to maximize social welfare. An example of the planned market approach is in the reforms adopted by Britain, shown below.

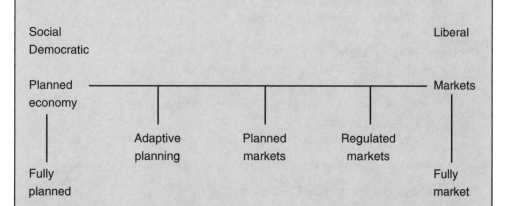

Planned markets: Intermediate position between command-and-control planning systems and pure market systems.
Regulated markets: State power limits certain socially disruptive behaviours that occurred previously.
Planned market: State uses select market instruments to achieve government policy objectives.
Adaptive planning: Management decentralized to regional planning bodies to enhance responsiveness to local needs. (Saltman and von Otter 1992: 16)

Britain's Internal Market: **"Purchaser Split from Provider"**
Health authorities (100 regions): Given fixed budget to purchase hospital care.
Hospitals (400) became providers: Self-financing trusts compete for contracts
Fund-holding family practices (100s): Given budget to buy specialist client care.
Specialist hospital doctors (providers): Work in public and private sector.

Britain's Internal Market:
Did not significantly reduce costs except by cutting services
Doubled administrative costs
Did not improve hospital care; budget pressure took precedence over patient needs
Reduced patient choice of hospitals (GPs)
Created two- to three-tiered care
- Private care
- Fund-holding practices
- Non-fund-holding practices

Problem: Waiting Lists
1. Hospital doctors on *minimum part-time* contract earn 90 percent of salary for half a week's work.
2. Hospital doctors can practise privately and earn as much or more from private practice.
3. Surgeons with the most private practice had the longest waiting lists.

"New Labour" Reforms (2000)
1. Increased NHS spending (6 percent per annum)
2. Expanded number of doctors and nurses
3. Prohibited senior NHS doctors from private practice in the first seven years after appointment
4. Increased role for nurses
5. Contracts with private acute and long-term care facilities for National Health Service patient beds

Portugal, and Greece), Britain and New Zealand have experimented with using primary care doctors as purchasers. In Britain, this has involved general practitioner fund holders who purchase specialist and hospital services on behalf of patients in their practice. However, evidence from Britain suggests such purchaser-provider arrangements have had little effect in changing patterns of service delivery (Docteur and Oxley 2003).

In summary, for *financing* medically required services, the best approach is public financing, as:

1. monopsony (single-payer) control over providers gives superior cost control
2. public financing avoids "cherry picking," where private insurers profit by refusing high-risk individuals

For *delivery* of medically required services, the best approach is private non-profit as:

1. public delivery often means less responsiveness to clients, and mixed incentives for cost-efficiency and quality
2. for-profit delivery is acceptable only when outcome standards can be clearly specified and monitored, which is difficult to develop for health care as it is a complex service

The lesson for Canada from this international comparison is that the public system should be well funded to maintain confidence in standards of care. Canadians should be cautious about allowing a parallel private system, as it siphons off the best practitioners, increases waiting lists, and reduces support for the public system. Moreover, a private system could not survive without the public system, which supports the patients the private system does not treat, and the full array of services the private system does not offer.

Recent Reforms

Medicare and Medicaid in the United States

Although the system of public health insurance in the U.S. has grown, the reforms have been modest. Medicare was expanded in 1972 to include people with end-stage renal disease and disabled beneficiaries of Social Security. Medicaid was first expanded to include children of lower-income employed parents, pregnant women in two-parent working families, and individuals with disabilities who could return to the workforce if provided with supports. A second phase of expansion in the 1980s and 1990s led to national income eligibility standards for children and pregnant women. The State Children's Health Insurance Program modestly increased the coverage for children in the late 1990s. *Medicaid* is thus largely geared toward low-income children and pregnant women. Although states have the option of covering both parents, in most states parents on minimum wage earn too much income to be eligible. Moreover, low-income people who are not parents of dependent children are not eligible for Medicaid (Feder 2004).

Medicaid is jointly funded and administered by the federal and state governments. Federal funding of the program comes with minimum national standards and accountability for the open-ended federal dollars spent (states cover 23–50 percent of Medicaid benefit costs). States are also given the flexibility to design their health service delivery systems according to local conditions, to set provider rates, and to impose cost-control mechanisms. States, however, vary in the proportion of the population they cover (from 28–59 percent of the low-income uninsured among 13 states assessed), and benefits provided: from $7,749 per beneficiary in New York to $2,334 in California in 2001 (Mann and Westmoreland 2004).

Some gradual expansion in the beneficiaries has occurred, as states have the option of expanding their program to cover people in eligible groups at higher incomes, and most have done so for some groups of beneficiaries. Medicaid was also expanded to pay for vaccines for uninsured and underinsured children who are not Medicaid beneficiaries. States could also expand eligibility to uninsured women diagnosed with breast or cervical cancer in a program initiated in 2000 by the Centers for Disease Control and Prevention. Medicaid accounts for about 16 percent of state budgets, second only to education (Mann and Westmoreland 2004).

Access to health care services under Medicaid also varies across states due to payment factors—low payment rates have in some cases compromised people's ability to access care. The breadth of services covered also varies. While Medicaid law requires states to offer nursing home services, home- and community-based long-term care services are not mandatory, and some states have not made them available as they believe they cannot afford their costs.

In terms of reforms, the federal government has made available "section 1115" waivers that allow states to use federal Medicaid funds in ways other than those specified in the legislation, to promote research and demonstration projects. States have used the provisions of the waiver to expand coverage, however, or to introduce other programmatic and financial changes. The federal Medicaid matching rate was increased through legislation in 2003, temporarily shifting a greater proportion of its costs to the federal government, which assisted states in averting eligibility rollbacks and reductions in coverage and benefits. Nevertheless, Medicaid essentially functions as a high-risk pool, covering people with disabilities and chronic illnesses that would otherwise not have access to insurance. Increasing budget pressures, however, threaten the viability of many state Medicaid programs, and suggest some future retrenchment. Medicaid is thus in need of reform, as it has been extremely flexible, growing in response to myriad needs in an incremental, piecemeal manner, but without the benefit of system-wide planning (Mann and Westmoreland 2004).

Medicare is also on the threshold of reform due to the rising cost of health care, and the rising proportion of the retired population. Problems, however, exist in the adequacy of its benefits. To provide some coverage for prescription drugs, the Medicare Prescription Drug, Improvement, and Modernization Act was enacted in 2003, and will take effect in 2006. The federal government's coverage of health care expenses for Medicare beneficiaries averages about 50 percent, and may reach 60 percent when the drug benefit is implemented. About 15 percent of Medicare beneficiaries are sufficiently impoverished to quality for Medicaid benefits.

Medicare as a public subsidy program, however, enjoys universal popularity, but only as long as administrative agencies limit the extent to which individual choice is narrowed. Cost-control measures within public programs have thus been limited to restraining physician payments instead of curtailing clinical services (Vladeck 2004).

Challenges to Managed Care

In the U.S., managed care was developed by the private sector as an alternative to government regulation. When employers were faced with covering increasingly high health insurance premiums, they shifted their employees to managed care programs. Although managed care has achieved economic success, patients have become disaffected with such gatekeeping aspects as "utilization review," which curtail the medical services they receive. The advantages managed care offers in terms of lower inflation for medical costs have been outweighed by the disadvantages of such cost-cutting care to employees, who seek litigation where limitations in medical care lead to adverse health consequences. "Investment analysts are downgrading stocks of firms that persist with narrow networks and capitation, while promoting stocks of those that offer the broadest panels with the least utilization review" (Robinson 2001: 2623). Managed care firms are thus moving from tightly managed to loosened utilization review, which in turn increases costs to employers. As a consequence, employees are being asked to pay a greater share of their health insurance premium.

Integrated Health Systems: Organizational Convergence

Although Canada and the U.S. diverge in how health care is financed and delivered, some common strategies have begun to emerge from an organizational perspective. One theme is the concept of integrated delivery networks (IDN), organized systems of care that reduce fragmentation among health care providers and promote greater continuity of care to enhance quality outcomes (Leatt, Pink, and Naylor 1996). Such integrated systems of care are recognized as being particularly important for managing chronic illness by coordinating multiple health professionals with different specialties. The intent of IDNs is to bridge care at different levels—from prevention, to acute, to rehabilitative and supportive home care—to ensure a seamless transition among the levels and to facilitate continuity of care. From an organizational perspective this involves *vertical integration and coordination* (Shortell et al. 2000).

Such *vertical integration* has varying forms in Canada and the U.S. Similarities are reflected in the merger of hospitals and other health care organizations with various specialties that can together offer a broader continuum of health care. It can alternatively involve *vertical coordination* where such organizations instead develop contracts or memorandums of agreement for sharing client referrals and information. The organizational and political forces guiding such mergers, however, vary across the two nations. In the U.S., *vertical integration* often occurs through private health insurance companies and health maintenance organizations (HMOs), which contract with an array of health care providers and organizations (hospitals, diagnostic clinics, and primary care clinics) to offer a comprehensive package of health care services. In Canada, *vertical integration* has been guided largely through the process of regionalization in all provinces (except Ontario). Regionalization involves the devolution of funding authority for health care services from a provincial Ministry of Health to a defined number of regional health authorities (RHAs). It also involves centralization at the local level through the integration of hospitals and other health care organizations under a regional board of governors and an overarching management structure (Kouri 2002).

Some critics, however, caution that organizational integration and coordination are not a panacea in terms of addressing cost and quality concerns related to health care systems. Developing integrated organizations can, for example, be costly and require years before efficiencies are realized. Integration also involves such challenges as melding organizational cultures and developing new operating processes across several organizations, which are often not easily achieved. Whether integrated systems lead to cost efficiencies is not clear. Evidence suggests integration and coordination efforts are most effective and efficient when focused on chronically ill patients through "disease management" or tailored to address patients with a complex set of conditions. Two types of care coordination programs have shown promise, focusing on (a) disease-management programs for patients with a particular chronic condition such as diabetes, with a common set of care needs, and (b) case-management programs for patients with a complex set of conditions (Burns and Pauly 2002). Such prevention programs are aimed at improving coordination of care, addressing health problems before they become more serious, and reducing costly hospitalizations (Wagner et al. 1999; Weisner et al. 2001).

Another way to integrate care is through information technology (IT), including electronic medical records (EMRs) that allow physicians and other health professionals to access patient information from a centralized medical record database through a communication network. A challenge, however, is that different providers use different information systems, such that information interfaces between organizations will likely be required to allow the providers within those organizations access to such information. While there is some convergence between Canada and the United States in terms of moving toward more integrated and coordinated health systems, divergence is, however, apparent with respect to access to pharmaceuticals, including the regulation of pharmaceutical prices.

Access to Pharmaceuticals: Health System Divergence

Canada and the United States differ in their approaches to ensuring access to pharmaceuticals, which is influenced by divergent perspectives within each nation on the extent to which the market allows access to pharmaceutical products. In Canada, provincial public health insurance includes drug benefits that facilitate access to medications for people 65 years and over, and those on social assistance. In some provinces, such as Quebec, the entire population has access to a subsidized drug benefit program, while other provinces such as Ontario make subsidized programs available to families with catastrophic drug costs. The remainder of the population attains access to drug insurance coverage largely through private employment benefit plans. This means that those employed in low-paying and part-time work do not normally gain access to such private insurance through employment, and are forced to pay for the medications they require.

By contrast, Medicare in the U.S. has not included insurance for medications, which made the elderly population vulnerable to covering their costs on an individual basis as most were unable to afford private insurance. An amendment to Medicare that takes effect in 2006, however, incorporates drug benefits that will subsidize about 50 percent of the costs of pharmaceuticals for seniors. However, the remainder of the population is expected to access coverage for pharmaceuticals through private insurance either through employment benefit plans or individually. Moreover, private insurance plans include variable coverage for pharmaceuticals, with co-payments often required even with insurance coverage. Of course the 15 percent of the population that are uninsured are forced to pay for their medications.

Another contrast between Canada and the U.S. concerns the regulation of pharmaceutical prices. In Canada, the prices of pharmaceuticals are regulated by the Patented Medicines Prices Review Board (PMPRB), which uses an index based on the average price of a specific pharmaceutical in seven industrialized nations, and its innovativeness to set its price in Canada. If a new medicine provides a novel and effective therapy for a condition with few therapies available, it would be considered a breakthrough product and granted a price higher than other new products on the market that provide no new breakthough in therapy. Increases in the prices of patented pharmaceuticals must also not increase beyond the rate of inflation. Companies that do not adhere to such regulations must pay penalties.

In the United States, in contrast, pharmaceuticals are not subject to price regulation, though individual drug companies will negotiate bulk discounts for their products with large insurers such as HMOs and the Veterans Administration. Such divergent processes have resulted in price differentials of up to 50 percent less for medicines in Canada than in the U.S. These price differences have sparked a movement in Internet pharmacy where Americans purchase their medicines in Canada. Cross-border purchase of drugs in Canada is allowed only if a Canadian physician writes the prescription. Internet pharmacies thus operate by having a Canadian physician review an American patient's file and issue a prescription for them. The Internet pharmacy business has grown in the order of $1 billion in trade per year. Such growth has led pharmaceutical firms to issue letters to provincial governments indicating they will limit supply of their drugs only to quantities sufficient for their population. The implicit threat is that if Internet pharmacies continue to supply Americans with drug products at reduced prices, provinces may lack supplies for their population. The federal government has indicated it would like to curtail the practice of Internet pharmacy.

The reasons such differences exist can be partially attributed to the perspective in Canada that medicines are subject to market failure due to price inelasticity (see Box 10.4), and therefore their prices should be regulated to ensure access. In the U.S., different concepts of the market and political pressure from pharmaceutical

> **Box 10.4: Market Failure and Pharmaceutical Price Regulation**
>
> One reason pharmaceutical prices are regulated in Canada is due to their price inelasticity. Price inelasticity refers to the concept that the demand for them is inelastic: if the price of these products rises sharply, most people would simply pay the extra cost because they require the product for health reasons. In time of need, the decision to purchase a medicine is insensitive to the cost of the product, even when a consumer pays directly. Since price competition for patented products does not exist, which normally decreases prices to competitive levels, profit-maximizing firms will charge prices that are too high and produce output levels that are too low from the allocational point of view (Brander 1992). Since increasing the price of pharmaceuticals has little effect on their demand, consumers and the public bear the consequences of high prices (Wiktorowicz 1995). In Canada, the Patented Medicines Prices Review Board (PMPRB) regulates the prices of pharmaceuticals to ensure their accessibility to the population and to public drug benefit plans. In contrast, medicines whose patents have expired are subject to competition from generic product manufacturers, which drives down their prices. For this reason, Canada does not regulate the prices of generic products.

companies, whose representative association is one of the most powerful, have ensured that pharmaceuticals are not subject to price regulation. Moreover, governments are also under pressure to ensure a competitive private sector that drives their economy (Hancher 1990). An analysis of regulatory measures must thus consider the government's competing imperatives of ensuring access to health care and preserving market competition. The divergent balances struck in Canada and the U.S. reflect their differing perspectives on how to address these important issues.

Conclusions

Canada has successfully attained universal coverage while containing the costs of health care, even though timely access to care has become an issue. The U.S. has not achieved universal access to health care, and instead relies on employer-based insurance coverage for its population aged under 65, leaving approximately 15 percent of Americans (45 million people) without health insurance coverage. Although health care reforms continue to be proposed in the U.S., the result has only led to "patchwork changes aligned to the demands of special interest groups representing consumers, pharmaceutical companies, health insurers and others" (Southby 2004: 442). A recent example is the amendments to Medicare that added prescription drug coverage for elderly and disabled beneficiaries. Enacting legislative changes in the U.S., however, entails addressing multiple institutional points that allow both access to myriad interest groups and veto for amendments that would expand coverage. Among the strongest opposition to proposals for universal coverage arise from private insurance companies and insured citizens who fear their level of choice or the quality of their health care plans will be diminished. Despite the areas of convergence and divergence in the health care systems of Canada and the United States, ongoing challenges remain for both in terms of meeting public expectations within public and private budgetary constraints.

References

Brander, J. (1992). *Government Policy toward Business*, 2nd ed. Toronto: Butterworths Canada Ltd.

Burns, L., and M.V. Pauly. (2002). "Integrated Delivery Networks: A Detour on the Road to Integrated Health Care?" *Health Affairs* 21(4): 128–143.

Deber, R.B. (2004). "Delivering Health Care: Public, Not-for-Profit, or Private?" In *The Fiscal Sustainability of Health Care in Canada*, edited by G.P. Marchildon, T. McIntosh, and P.G. Forest, 233–296. Toronto: University of Toronto Press.

Devereaux, P.J., H.J. Schunemann, N. Ravindran, M. Bhandari, A.X. Garg, P.T. Choi, B.J. Grant, T. Haines, C. Lacchetti, B. Weaver, J.N. Lavis, D.J. Cook, D.R. Haslam, T. Sullivan, and G.H. Guyatt. (2002). "Comparison of Mortality between Private For-Profit and Private Not-for-Profit Hemodialysis Centers: A Systematic Review and Meta-analysis." *Journal of the American Medical Association* 288(19): 2449–2457.

Docteur, E., and H. Oxley. (2003). *Health Care Systems: Lessons from the Reform Experience*, OECD Health Working Papers 9. Paris. Available on-line at www.oecd.org/dataoecd/5/53/22364122.pdf.

Doern, G.B., and R.W. Phidd. (1988). *Canadian Public Policy: Ideas, Structure, Process*. Scarborough: Nelson Canada.

Dyson, K.P. (1980). *The State Tradition in Western Europe*. Oxford: Basil Blackwell.

Feder, J. (2004). "Crowd-out and the Politics of Health Reform." *Journal of Law, Medicine and Ethics* 32(3): 461–464.

Hacker, J. (2002). *The Divided Welfare State*. New York: Cambridge University Press.

Hancher, Leigh. (1990). *Regulating for Competition: Government, Law and the Pharmaceutical Industry in the United Kingdom and France*. Oxford: Clarendon Press.

Kouri, D. (2002). "Is Regionalization Working?" *Canadian Healthcare Manager*. Available on-line at www.chmonline.ca/chmonline/story.asp?Article ID=645.

Leatt, P., G. Pink, and D. Naylor. (1996). "Integrated Delivery Systems: Has Their Time Come in Canada?" *Canadian Medical Association Journal* 154(6): 803–809.

MacLean, G.A., and D.R. Wood. (2002). *Introduction to Politics, Power, Participation and the Distribution of Wealth*. Toronto: Pearson Education Canada.

Maioni, A. (1998). *Parting at the Crossroads, the Emergence of Health Insurance in the United States and Canada*. Princeton: Princeton University Press.

Mann, C., and T. Westmoreland. (2004). "Attending to Medicaid." *The Journal of Law, Medicine and Ethics* 32(3): 416–425.

Rawls, J. (1971). *A Theory of Justice*. Cambridge: Harvard University Press.

Robinson, J.C. (2001). "The End of Managed Care." *JAMA* 285(20): 2622–2628.

Saltman, R.B., and C. von Otter. (1992). *Planned Markets and Public Competition: Stratgic Reform in Northern European Health Systems*. London: Open University Press.

Sandier, S., V. Paris, and D. Polton. (2004). "Health Care Systems in Transition: France." Copenhagen: WHO Regional Office for Europe on behalf of The European Observatory on Health Systems and Policies. Available on-line at www.euro.who.int/document/e83126.pdf.

Shortell, S.M., R.R. Gillies, D.A. Anderson, and J.B. Mitchell. (2000). *Remaking Health Care in America: The Evolution of Organized Delivery Systems*, 2nd ed. San Francisco: Jossey-Bass.

Simeon, R. (1976). "Studying Public Policy." *Canadian Journal of Political Science* 9(4): 548–580.

Southby, R.F. (2004). "Where Do We Go from Here: Is There Any Hope for Real Health Care Reform?" *The Journal of Law, Medicine and Ethics* 32(3): 442–445.

Stone, D.A. (1988). *Policy Paradox and Political Reason*. Glenview: Scott Foresman.

Tuohy, C. H. (1999). *Accidental Logics: The Dynamics of Change in the Health Care Arena in the United States, Britain, and Canada*. New York: Oxford University Press.

Vladeck, B.C. (2004). "The Struggle for the Soul of Medicare." *The Journal of Law, Medicine and Ethics* 32(3): 410–415.

Wagner, E.H., C. Davies, J. Schaefer, M. Von Korff, and B. Austin. (1999). "A Survey of Leading Chronic Disease Management Programs: Are They Consistent with the Literature?" *Managed Care Quarterly* 7 (3): 56–66.

Weimer, D.L., and A.R. Vining. (1989). *Policy Analysis, Concepts and Practice*. Englewood Cliffs: Prentice Hall Inc.

Weisner, C., J. Merters, S. Parthasarathy, C. Moore, and Y. Lu. (2001). "Integrating Primary Medical Care with Addiction Treatment." *Journal of American Medical Association* 286(14): 1715–1723.

Wiktorowicz, M. (1995). "Regulating Biotechnology: A Model of Rational-Political Policy Development." Ph.D. dissertation, University of Toronto.

● ●

Critical Thinking Questions

1. On which aspects do liberalism and socialism differ?
2. Consider the different processes through which laws are passed in Canada and the U.S. Why is it more difficult to pass laws in general, and laws concerning health care in particular in the U.S. than in Canada?
3. In countries with a publicly insured universal health care system, what inequities result from allowing a parallel private system?
4. Why is public financing considered the optimal form of health care financing? Why is the optimal mode of health care delivery considered to be private not-for-profit?
5. What challenges are faced by Medicare, Medicaid, and managed care?

Further Readings

Deber, R.B. (2004). "Delivering Health Care: Public, Not-for-Profit, or Private?" In *The Fiscal Sustainability of Health Care in Canada*, edited by G.P. Marchildon, T. McIntosh, and P.G. Forest, 233–296. Toronto: University of Toronto Press. Raisa Deber provides an overview of the terms and debate concerning private and public delivery. This includes the strengths and weaknesses of the various modes of health care financing and delivery.

Feder, J. (2004). "Crowd-out and the Politics of Health Reform." *Journal of Law, Medicine and Ethics* 32(3): 461–464.
Judith Feder provides political and historical analysis of the resistance to universal public health insurance in the U.S. She provides a pithy analysis of the challenges to universal health care coverage in the U.S.

Maioni, A. (1998). *Parting at the Crossroads, the Emergence of Health Insurance in the United States and Canada.* Princeton: Princeton University Press.
The differences in the historical and political trajectories for the development of health care insurance in Canada and the U.S. are analyzed. Maioni's historical analysis also clarifies the differences in the political contexts of the two nations.

Tuohy, C. Hughes. (1999). *Accidental Logics: The Dynamics of Change in the Health Care Arena in the United States, Britain, and Canada.* New York: Oxford University Press.
A comparative political analysis that draws on the theory of path dependency to clarify how past choices in the development of health insurance in U.S., Canada, and Britain shape these nations' responses to the current challenge of escalating costs. Provides an understanding of the forces leading to change in different national contexts.

Relevant Web Sites

Centers for Medicare and Medicaid Services
www.cms.hhs.gov/
   Provides information on changing provisions in the benefit plans associated with Medicare and Medicaid. Links to related research and information sites on Medicare and Medicaid are also included.

Kaiser Family Foundation
www.kff.org/healthpollreport/archive_aug2004/index.cfm
   The Kaiser Family Foundation provides analysis of managed care. It also provides access to papers offering evidence-based analysis of different types of health care plans in the U.S.

Organisation of Economic Co-operation and Development
www.oecd.org
   The Organization of Economic Co-operation and Development (OECD) Web site provides access to their overviews of national health care systems. Provides analysis of national health care systems from a comparative perspective.

WHO Regional Office for Europe on behalf of the European Observatory on Health Systems and Policies
www.euro.who.int/document/e83126.pdf
   The European Observatory provides in-depth analysis of national health care systems from both individual nations and comparative perspectives.

Glossary

Case manager: A nurse, doctor, or social worker who works with patients, providers, and insurers to coordinate all services deemed necessary to provide the patient with a plan of medically necessary and appropriate health care.

Health maintenance organization (HMO): An entity that provides or arranges for coverage of health services needed by members for a fixed, prepaid premium.

Integrated delivery systems: Organized systems of health care that reduce fragmentation among health care providers and promote greater continuity of care to enhance quality outcomes.

Managed care: A system of health care that combines delivery and payment and influences utilization of services by employing management techniques designed to promote the delivery of cost-effective health care.

Managed health care plan: An arrangement that integrates financing and management with the delivery of health care services to an enrolled population. It employs or contracts with an organized system of providers who deliver services and frequently share financial risk.

Utilization review: A formal review of utilization for appropriateness of health care services delivered to a member on a prospective, concurrent, or retrospective basis.

CHAPTER ELEVEN

THE PROVISION OF CARE

Professions, Politics, and Profit

Ivy Lynn Bourgeault

Learning Objectives

At the conclusion of this chapter, the reader will be able to
- understand the health care division of labour in Canada and how this has evolved
- identify different types of health care providers
- understand the various elements of health human resource management
- understand the impact of health care reforms and cutbacks on *who* provides *what* various forms of health care
- understand what is meant by the term "managed care"
- identify the various ways that health care is being privatized and profitized

---

Introduction

The National Film Board documentary *Bitter Medicine* (1983), which details the birth of Medicare in Saskatchewan, describes the key outcomes of the struggle for Canadian health care as being the coverage of those health care services deemed most expensive—hospitals and physicians. It is not surprising, therefore, that rising costs of health care have become a problem, and that hospitals and physicians have been the primary target of efforts to control costs. In the first part of this chapter, I address which health care providers are called upon to provide what sorts of care, including how this has evolved historically. This is followed by a discussion of how the health care division of labour is managed, and the impact of cost controls on both who provides care and what care they provide.

But it is not only that the most expensive services are covered, but that they continue to be provided largely in privately owned facilities. Naylor (1986) described this situation in medicine as public payment for private practice. Many advocates of further privatization of the Canadian health care system often emphasize that our system is already based on private delivery. Indeed, the continuity of private provision of health care services in Canada has not only made it vulnerable to increased privatization—much of which has been insidious—but also to the intrusion of for-profit care models and motives. These are addressed directly in the second part of this chapter.

In both cases, the policies to curb rising health care costs and the expansion of private, for-profit provision have been imported from the United States, a much more expensive (per capita) and highly privatized system. In light of this, it is imperative to look at the dynamics of professions, profit, and care in Canada in this comparative context. In addition to drawing upon a comparative lens, this chapter will also take a critical perspective by teasing apart the rhetoric from the reality, exposing the broader structural forces that impinge upon the provision of care, and emphasizing the impact that gender has played on these processes.

Evolution of the Health Care Division of Labour

As noted in the historical essay by Feldberg and Vipond (Chapter 9), the health care systems—and, by extension, the *health care divisions of labour*—in Canada and the United States developed along very similar lines. The provision of care was initially quite eclectic, sometimes including care by Aboriginal healers, religious orders (usually nuns as nurses), barber surgeons, and various forms of midwives (Connor 1989; Laforce 1990; Mason 1988). There were large differences between urban centres in Upper and Lower Canada and the "Western Territories," the latter being largely either self-sufficient or reliant on lay models of care. Lay or self-provision of care also reflected class and urban and rural differences as well (Mason 1988). Waves of immigration also brought health care providers trained in other jurisdictions, some of whom initially practised only in their cultural community, but later among the larger population (Biggs 2004). Local educational and training programs were established beginning with the first medical school in Montreal in 1824 and the first nursing school in St. Catharines, Ontario, in 1874 (Coburn 1988; Coburn, Torrance, and Kaufert 1983). These various developments not only increased the numbers but also in some areas the competition among health care providers.

Due to a variety of factors, the medical profession emerged as the dominant health occupation in Canada in the late 19th and early 20th centuries, consolidating its power between the First World War and the Saskatchewan doctors' strike of 1962 (Coburn et al. 1983). Its dominance was attained first by establishing powerful professional organizations that successfully lobbied for protective legislation to place limits on who would be officially allowed to practise medicine. These organizations and their leaders also began to exert control over the production of medical knowledge and, by extension, entrance to medical schools and who would ultimately practise as physicians. It was particularly critical that the profession begin to appeal to elite members of society to support the professions' overall lobbying efforts. Perhaps most critically, the medical profession sought sponsorship by state officials and by wealthy patrons. This was most clearly exemplified in the Carnegie Foundation sponsorship of medical school reform in the U.S. and Canada in the early 20th century through the Flexner Report.[1]

One of the key consequences of the strategies to achieve medical dominance has been the gendered exclusion and segregation of the health care division of labour assigning a secondary status to women.[2] Historically, gender was used as an exclusionary criteria by the medical profession in its quest for professional status. This began with the efforts to exclude women from medical school and, failing that, from medical practice and/or hospital admitting privileges. Prior to the mid-20th century, only a handful of women under the most unusual circumstances managed to receive medical training in Canada (Strong-Boag 1979). Even when female students were admitted, they were made to feel very uncomfortable, there was a lack of female role models, and many experienced subtle and not-so-subtle sexual harassment.

Women's involvement in the health care division of labour was largely channelled into support occupations—such as nursing, dental hygiene, and dental and legal assistant work—with limited scopes of practice, lower status, and little autonomy (Adams and Bourgeault 2003; Valentine 1996). Indeed, female-dominated professions have been regarded by some as achieving only "semi-professional" (Etzioni 1969) or subordinate (Willis 1989) status, often functioning only under the direct supervision of more powerful professions dominated by men (see Box 11.1). Thus, while women make up the bulk of health care providers, their employment is not evenly distributed.

Box 11.1: Types of Health Care Providers

Wardwell (1981) and Willis (1989) both define the three different kinds of professions in terms of their relationship to the dominant medical profession:

- *ancillary or subordinate professions* that are different as ... *under the direct control of supervision by medicine*
- *limited professions* that are defined as ... *practicing independently of medicine but with a limited scope of practice (in terms of patient or treatment modality)*
- *marginal or excluded professions* which are defined as ... *practicing outside of the mainstream medical system and denied official legitimacy*

Some female professions, such as midwifery, were excluded altogether from many segments of the Canadian health care division of labour. Indeed, another consequence of medicine's quest for dominance has been the exclusion of health care provider groups altogether. In addition to midwifery, many provider groups that are now considered to be complementary or alternative medical practitioners—such as homeopaths and herbalists—were also excluded from the Canadian health care landscape (Connor 1994).

When the efforts arose to reshape the health care division of labour following the inception of Medicare, the various professional groups were at very different starting points. Medical dominance, as Coburn et al. (1983) argue, was beginning to decline. The status of largely female health professions, such as nursing, was just beginning to climb, propelled in part by the women's movement and labour movements. All professions, however, were and continue to be subject to the *rationalization* process, which focuses on the most efficient use of health care resources, or the assignment of tasks to the "most appropriate" professional. Two key issues involved in the rationalization process include a focus on *flexibility* and the ability to respond to shortages and surpluses through the substitution of health labour. The second, and some would argue primary, concern is with *keeping costs low* so that the least expensive worker performs tasks at the lowest unit cost. These reforms have led to some dramatic changes in *who* does *what* in the provision of health care.

Reforms Directed toward Who Provides Care

Efforts to rationalize the health care division of labour is often considered synonymous with the term "health human resource planning." This involves preparing, regulating, deploying, and assigning tasks to people who work in health care. The key questions posed include:

- What types of workers should exist?
- What will each type of worker do?
- What training and educational requirements are required for these workers to accomplish their tasks?

When Medicare came into effect, several provincial governments sponsored reviews of the health care division of labour. Many of these addressed the key problems of the supply, mix, and distribution of health care providers (see Box 11.2). In Ontario, this was accomplished by the Ontario Committee of the Healing Arts, which was struck in 1966. In its 1970 report to the provincial government, it made several recommendations, some of which addressed increasing medical school enrolment whereas others addressed the issue of expanding the scope of practice of such professions as nurse-midwives and nurse practitioners. It is important to note that these recommendations were made in a context of a perceived physician shortage. Although nurse practitioners experienced a short-lived surge of interest

> **Box 11.2: Health Human Resource Issues**
>
> Health human resources addresses three basic problems:
> - *Problems with supply*: The numbers of health care professionals providing services to a population
> - *Problems with mix*: The relative numbers of health care professionals providing various types of specialty services
> - *Problems with distribution*: The location or deployment of health care professionals across geographic areas

between the early 1970s to early 1980s (Angus and Bourgeault 1988–1989), nurse-midwifery failed to capture enough political support at that time to become more fully integrated into the publicly funded health care system (Bourgeault 2005b).

Some 10 years later, the Ontario government appointed a Health Professions Legislation Review (HPLR) in 1982 to respond to various pressures for change in the way health professions were regulated. The mandate of the HPLR was to make recommendations to the Minister of Health in the form of draft legislation with respect to which health professions should be regulated and a new structure for the legislation governing the health professions in the province (Health Professions Legislation Review 1989). Although the primary objective of the review was to design a new regulatory framework that would more effectively advance and protect the public interest, it also attempted to increase the flexibility of the health care division of labour through this framework. The way this was to be achieved was by regulating health care providers through 13 controlled acts rather than through exclusive scopes of practice. Some of the controlled acts include:

- communicating a diagnosis
- performing a procedure on tissue below the dermis
- administering a substance by injection or inhalation
- applying or ordering the application of a form of energy (e.g., such as X-rays)

One or more professions are allowed to undertake particular controlled acts allowing for overlapping scopes of practice. For example, both midwives and physicians are able to manage labour or deliver a baby, another one of the controlled acts under this legislation.

But this attempt to increase the flexibility of the health care division of labour was not simply an Ontario phenomenon. Similar legislation exists in British Columbia. Further, the 1991 report by health economists Morris Barer and Greg Stoddart for the federal/provincial/territorial Ministers of Health also addressed the issue of eliminating exclusive scopes of practice and replacing these with a more circumscribed set of controlled acts and reserved titles through legislation similar to the HPLR recommendations (Barer and Stoddart 1991; Scully 1999). Several of these recommendations were directed toward managing what was at that time perceived to be an oversupply of physicians. In addition to recommending strategies to curb the medical human resources, it also addressed the mix of providers, particularly in primary care. Key among these recommendations addressed the expanded use of nurse practitioners in primary care.

Primary care has historically been the most highly sought after and fiercely defended of all health care domains. More recently, however, general medical practice has become less attractive (Cesa and Larente 2004). In Canada, for example, whereas family physicians make up approximately 48 percent of practising physicians, less than 40 percent of new practice entrants since 1993 are in family medicine (Hawley 2004; Kralj 1999).[3] In the U.S., this is even lower with some states having only 11 percent of their complement of physicians in family practice. This has created a strong impetus for the expansion of a variety of both medical and non-medical primary care providers (see Box 11.3) in order to meet patient needs.

But this begs the question as to whether non-medical primary care providers are alternatives to medical providers or complementary. Both perspectives are evident in the Canadian context. Prior to the Barer-Stoddart report, Lomas and Stoddart (1985) estimated that between 20 percent and 32 percent of general practitioners in Ontario could be replaced by a nurse practitioner. A complementary approach, however, is most salient, particularly at the political level. For example, one family physician who has worked extensively with NPs notes:

> The family practice and nursing models should mesh very nicely to fulfil the demand that Nurse Practitioners' strengths in patient education, counselling and health promotion be linked with family physicians' strengths in diagnosis, treatment and prevention of disease. (Dr. Daniel Way in Birenbaum 1994: 77)

Representatives from medical associations have been more forceful, stating that "physicians cannot be expected to accept the proposal to create another health care provider when that creation is based on their own devaluation" (Dr. Ted Boadway in Birenbaum 1994: 77).

The trend toward expanding the deployment and scope of practice of nurse practitioners has an interesting gender dimension because most tend to be female. Some have argued that the reasoning behind the notion that non-physician providers are cheaper than physicians can be related to societal notions of skill, which have been argued to be inherently gendered. For example, the delegation of technical skills to women has long been justified on the basis of driving down the cost of labour (Wajcman 1991), and female health professions are no exception to this observation. Historically, the poorly rewarded work of nurses, for example, was viewed as a natural extension of the caring services that women provided for their families in the private sphere; it was therefore not seen as the product of rigorous

Box 11.3: The Primary Health Care Division of Labour in Canada and the U.S.

Canada	United States
Family physicians	Family physicians
Primary care specialists	
Gynecologists for women	
Internists for men	
Pediatricians for children	
Nurse practitioners	Nurse practitioners
Physician assistants	

Nurse practitioners are advanced practice nurses who provide a broad range of health care services, including: taking the patient's history, performing a physical exam, and ordering appropriate laboratory tests and procedures; diagnosing, treating, and managing acute and chronic diseases; providing prescriptions and coordinating referrals; and promoting healthy activities in collaboration with the patient (www.nlm.nih.gov/medlineplus/ency/article/009134.htm).

Physician assistants are health care professionals licensed to practise medicine with physician supervision. Common services provided by a PA include taking medical histories and performing physical examinations; ordering and interpreting lab tests; diagnosing and treating illnesses; assisting in surgery; prescribing and/or dispensing medication; and counselling patients (www.asapa.org/definition.htm).

training (Coburn 1987; Kazanjian 1993). But the notion that people are paid on the basis of their skills obscures the very nature of skilled work as a socially defined and socially evaluated set of characteristics that varies according to the gender, ethnicity, and power of workers, as well as with historical and economic context (Gaskell 1987). Specifically, female health care providers operate within a social system of health care that devalues their skills and knowledge.

In part because of this devaluation of nursing work, the nursing profession has also been subjected to similar kinds of "substitution" as have primary care providers (Bourgeault 2005a). As nursing human resources are one of the primary budgetary items for hospitals, they are clearly targeted for cost-cutting measures in times of fiscal restraint. As a direct result of hospital cost cutting, the nursing profession has experienced a dramatic loss of jobs and replacement of RNs by lesser-trained nursing staff. Concurrent with these changes, more full-time positions were converted to part-time as a means of increasing the flexibility of the nursing workforce. Nursing layoffs were exacerbated by the trend toward the replacement of RNs with registered practical nurses (RPNs) and unregulated care providers (UCPs). For example, one hospital in Toronto replaced almost 100 full-time RN jobs with RPNs and unregulated generic health care workers, who, with as little as three weeks of on-the-job training, were being assigned direct patient care. Similar policies have also been implemented in American hospitals.

Provincial nursing organizations in Canada have responded to these initiatives with strong opposition. They argue that the increased acuity of patients in hospitals and the decreased length of hospital stays require nurses with a higher rather than a lower level of knowledge, and a broader range of skills and competency. The cost-effectiveness of replacing RNs has also been called into question by several recent studies suggesting the opposite (Aiken et al. 2001, Norrish and Rundall 2000). They claim that it is a misconception that RNs are too expensive, and moreover that it is illogical to blame nurses' present situation on their previously successful negotiations for a fair wage (c.f. Shamian 1993).

So there have been a variety of policies directed toward the rationalization of the health care division of labour, most of which address the supply and, to a lesser extent, the mix aspects of the situation. Far less attention has been paid to the consideration of the needs that this supply is supposed to meet. Tomblin Murphy et al. (2003), for example, argue that:

> Decisions about the level and deployment of health human resources are often made in response to short-term financial pressures as opposed to evidence of the effect healthcare staff have on health outcomes.... While the stated goal of health human resources planning is to match human resources to *need* for services, decisions on how to allocate healthcare staff are primarily based on *demand* for services. (Tomblin Murphy et al. 2003: 1)

Newer approaches to health human resource issues highlight the importance of taking a broader perspective. O'Brien-Pallas et al. (2001) present a broad conceptual framework for making sound health human resource decisions that highlight the importance of population health needs; how supply, production, financial, and management factors should all feed into planning and forecasting; how utilization should be measured in terms of health outcomes, provider outcomes (such as workload and prevention of burnout), and system outcomes to ensure an efficient and effective mix of health human resources (see Box 11.4).

Reforms have also not only focused on who is providing care as policies have also been developed and implemented regarding what or how care is to be provided. Care is increasingly becoming managed and those doing the managing have

Box 11.4: Conceptual Framework for Understanding Health Human Resources

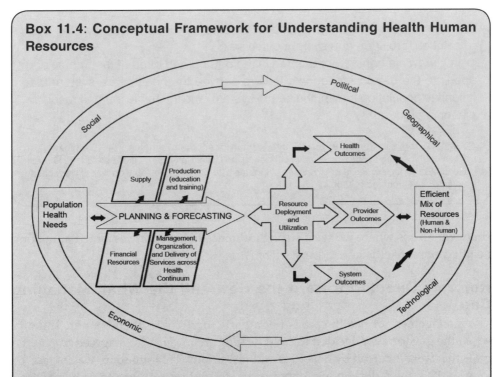

Elements of the Framework

Population health needs reflect people's various characteristics that create the need for curative as well as preventive health services. Addressing the health needs of the population provides the motive, context, and justification for health human resources planning practices.

The *production* element of the framework highlights the fact that future population health needs must be considered when setting targets for health education and training programs.

The *supply* element reflects the actual number, type, and geographic distribution of health-care providers. It recognizes that supply is fluid and is related to production elements, as well as to factors such as recruitment/retention, licensing, regulation, and scope of practice.

Planning and forecasting reflects the varieties of available health human resources planning practices and models, their assumptions, methods, data requirements, and limitations.

Health, provider, and system outcomes refer to establishing the effectiveness and quality of health human resource practices by examining the effect on population health, provider health, job satisfaction, etc., and system costs and efficiencies.

Efficient mix of human and non-human resources (such as fiscal resources, physical plant, space, supplies, equipment, and technology) reflects the number and type of resources that must be developed in order to achieve the best population, provider, and system outcomes.

Context elements (represented in the outer broad band of the framework) speak to the need to recognize factors outside the health care system that influence population health, the health system, and the health human resource planning process.

Source: G. Tomblin Murphy et al., "Health Human Resources Planning : An Examination of Relationships among Nursing Service Utilization, an Estimate of Population Health and Overall Health Status Outcomes in the Province of Ontario" (2003: 2–4). Available on-line at www.chsrf. ca/final_research/ogc/pdf/toblin_final.pdf.

changed. This is where we see a strong influence of U.S. policies aimed at making health care more efficient and cost-effective.

Reforms Directed toward the How and the What: Managing Care

The management of health care is not a particularly new phenomenon. Initially when the government decided to fund health care in Canada, it agreed to pay the costs that were incurred by hospitals and physicians. This situation did not last for long. In 1978 the federal government began to set limits on health care spending because the costs of providing health care far outstripped indicators of economic growth. This resulted in a cascade of economic constraints that have trickled down from provincial governments to hospitals to the day-to-day practices of health care providers.

Reforms to the hospital sector have included shorter hospital stays, more out-patient services and day surgery, cutting beds and staff, contracting out, standardization of care, and deinstitutionalization. Such reforms focus primarily on getting people out of health care institutions or not letting them enter in the first place (or delaying them from accessing care). But reforms not only focus on utilization. Many are focused on rationalizing the organization of health care work. This includes such policies as total quality management, patient-focused care, and other models developed in the for-profit, goods-producing sector, which have had a negative impact on hospital-based work, particularly nursing (Armstrong and Armstrong 2002). For example, Armstrong and Armstrong (2002) argue that although the total quality approach is portrayed as building on and strengthening nurses' approach to care, the consequences of these reforms have been an increasing fragmentation and quantification of nursing work. They describe further that "care disappears, in part because it is less visible and easy to measure, in part because it is mainly done by women.... Meanwhile, work for providers becomes more intensive, less satisfying, and less secure" (Armstrong and Armstrong 2002: 226).

The origin of many of these new managerial strategies can be traced to the United States. Similar to Canada, the management of health care in the United States has also emerged slowly in the last couple of decades so as to reduce unneeded services and constrain cost (Mechanic 2004). The most recent umbrella term used for a wide range of largely market-based organizational forms to the allocation of care is "managed care" (see Box 11.5). Managed care has a variety of definitions, but usually involves:

> The provision of health services through a single point of entry and formal enrollment where patient care is managed to ensure an emphasis on quality preventive and primary care, a reduction in inappropriate use of services, control of costs, and management of risk.[4]

Its origins can be drawn from industry-based health programs where companies contract with physicians to provide basic medical care for their employees through a capitation arrangement (Mechanic 2004). In the last two decades, both private and public health care providers have incorporated various aspects of managed care. Further, although many managed care organizations were largely non-profit organizations in the early 1980s, by the end of that decade more than two-thirds of them were for-profit (Armstrong et al. 2000). Not surprisingly, the for-profit organizations have become powerful voices in setting the American health care agenda.

Based on some key indicators, some could say that managed care has been successful in containing health care costs, but as Mechanic (2004: 77) notes, "Many of the cost reductions came by negotiating, some would say dictating, lower rates of reimbursement for hospitals, doctors, other professionals, and a variety of ancillary services." Indeed, a constant state of negotiation is a salient theme in how health care providers in the U.S. view managed care. Physicians and nurses tell of an increasing burden of negotiating care for patients—particularly textually mediated negotiations—as the access to and amount of care are increasingly limited through managed care policies (Bourgeault et al. 2004). Providers particularly complain about the myriad of plans and insurers that they need to negotiate with; constantly changing criteria for inclusions and exclusions; equally changing drug formularies; and changing networks of decision makers. The amount of time devoted to negotiating care is also salient in Canada, particularly where the hospital sector has been restructured through mergers and closures. Health care providers in the U.S., however, were particularly concerned about the audience for negotiations—which in their case are insurers as opposed to other care providers as is the case in Canada—and the purpose of the negotiations—securing payment and not just care.

Managed care is ultimately a means of rationing care both in terms of access and amount (Bourgeault et al. 2001). As Mechanic (2004: 77) states, "Managed care … was rationing in your face." Access is clearly rationed in the U.S. with more

---

Box 11.5: Principles of Managed Care

Any system that controls costs through closely monitoring and controlling the decisions of health care providers, which includes:
- a clearly differentiated and carefully examined member population
- a central management structure that controls costs
- a known group of physicians on fixed salary or capitation
- general practitioners as gatekeepers
- specific sets of services/benefits
- an identified and limited supply of hospital beds
- an annual budget based on subscription fees

Intended outcomes are supposed to include:
- more integrated systems with greater continuity of care to help reduce duplication and gaps in the system
- increased accountability for providers and patients leading to more appropriate, higher quality care
- increased emphasis on illness prevention and health promotion to help ensure that people stay healthy

---

than 46 million Americans having no health care insurance. Access is not so much denied in the Canadian context—due in large part to its publicly funded health care system—as it is delayed through the sometimes lengthy waiting lists we have for a variety of health care, particularly surgical procedures. Many more similarities are revealed when we examine how the amount of care is rationed in the U.S. and in Canada. Various tools, such as policies that mandate shorter times for hospital stays and increasing the number of patients for which health care providers are responsible, have been adopted on both sides of the border with the criteria for adoption being based more on their ability to control costs than on evidence of improved quality.

The Privatization and Profitization of Care

Many of the practices of managed care have resulted in an insidious *privatization* of health care (see Box 11.6). According to Armstrong et al. (2003), privatization can take many forms, including: the introduction of for-profit practices into public systems of provision; the replacement of public payment for services with private payment, whether directly by individuals or through private insurance; the shift from publicly funded services to private, for-profit provision; the transfer of work—primarily care work—to the home, where the responsibility is disproportionately borne by women working without pay. This latter more invisible form of privatization is particularly problematic because women are increasingly involved in paid employment, hence are not readily available to care for sick relatives. If they do take on care, both their paid work and their unpaid caring work are compromised. This can in turn result in greater stress and negative health consequences for the provider, and often also greater risks for those being cared for as they may not be receiving the most appropriate care. There is also the added burden of greater financial costs for the entire household.

Box 11.6: The Case against Privatization

Armstrong et al. (1999) highlight that there are at least three major differences between health care delivery and goods production, differences that raise significant questions about how appropriate market-based techniques are for the provision of health care.

First, care providers assume and demand autonomy in making decisions based on their assessments of complex individual needs. This is particularly the case with doctors, who determine many of the health care expenditures. In contrast, *strategies in the for-profit sector assume and demand managerial control over processes and decision making.*

A second major difference between the two sectors relates to sales. *In the for-profit sector, selling more is critical to maintaining profit growth.* Customers are encouraged to spend and use more. In health care reform, however, the stated purpose is to spend and use less. Utilization reviews are intended to reduce the number of procedures and processes to lower costs and improve care.

This is related to a third major difference between health care delivery and for-profit production. *Customer choice is defined as a primary basis for competition in the market*, but many patients lack the knowledge, the capacity, or the time to decide among alternatives. In other words, many are not in a position to exercise the choice that is seen as a fundamental basis for efficiency in for-profit settings. This unpredictability makes care delivery less amenable than goods production to managerial planning and costing based on assumptions about regularity and uniformity among products.

Although some argue that the only conceivable solution to rising costs in health care and other public services is thought to be further market penetration and the adoption of more for-profit practices, Armstrong et al. (2003) argue that mixing public and private, for-profit partnerships squeezes out public values and practices. What are left are corporate, for-profit values and methods combined with limited choice. In its worst form, it substitutes profit maximization for essential care, it can limit access to critically needed services, it can deliver substandard services to consumers, and/or sets inadequate reimbursement rates for care providers.[5] Further, what is lost is "the efficiency of a public system, the social solidarity created by shared responsibility and rights and the democratic accountability that is possible in a public system" (Armstrong et al. 2003: 16).

Conclusions

At the outset of this chapter, I intended to shed some light on how the health care division of labour in Canada developed, how it has evolved, and how it has been differentially affected by recent reforms that have increasingly managed care. The management strategies we have examined here address not only who provides care in terms of health human resources, but also how that care is provided. The critical perspective taken in this examination should not be viewed as a general unquestioning criticism of all forms of health care reforms. Rather, this perspective, I hope, helps to reveal what some of the consequences of these reforms—both intended and unintended—have been for the people who provide care within our health care system.

References

Adams, T., and I.L. Bourgeault. (2003). "Feminism and Female Health Professions." *Women's Health* 38(4): 73–90.

Aiken, L.H., S.P. Clarke, D.M. Sloane, J.A. Sochalski, R. Busse, H. Clarke, P. Giovannetti, J. Hunt, A.M. Rafferty, and J. Shamian. (2001). "Nurses' Reports on Hospital Care in Five Countries: The Ways in Which Nurses' Work is Structured Have Left Nurses Among the Least Satisfied Workers, and the Problem is Getting Worse." *Health Affairs* 20(3): 43–53.

Angus, J., and I.L. Bourgeault. (1998–1999). "Medical Dominance, Gender and the State: The Nurse Practitioner Initiative in Ontario." *Health and Canadian Society* 5(1): 55–81.

Armstrong, P., H. Armstrong, I.L. Bourgeault, J. Choinière, E. Mykhalovskiy, and J. White. (1999). *Managed Care: The Experience of Nurses in California*. Sacramento: California Nurses Union.

_____. (2000). *Heal Thyself: Managing Health Care Reform*. Toronto: Garamond Press.

Armstrong, P., and H. Armstrong. (2002). *Wasting Away: The Undermining of Canadian Health Care*, 2nd ed. Toronto: Oxford University Press.

Armstrong, P., H. Armstrong, I.L. Bourgeault, J. Choinière, J. Lexchin, E. Mykhalovskiy, S. Peters, and J. White. (2003). "Market Principles, Business Practices and Health Care: Comparing the U.S. and Canadian Experiences." *International Journal of Canadian Studies* 28: 13–38.

Barer, M.L., and G. Stoddart. (1991). *Toward Integrated Medical Resource Policies for Canada*. Winnipeg: Manitoba Ministry of Health.

Biggs, C. Lesley. (2004). "Rethinking the History of Midwifery in Canada." In *Reconceiving Midwifery*, edited by I. Bourgeault, C. Benoit, and R. Davis-Floyd, 17–45. Kingston and Montreal: McGill Queen's University Press.

Birenbaum R. (1994). "Nurse Practitioners and Physicians: Competition or Collaboration?" *Canadian Medical Association Journal* 151(1): 76–78.

Bourgeault, I.L. (2005a). "Gendered Professionalization Strategies and the Rationalization of Health Care: Midwifery, Nurse Practitioners, and Hospital Nurse Staffing in Ontario, Canada." *Knowledge, Work and Society* 3(1).

_____. (2005b). *Push! The Struggle for Midwifery in Ontario*. Kingston and Montreal: McGill-Queen's University Press.

Bourgeault, I.L., P. Armstrong, H. Armstrong, J. Choinière, J. Lexchin, E. Mykhalovskiy, S. Peters, and J. White. (2001). "The Everyday Experiences of Implicit Rationing: Comparing the Voices of Nurses in California and British Columbia." *Sociology of Health and Illness* 23(5): 633–653.

Bourgeault, I.L., S. Lindsay, E. Mykahalovskiy, P. Armstrong, H. Armstrong, J. Choinière, J. Lexchin, S. Peters, and J. White. (2004). "At First You Will Not Succeed: Negotiating Care in the Context of Health Reform." *Research in the Sociology of Health Care* 22: 261–276.

Cesa, F., and S. Larente. (2004). "Work Force Shortages: A Question of Supply and Demand." *Health Policy Research Bulletin* 8: 12–16.

Coburn, D. (1988). "The Development of Nursing in Canada: Professionalization and Proletarianization." *International Journal of Health Services* 18: 437–456.

Coburn, D., G. Torrance, and J. Kaufert. (1983). "Medical Dominance in Canada in Historical Perspective: The Rise and Fall of Medicine?" *International Journal of Health Services* 13: 407–432.

Coburn, J. (1987). "'I See and Am Silent': A Short History of Nursing in Ontario 1850–1930." In *Health and Canadian Society*, 2nd ed., edited by D. Coburn, C. D'Arcy, G. Torrance, and P. New, 441–462. Markham: Fitzhenry and Whiteside.

Connor, J.T.H. (1989). "Minority Medicine in Ontario, 1795–1903: A Study of Medical Pluralism and Its Decline." Ph.D. dissertation, University of Waterloo.

_____. (1994). "'Larger Fish to Catch Here Than Midwives': Midwifery and the Medical Profession in Nineteenth-Century Ontario." In *Caring and Curing: Historical Perspectives on Women and Healing in Canada*, edited by D. Dodd and D. Gorham, 103–134. Ottawa: University of Ottawa Press.

Etzioni, A., ed. (1969). *The Semi-professions and Their Organization: Teachers, Nurses, and Social Workers*. New York: Free Press.

Gaskell, J. (1987). "Conceptions of Skill and the Work of Women: Some Historical and Political Issues." In *The Politics of Diversity*, edited by R. Hamilton and M. Barrett, 361–380. London: Verso.

Hawley, G. (2004). "Canada's Health Care Workers: A Snapshot." *Health Polity Research Bulletin* 8: 8–11.

Health Professions Legislation Review. (1989). *Striking a Balance*. Toronto: Queen's Park Printers.

Kazanjian, A. (1993). "Health Manpower Planning or Gender Relations? The Obvious and the Oblique." In *Gender, Work and Medicine: Women and the Medical Division of Labour*, edited by E. Riska and K Wegar, 147–171. Newbury Park: Sage.

Kralj, B. (1999). "Physician Human Resources in Ontario: A Looming Crisis." *Ontario Medical Review* 66(4): 16–20.

Laforce, H. (1990). "The Different Stages of the Elimination of Midwives in Quebec." In *Delivering Motherhood: Maternal Idceologies and Practices in the 19th and 20th Centuries*, edited by K. Arnup, S. Levesque, and R. Roach Pierson, 36–50. New York: Routledge.

Lomas, J., and G. Stoddart. (1985). "Estimates of the Potential Impact of Nurse Practitioners on Future Requirements for Physicians in Office-Based General Practice." *Canadian Journal of Public Health* 76: 119–123.

Mason, J. (1988). "Midwifery in Canada." In *The Midwife Challenge*, edited by S. Kitzinger, 99–133. London: Pandora.

Mechanic, D. (2004). "The Rise and Fall of Managed Care." *Journal of Health and Social Behavior* 45(Extra Issue): 76–86.

National Film Board of Canada. (1983). *Bitter Medicine: The Birth of Medicare*. Directed by Tom Shandel; produced by G. Johnson and T. Shandel.

Naylor, C.D. (1986). *Private Practice, Public Payment: Canadian Medicine and the Politics of Health Insurance, 1911–1966*. Kingston and Montreal: McGill-Queen's University Press.

Norrish, B.R. and T. Rundall. (2002). "Hospital Restructuring and the Work of Registered Nurses." *The Milbank Quarterly* 79(1): 55–60.

O'Brien-Pallas, L., G. Murphy, S. Birch, and A. Baumann. (2001). "Framework for Analyzing Health Human Resources." In *Canadian Institute for Health Information. Future Development of Information to Support the Management of Nursing Resources: Recommendations* 6. Ottawa: Canadian Institute for Health Information.

Scully, H. (1999). "Building on One of the Best Delivery Systems in the World." *Healthcare Papers* 1(1). Available on-line at www.longwoods.com/hp/winter99/2.html.

Shamian, J. (1993). *ONA News* (March 4-5): 2.

Strong-Boag, V. (1979). "Canada's Women Doctors: Feminism Constrained." In *A Not Unreasonable Claim: Women and Reform in Canada*, edited by L. Kealey, 109–129. Toronto: Women's Press.

Tomblin M., G.L. O'Brien-Pallas, C. Alksnis, S. Birch, G. Kephart, M. Pennock, D. Pringle, I. Rootman, and S. Wang. (2003). "Health Human Resources Planning: An Examination of Relationships among Nursing Service Utilization, an Estimate of Population Health and Overall Health Status Outcomes in the Province of Ontario." Available on-line at www.chsrf.ca/final_research/ogc/pdf/tomblin_final.pdf.

Valentine, P.E. (1996). "Nursing: A Ghettoized Profession Relegated to Women's Sphere." *International Journal of Nursing Studies* 33(1): 98–106.

Wajcman, J. (1991). "Patriarchy, Technology, and Conceptions of Skill." *Work and Occupations* 18(1): 29–45.

Wardwell, W.I. (1981). "Chiropractors: Challengers of Medical Dominance." *Research in the Sociology of Health Care* 2: 207–250.

Willis, E. (1989). *Medical Dominance: The Division of Labour in the Australian Health Care System*, 2nd ed. Sydney: George Allen and Unwin.

Notes

1. Although no medical schools in Canada were closed as a result of this review, several schools in the U.S. were recommended for closure, primarily those for women and ethnic and visible minorities.

2. It is important to note that there were also racial dimensions to the exclusion of particular forms of care (i.e., Aboriginal healers); albeit important, it is beyond the scope of this discussion here, which is focused on the evolving "official" health care division of labour.

3. The terms "general practice," "family physicians," and "primary care physicians" are treated synonymously here, although there are some distinctions between entry to practice requirements for each of these.
4. Available on-line at www3.uta.edu/sswtech/sapvc/information/teens13_15/Teens_(ages13-15)_Glossary.htm.
5. "The Profitization of Social Services: Where Do We Set Limits on a Market-Driven Social Service System?" Available on-line at www.catholiccharitiesusa.org/news/opinion/2000/profitization.htm.
6. Available on-line at www.answers.com/privatization.
7. Rationalization is the organization of a business according to scientific principles of management in order to increase efficiency. Available on-line at www.answers.com/rationalization&r=67.

• •

Critical Thinking Questions

1. How has the rationalization of the health care division of labour differentially affected the medical profession versus predominantly female health professions such as nursing?
2. Why do you think so many health human resource policies deal with the issue of *supply*?
3. What is the difference between *rationalizing* and *rationing* when it comes to health care?
4. What might be some of the problems in transferring policies created to solve problems in the American health care system to Canada?
5. What is the impact of the profit motive on the provision of health care in Canada and the United States?

Further Readings

Armstrong, P., and H. Armstrong. (2002). *Wasting Away: The Undermining of Canadian Health Care*, 2nd ed. Toronto: Oxford University Press.
This text provides an excellent description of the development of the health care system and recent reforms to it. Particularly useful for this topic are Chapter 3, "Who Provides: The Institutions," and Chapter 4, "Who Provides: The People."

Armstrong, P., H. Armstrong, I.L. Bourgeault, J. Choinière, J. Lexchin, E. Mykhalovskiy, S. Peters, and J. White. (2003). "Market Principles, Business

Practices and Health Care: Comparing the U.S. and Canadian Experiences."
International Journal of Canadian Studies 28: 13–38.
This article provides a critical comparison of the provision of care in Canada
and the United States.

Barer, M.L., and G. Stoddart. (1991). *Toward Integrated Medical Resource
Policies for Canada.* Winnipeg: Manitoba Ministry of Health.
This provides an excellent summary of the state of the health care division of
labour at the time. It is also a key document in the literature on health human
resources highlighting the importance of integrated policy.

Coburn, D., G. Torrance, and J. Kaufert. (1983). "Medical Dominance in Canada
in Historical Perspective: The Rise and Fall of Medicine?" *International Journal
of Health Services* 13: 407–432.
This is a classic reading on the history of the Canadian medical profession.

Light, D.W., and I. Bourgeault, eds. (2004). "Health and Health Care in the
United States: Origins and Dynamics." Special Issue of the *Journal of Health
and Social Behavior.*
This special issue contain original essays by scholars showing how sociological
concepts and research can help us to better understand the American health
care system. Each paper analyzes how past or current theories or explanations
need to be changed, and each outlines the most promising directions for future
research.

Relevant Web Sites

Canadian Health Services Research Foundation, Health Human Resources
www.chsrf.ca/research_themes/hhr_e.php
   This includes a variety of reports from CHSRF-funded research on this
issue.

Canadian Institute for Health Information
http://secure.cihi.ca/cihiweb/dispPage.jsp?cw_page=AR_35_E
   In November 2001, CIHI released a special report entitled *Canada's Health
Care Providers.* This report presents a fact-based compilation of current
research, historical trends and data, findings, and analysis on what we know
and don't know about Canada's health care providers as a foundation for
understanding some of today's most critical and complex issues in health
care.

Canadian Policy Research Networks: Health Human Resource Planning
www.cprn.org/en/theme.cfm?theme=39
   In 2002, CPRN released *Health Human Resource Planning in Canada:
Physician and Nursing Work Force Issues, a Summary Report,* prepared

for the Commission on the Future of Health Care in Canada (the Romanow Commission).

This report cites a number of barriers to implementation of reform, including the historic separation of health human resource planning from other health system issues.

Health Canada: Health Human Resources
www.hc-sc.gc.ca/hppb/healthcare/health_resources.htm

This site brings together materials addressing a range of health human resources issues, including physician supply, medical licensure, and mobility and training of health service providers.

Human Resources for Health
www.human-resources-health.com/home/

This is an open access, peer-reviewed, on-line journal covering all aspects of planning, producing, and managing the health workforce—all those who provide health services worldwide. It is edited by Orvill Adams, director of the World Health Organization's Department of Human Resources for Health.

Glossary

Deinstitutionalization: The movement of care from institutional to community-based settings, including the home; it is often used to refer to the movement of institutionalized people, particularly mental health patients.

Health care division of labour: All of the various groups of providers who interact in the provision of health care to a specified population.

Managed care: The provision of health services through a single point of entry and formal enrolment where patient care is managed to ensure an emphasis on quality preventive and primary care, a reduction in inappropriate use of services, control of costs, and management of risk. It does so through closely monitoring and controlling the decisions of health care providers.

Privatization: The process of transferring property from public ownership to private ownership and/or transferring the management of a service or activity from the government to the private sector.[6]

Profitization: A form of privatization that gives primacy to profit ahead of individual and community need.

Rationalization: In the context of the health care division of labour, it is the process of assigning tasks to the "most appropriate" health care provider and an overall focus on the most efficient use of health care human resources, with the implicit or explicit purpose of controlling rising health care costs.[7]

Rationing: The process of apportioning care according to some plan; rationing of care comes in a variety of forms, including more implicit, upstream forms of rationing, or *macro*allocation, which include government policy, funding decisions, and distribution of services; and the more explicit, downstream rationing, or *micro*allocation, which occurs at patients' bedside.

PART IV
....

CRITICAL ISSUES IN HEALTH, ILLNESS, AND HEALTH CARE

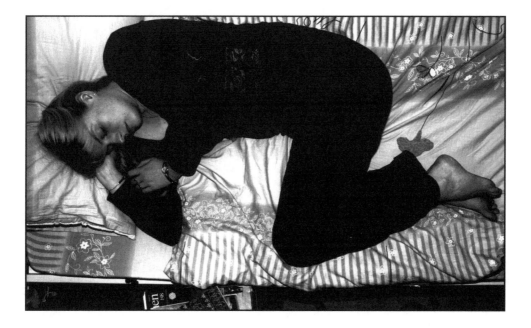

This section explores some of the current issues in health care. Politicians and the public perceive a health care crisis usually defined in terms of long waiting lists for treatment or a shortage of general practitioners in either urban or rural areas. While these are important issues, also of importance are more difficult to define issues of how and why different groups are treated differently by the health care system, how health care professionals and the public understand illness and disability, and the appropriate and most effective response to such issues.

Also of great importance is the role that political and economic forces play in the treatment of disease and illness. The issue of pharmaceuticals—the drugs used to treat illness and disease—is a potent example of such influences. And the understandings that citizens have concerning the sources of health and disease are critical in that they both reflect and contribute to the emphasis societies place on providing living conditions that support health versus emphasis upon curative medical care provided by health care professionals. The chapters in this section address these issues and illustrate the value of each of the broad approaches to understanding health, illness, and health care in Canadian society.

In Chapter 12, Pat Armstrong explores the centrality of gender to understanding and delivering health care. The centrality of gender recognizes women as the primary caregivers both within their families and in the health care system. She illustrates this concept with nurses' experiences as workers and caregivers. She also examines gender as a determinant of health and why health and health care are women's issues. It is also important to consider differences among women. She explores the differences in health care treatments administered to men and women, differences in symptoms, experiences, and outcomes. Armstrong identifies the gaps in understanding that result from failing to apply a gendered analysis to health care issues.

In Chapter 13, Marcia Rioux and Tamara Daly examine different theoretical approaches to understanding disability and illness and how social structures determine how professionals and the public construct disability. In particular, they discuss how disability is experienced by women, as an experience associated with aging, and by those living in different parts of Canada. The authors consider critical appraisals of the disability adjusted life years (DALYs) measurement concept, which is compared with statistical analyses of people's experiences of disability or illness.

They also consider some ethical and legal issues related to disability and examine the role played by the Canadian Charter of Rights and Freedoms in ensuring the equality of disabled people.

In Chapter 14, Joel Lexchin examines the tensions between corporate and public health viewpoints in relation to pharmaceutical issues in Canada. He is especially concerned about the drug regulatory system in Canada and the differing priorities of those producing the drugs and those who may benefit from them. Lexchin explores the industry's promotion of medications and considers the relation of these activities to rising drug costs that threaten the viability of the health care system. The author also considers how the patent system influences drug spending, the interactions between Health Canada and the pharmaceutical industry, and the effects of recent trade agreements upon these issues.

In Chapter 15, Dennis Raphael and Toba Bryant examine public health approaches in Canada, the U.S., the United Kingdom, and Sweden. Despite three decades of Canadian government and public health statements on the importance of broader determinants of health, governmental and public health practice—with a few notable exceptions—is firmly focused on behavioural approaches to health promotion. In the U.S., there is virtually no penetration of broader concepts of health into public health discourse or practice, which is firmly focused on assuring access to health care and individual risk factor management. In the U.K., the government's systematic efforts are addressing determinants of health inequalities with early evidence of effectiveness. In Sweden, broader approaches to public health are firmly established and represent a continuation of Swedish approaches to public policy that ensure equitable distribution of resources among the population.

In the concluding chapter, Toba Bryant, Dennis Raphael, and Marcia Rioux outline future directions for health research and practice. The key themes they identify that emerge from the contributions to this volume include the definition of the field of health studies, models of understanding health, illness, and health care, power and influence, the importance of public policy, and public versus private governance, among others. Bryant, Raphael, and Rioux emphasize the importance of developing and applying innovative theoretical and conceptual approaches to the health field that draw upon principles of justice, equity, and democratic participation.

CHAPTER TWELVE

. . . .

GENDER, HEALTH, AND CARE

Pat Armstrong

. . . .

Learning Objectives

At the conclusion of this chapter, the reader will be able to
- understand the centrality of gender to understanding and delivering health care
- review how gender has been considered as a determinant of health
- consider the specific example of nurses' experiences as workers and caregivers
- examine health and health care issues specific to women
- show the gaps in understanding that result from failing to apply a gendered analysis to health care issues

---

Introduction

Health care is profoundly gendered. Women and men use the health care system differently and are treated differently once they enter it. Women also provide the overwhelming majority of care, although they are a minority of those in positions of power within health care services and policy organizations. As a result, many health care reforms and government reforms more generally have a different impact on women and men.

Bodies, and ideas about bodies, contribute to these patterns. However, neither bodies nor ideas about them can provide an adequate explanation for the unequal distribution of care work and the treatment women receive in health care. Policies, practices, and structures all contribute to these patterns that put the burden of care on women while often failing to respond to their needs or provide access to appropriate care.

But these policies and practices are not simply neutral or evidence-based. For feminist political economists, profits, power, contradictions, and inequalities frame the conditions for health and care. Contexts are critical, as are relations not only between women and men but also between employers and employees, among household members and racialized groups, to name only some of the many that matter.

This chapter begins by explaining why a focus on women is critical to understanding and improving health care. It then looks at women's access to care and at the treatment they receive in care. It explores the ways reforms in health care are simultaneously working to provide more appropriate care and limiting women's access to care. The final sections examine women's care work, both paid and unpaid. While women have struggled hard to make health care work both visible and valued, their gains are rapidly being undermined by reforms that shift care to the home and redefine what is paid work in care.

Why Women?

All populations are gendered. Of course, other social locations linked to age, culture, income, disability, and racialization—to name only some—also matter. But these, too, are divided by gender, intersecting with other social and physical locations. Being gender-sensitive means much more than analyzing data by sex; it means recognizing how gender shapes and is shaped by conditions, practices, and relations, including relations of markets, of power, and of inequality. It means as well how gender intersects with other locations. A gendered analysis in health and health care requires the assessment of causes, processes, and consequences by gender, "taking into account the context of individual's lives" (DesMeules, Turner, and Cho 2003a: 2). The impact may be contradictory for women, simultaneously or alternatively improving and challenging their health and capacity to provide care. And the impact may vary among women, depending on their location.

Not surprisingly, much of the gender-sensitive research and policy in Canada has focused on women. It is not surprising because it was the women's movement that began demonstrating how gender and assumptions about gender permeate policy and practice, and do so in ways that assume male norms, standards, and subjects. The consequences of what Karen Messing (1998) has called "One-Eyed Science" are particularly harmful for women. As the authors of *The Politics of Women's Health* put it, medicine has played "an active role in perpetuating some aspects of women's oppression while helping to reduce other dimensions" (Sherwin et al. 1998: 6). Inequalities perpetuated by such structural factors as differential access to education, income, benefits, and personal security along with the organization of paid work and of the professions, the absence of public day care, and limited public transit play important roles as well. More women than men are poor and fewer women than men have access to the kinds of resources that provide them with choices (Desmeules et al. 2003b). In other words, the causes, processes, and consequences of health care are not only different for women and men. They also contribute to inequality both between women and men and among women.

It is also not surprising that such analysis focused on women because in Canada, at least more than 80 percent of paid care providers are women and women account for a similar proportion of those providing unpaid care in the home and community (Armstrong et al. 2002a). As women moved into the labour force, they became more vocal not only about the nature and conditions of this work, but also about the negative consequences of the gender assumptions imbedded in them. And women use the health care system more than men, and in different ways than men, further contributing to their activism. For example, although women's rate of hospitalization has been decreasing, it is consistently 20 percent higher than that of men (DesMeules, Turner, and Cho 2003b). This is the case even though hospitalization is less likely for women than for men with chronic conditions such as diabetes, asthma, and drug dependency. Women, however, are more likely than men to experience severe disability (DesMeules, Turner, and Cho 2003b). The use of emergency varies as well. Until age 15, there are more male visits to emergency, but then women's visits rise significantly above those for men until the mid-forties, when visits by men once again outnumber those by women (CIHI 2004c). Moreover, it is women who take care of the children and often the elderly as well. Thus, health and health care have clearly emerged as women's issues and women have played an active role in revealing how gender matters. This effort to have gender taken into account in ways that serve women has not been an easy process, however, and is far from complete.

Does this mean that gender-sensitive research is just about women, and serves only their interests? Although gender-sensitive analysis emerged within and from the women's movement, it has neither excluded men nor been irrelevant to men. Indeed, much of the research intended to demonstrate the importance of gender required comparative data on women and men. Moreover, a great deal of health behaviour, of health care, and of other health processes involves relations between women and men, a fact not lost on those beginning from a women's perspective. Power relations in particular have played a major role in the analysis, with an emphasis on the subordination shared by most women. It should be noted, however, that gender-sensitive research is not necessarily comparative. It can study women or men without searching for comparisons or emphasizing gender relations. Yet even those who have been most concerned with women's issues and who see women as subordinate in terms of both health and care recognize that strategies for change cannot be developed in many areas without understanding what is happening with men. Perhaps more critically, this women's research developed many of the tools of analysis that allow us to see gendered causes, consequences, processes, and contexts. What works for women does not necessarily work for men, just as what works for men does not necessarily work for women. In fact, that is a major point of gender-sensitive research.

It was evidence and pressure from the women's movement that led Canada to adopt a federal plan for gender equality in 1995, a plan that requires legislation and policy to include an analysis of the potential for differential impacts on women and men. Canada has also established a Women's Health Bureau within Health Canada, a Centres of Excellence Programme for Women's Health, and a Canadian Women's Health Network. Materials produced by these agencies and groups can be found at www.cewh-cesf.ca or www.cwhn.ca. To find the publications of the Coordinating Group on Health Care Reform and Women, click on "Health Reform."

All these initiatives were based on the recognition that gender differences are critical in health and care; and that women were often excluded from research and treated inappropriately in practice. All include gender-sensitive research, policy, and practice in their mandate. Most recently, the federal government has funded a Canadian Institute of Health Research Institute of Gender and Health with a mandate "to support research to address how sex and gender interact with other factors that influence health to create conditions and problems that are unique, more prevalent, more serious or different with respect to risk factors or effective interventions for women and men" (Health Canada 2003: 7). In short, it is devoted to research that focuses on either women or men, or each in relation to the other. The Institute of Gender and Health (2003) has funded research on men's issues such as hormone treatment for prostrate cancer, the service needs of elderly gay men, and Black men's experience of violence, as well as many comparative projects such as the role of women and men in unpaid caregiving.

Health Canada now recognizes 12 distinct determinants of health, having expanded the list beyond biological and genetic endowments to include gender. Even the traditional focus on reproductive health is shifting. The range of sex issues is understood to be much broader and biology is increasingly understood as influenced by social contexts while gender is used to draw particular attention to the social construction of female/male differences.

The inclusion of gender as a health determinant marks a major advance. However, it is equally important to examine how gender pervades all the other determinants. Income and social status, employment and education, physical environments and social environments, social support networks and healthy child development, personal health practices and coping skills, culture and health services are all gendered. Too often, however, gender and sex are considered independent variables, while gender is controlled for and thus eliminated from the examination of other health determinants. And too often gender is left to the women's centres, with the rest getting on with what they regard as the real scientific or policy work. The other 12 Institutes for Health Research do not make gender a central concern, in spite of the federal policy, which should cover such federally funded programs. Equally important, the global, national, regional, and local political economies that set the conditions for care are too often ignored, as are differences linked to other social locations such as race.

The Report of the Royal Commission on the Future of Health Care in Canada (Romanow 2002), more popularly known as the Romanow Report, provides an example of both why women should be a focus and the failure to provide a gender-sensitive analysis. This report was prepared after the federal policy requiring a gender-sensitive analysis was in place.

Box 12.1: The Romanow Report: What Does It Mean for Women?

We applaud Romanow for demonstrating the sustainability of Medicare. A publicly funded system delivered through non-profit services is crucial for all women in Canada. But like other reports on health care reform in the last decade, this report fails to recognize the significant ways in which health care is an issue for women. Women are 80% of paid health care providers, a similar proportion of those providing unpaid personal care and a majority of those receiving care, especially among the elderly.

The sustainability of the system is not just about finances—it's about women's work. As paid workers women provide medical, nursing and diagnostic care as well as cleaning, cooking and laundry services that are essential determinants of health in the delivery of care. By drawing a distinction between "direct" and "ancillary" health care services, Romanow ignores the skilled nature of women's paid work and their contributions to care. Moreover, he fails to make recommendations to address the deteriorating conditions women face in providing care.

Women also sustain the system as unpaid health care providers. Romanow's report fails to adequately address the full range of home care women provide, especially long-term and chronic care. While he reports "that caregiving is becoming an increasing burden on many in our society, especially women," his recommendation for caregiver leave through the Employment Insurance Program will not benefit the many women who do not have forms of paid work that would make them eligible for such leave.

Romanow recognizes gender as a determinant of health. He also offers valuable recommendations for primary health care reform that could benefit women, but only if attention is paid to women's particular needs. Finally, although women constitute up to 3/4 of those in long-term care facilities, the report is virtually silent on these services.

Sustaining an efficient, affordable and effective health care system must mean sustaining women in providing and receiving care. Like Romanow, we agree that "we need more than rhetoric; we need action." *We need to make the health care system work for women.*

Source: National Coordinating Group on Health Care Reform and Women, The Centres of Excellence for Women's Health Program, November 28, 2002. Available on-line at www.cewh-cesf.ca/healthreform/news/releases.html.

Our National Coordinating Group on Health Care Reform and Women has provided a detailed gender-sensitive analysis of this report (Armstrong et al. 2002b). I want to highlight just one aspect here, the human resources question. I am drawing on both my own research and the analysis undertaken by the Coordinating Group.

Although several presentations at the commission's public hearings stressed the importance of providing such an analysis, the report considers gender only in relation to home care. And even then, the excessive burdens on women are mentioned, but not addressed in the recommendations.

Yet the report stresses the very high illness and injury rate among health care providers and the "decline in morale" apparent in health services (Romanow 2002: 96). Indeed, health care has emerged as a high-risk industry and nursing has emerged as the most dangerous occupation (CIHI 2001). The report considers this issue without mentioning that more than 9 out of 10 registered nurses are women and more than 80 percent of other categories of nurses. Why is this relevant?

Because nurses are women, we now have a majority who are over age 40 (CIHI 2003). This has never happened before because they are women. Until this generation of nurses, women were forced to leave when they got married, and somewhat later they were allowed to stay in their jobs after marriage, but had to leave when they became pregnant. As a result, nurses in the past were either young or single and senior, with the senior nurses much less likely to undertake regular bedside care. Nevertheless nursing work organization often still assumes young, fit women are doing the bedside care. Indeed, the workload in this very physically demanding job has increased along with the age of the nurses.

Because nurses are women, we have not understood the work as physically demanding in the same way we see much of men's labour as physically demanding. This, too, contributes to the failure to develop policies that adequately take these demands into account. Women have often been loath to stress the physical demands because they were trying to establish nursing as a profession and because they did not want to appear as weak females.

Because nurses are women, they feel responsible and are held responsible for care. New managerial strategies designed to shorten patient hospital stays and provide more care on an out-patient basis have dramatically increased the pace of nursing work. The result is not only a speed-up in the work but also a severe reduction in the time available to provide the kind of care nurses have learned to provide. Nurses tell us they still scramble to make up for the care deficit and they are expected to do so. The expectations they have of themselves and that others have of them are directly linked to gendered assumptions of nursing work (Armstrong et al. 2000).

Because nurses are women, many of the skills are assumed to come naturally. In practice, many of the skills are learned informally from other women in the process of doing the work. Such learning takes time as well as effort, but the time for continual learning interchange is disappearing as the focus on measurable tasks increases.

Finally, because they are women they are doing more than one job. When they go home at night, they take up very similar work in the household. Increasingly, they are looking after family, friends, and relatives who need home care. The pressure to provide the care that is being sent home is particularly heavy on women with nursing experience.

In short, older nurses are working much harder at a double or triple shift in ways that make them more vulnerable to illness and injury. The high rates of illness and injury are not only a concern to nurses but also to their patients and to the system as a whole. Injury and illness cost us all. If the absenteeism rate of RNs were reduced to that of all other workers, the equivalent of almost 5,500 more would be at work full-time each year (CIHI 2001). Gender is a critical component in understanding the increases and thus in addressing these outcomes. Indeed, gender is critical to understanding health care, reforms, and consequences.

Box 12.2: Medication and Women

"Women respond to certain drugs differently from men, use more medications than men, and are more likely to experience adverse drug reactions."

This underscores the need for targeted studies to understand these gender differences and identify ways to improve the safety of medication use in women, as described in the January/February 2005 Special Issue of the *Journal of Women's Health* 14(1), a peer-reviewed journal published by Mary Ann Liebert, Inc. (www.liebertpub.com). The entire issue is available free on-line at www.liebertonline.com/toc/jwh/14/1;jsessionid=jBJw7TQTGmDe.

Accessible, Appropriate Care

There is little dispute that men and women have different health care needs, at least when it comes to reproductive aspects of their health. The issue is how gender does and should matter in understanding causes, processes, treatments, and consequences. Until recently, research on women has focused primarily on breasts and babies, and women's health has been defined primarily in these terms. Women have too often been treated in ways that not only equate them with their reproductive capacities but that also limit their power.

Women have struggled with some success to gain control over their reproductive health. Midwifery provides a particularly good example. As Benoit (1991) points out, midwifery has a varied history across Canada and was never completely eliminated in Aboriginal and remote communities, in spite of pressure from both nurses and doctors. Although often idealized, "the difficulties of 'independent' practice in the past far outweighed any social prestige they achieved during their careers" (Benoit 1991: 98). The revival of midwifery in the last quarter of the 20th century was not only about women resisting the medical takeover of birth and the desire to restore women's control over the birth process. It was also about redefining midwifery to fit with current knowledge and to gain acceptance as health professionals for those providing women-centred care based on health rather than illness models.

After considerable effort, midwives have been integrated into health systems across Canada and are offering women alternatives to medicalized care, yet "5 provinces/territories have no midwifery legislation or funding, 2 provinces have legislated midwifery but have not provided funding, and Quebec does not sanction homebirth, making this safe and inexpensive option nearly impossible for women who want reliable care" (Hawkins and Knox 2003: 1). Thus, the midwifery alternative remains beyond the reach of the many who do not have the money to pay for this care and for those in regions of the country where midwifery is not a regulated profession.

Meanwhile, fewer family physicians now provide obstetrical care. Family physicians are more likely than specialists to know their patients and less likely to use interventionist techniques, practices made evident in recent research showing a significant rise in the number of Caesarian births accompanying this increasing specialist care (CIHI 2004a, 2004b). In other words, for a growing number of women, childbirth is treated as a medical event in spite of the reintroduction of midwifery.

But the question of appropriate treatment is much larger than childbirth or reproductive matters more generally. Too often, other aspects of health have been treated as if they were the same for both sexes (Laurence and Weinhouse 1997). Research is much more likely to be carried out on men and the evidence thus gathered is assumed to apply to women. Searching for the same symptoms in women often means women's illnesses are treated as merely female complaints or imaginary problems while providing the same treatment for women as for men may be harmful to their health. The consequence of leaving women out of the research and analyzing data by sex has frequently been inappropriate care for women and greater costs to the system resulting from poor diagnosis.

Gender-sensitive analysis has made a difference in some treatments for women. Cardiovascular disease (CVD) provides a good example. A case study is developed in some detail in Health Canada's recent publication *Exploring Concepts of Gender and Health* (Health Canada 2003) and is worth summarizing briefly here.

As this study points out, until the last decade, the overwhelming majority of research in CVD was done on men, both because it was assumed this was a men's disease and because it was assumed that what was true for men was true for women. The initial Aspirin trials, for instance, were done on men, and then Aspirin was prescribed to both women and men. Yet more recent research has demonstrated that Aspirin is not effective for this indication in women. Research over the last five years has also shown that the causes and risk factors are different for women and men. For instance,

- men suffer heart disease at an earlier age than women
- high blood pressure is two to three times more common in women
- while high levels of bad cholesterol are a risk factor for men, low levels of good cholesterol are a bigger risk factor for women
- diabetes is a greater risk factor for women than for men
- women and men have different smoking patterns and activity patterns

The causes and risks differ by racialized groups, income, and culture as well. Aboriginal women are more likely than their male counterparts to develop diabetes and are more likely than other women to die from heart disease.

Research has also shown that the processes of the disease and the treatment differ by gender. For instance,

- women are more likely to have subtle symptoms of heart attack, such as indigestion, abdominal or mid-back pain, nausea, and vomiting
- women are less likely than men to be offered invasive procedures and clot-buster medicine
- women are less likely to be hospitalized, but stay longer than men when they do enter the hospital
- between 80 and 90 percent of heart transplant recipients are male

Research indicates different consequences as well.

- women are more likely to have a second heart attack within six months
- women fare less well after heart surgery

And, finally, and at least as significantly, research indicates that the context of women's lives differs from those of men in ways that influence their likelihood of suffering from cardiovascular disease, of being treated for the disease, and of surviving the disease.

As a result of such gender-sensitive research, protocols are changing. New guidelines are developing for treatment that may well start to show up in outcomes. There is a move beyond thinking about gender differences simply in terms of reproductive issues to the inclusion of other biological processes. Some of the social factors that contribute to differences in health and care are being considered, such as the different reasons why young men and women take up smoking. These gender-sensitive strategies can mean not only more equal and appropriate treatment and outcomes; they can mean cost savings as well.

But there is still a long way to go before gender sensitivity is a feature of practice. A 1998 article in the *Canadian Medical Association Journal* reported that "women were poorly represented in the randomized control trials" in their sample of leading medical journal articles on myocardial infarction, "regardless of whether the trials were funded by an agency with a gender-related policy" (Rochon et al. 1998: 321). An even more recent article linked to CVD featured on the Web site for the Ontario Institute for Clinical Evaluative Sciences makes "adjustments for age and sex differences" to groups of patients, thus eliminating gender as a category for analysis (McAlister et al. 2000: 405).

Moreover, the emphasis remains on biology, albeit an expanded notion of biology, in spite of the fact that the recent *Women's Health Surveillance Report* suggests that context, relations, and behaviour are critical to understanding differences (DesMeules et al. 2003a). Significant gaps remain even in this CVD research and the new emphasis on a broader notion of sex differences may be more a reflection of the growing interest in genetic research than it is of a commitment to gender-sensitive research in all aspects of policy. And research into many areas provides no analysis of the specificity of women and men's diseases.

Thus, research that recognizes not only physical differences but also how these differences are shaped by environments and relations are characterized by inequality is essential. So is education for practitioners on these differences. However, the move to apply managerial techniques taken from the for-profit sector can challenge this recognition. Strategies are designed to increase managerial control over providers, in large measure by standardizing treatment protocols and the timing of care. For example, care pathways that set out to describe and prescribe the trajectory for an illness implies sameness rather than difference. Indeed, the intent is to make the treatment of each person and the timing of the care as similar as possible. As feminists have long pointed out, same treatment does not necessarily mean equitable treatment because it fails to take into account both differences among groups of people in different social locations and the specificity of individual lives.

These examples of research and practice are concerned with appropriate care. But even appropriate care needs to be accessible. The introduction of universal public health care in Canada for hospital and doctor services made a tremendous difference in access for marginalized groups. The Canada Health Act clearly states that provinces and territories must work to eliminate financial or other barriers to such care. And these governments initially did make significant progress in this direction. The number of doctors and hospitals grew and fees for these medically necessary services were virtually eliminated. Obviously these developments were important for women, given that they use the system more than men and that they are responsible for taking care of children and many of the elderly. Equally important, many more women than men lack the resources with which to purchase care or the workplace health coverage that could pay for their care. Of course, barriers remained and marginalized groups were still at a disadvantage especially in terms of services and treatments such as medications, tests, and homemaking not covered by the Canada Health Act. Nevertheless, public health insurance did significantly improve access to care for marginalized groups.

Reforms over the last decade have been reversing this trend, however. Patients are sent home from hospital quicker and sicker or they never stay at all because they have day surgery and out-patient care. The Canada Health Act ensures that all necessary drugs, tests, treatments, and personnel are provided without fees within hospitals, but as soon as patients leave the hospital, fees can be charged. And as soon as fees are charged, there are two kinds of services and significant differences in access to care. Money then plays an important role in both access and quality. The marginalized often end up with poorer care and less care or no care. Provinces and territories have also been delisting services, treatments, and drugs. Removing them from coverage under the public plan has even greater consequences for the marginalized because then the entire costs must be assumed by individuals or families. As Guruge, Donner, and Morrison (2000: 235) point out about immigrant families, paying for rent and food must take priority over paying for prescriptions, tests, therapy, or long-term institutional care.

Following a for-profit business model, governments across Canada have also been consolidating services into giant hospitals and closing small community ones. Many more women than men rely on public transport. And many more women than men have limited mobility because they have to care for children and others at home. Centralized services take people out of their social support networks, placing them far from those who provide daily connections. With centralization, then, women in particular have difficulty travelling to these centres to get care or provide care for friends and relatives, but the consequences are felt by both women and men.

A gender-sensitive analysis is equally absent from the Romanow Report's discussion of the rest of the health care labour force. The report separates ancillary services from direct health care services, suggesting that it is appropriate to contract out such services as cleaning, cooking, and laundry for delivery by for-profit concerns because quality is "relatively easy to judge" and "competitors in the same business" could provide appropriate ancillary services (Romanow 2002: 6). No evidence is provided to support the claim that quality is evident or that such work in health care is equivalent to similar work in other sectors. A gender-sensitive analysis might come to different conclusions.

Like nursing, cleaning, cooking, and laundry work are female-dominated jobs long associated with skills that come with the genitalia. Cleaning, cooking, and laundry seem like jobs any woman can do, but we may be ignoring the hidden gender assumptions at our peril. British research is starting to show how important these services are to care and how the quality tends to decline with privatization. The U.K. House of Commons Health Select Committee (1999) warned that "the often spurious division of staff into clinical or non-clinical groups can create an institutional apartheid which might be detrimental to staff morale and to patients" (quoted in Sachdev 2001: 33). In Taiwan, the Center for Disease control has argued that the outsourcing of nursing aides, cleaners, and laundry workers contributed to the transmission of SARS in that country (Chen 2003).

Equally important, these strategies tend to exacerbate gender equality. Again we need to rely on the U.K. because Canada is just introducing these strategies. Case studies in the United Kingdom and Northern Ireland "found that exposure to tendering led to the, often dramatic, erosion of terms and conditions of employment.... Estimates state that some 40 per cent of the NHS ancillary jobs were lost" (Sachdev 2001: 5). Moreover, the impact on women was more extensive, resulting in a widening of the gender gap. According to the Equal Opportunities Commission of Northern Ireland (1996), most work contracted out was female-dominated. The rate of female job loss was more than double that of men. While both women and men experienced wage reductions, the proportionate reduction was larger for women. Some benefits disappeared, along with some entitlements. There are new rules under the European Union designed to address some of these consequences, but I would suggest that a gender-sensitive analysis before the fact could prevent them from developing in the first place. A lower court refused to hear a case against the government in British Columbia that argued such a strategy for ancillary workers discriminates against women, although U.K. evidence suggests this is likely to be the case. Under the North American Free Trade Agreement (NAFTA), once privatized, these services will be difficult to bring back into the public sector or even to make subject to new rules such as those in the E.U. The Canadian Supreme Court has granted leave to appeal this B.C. case, leaving the possibility that more recent Canadian evidence will establish the claim for women and health (Cohen 2003; Hospital Employees' Union 2005).

Box 12.3: Benefits of a Gender-Sensitive Approach

Gender-sensitive research, policy and practice can:
- lead to more effective disease prevention and health promotion strategies
- encourage more appropriate treatment
- help produce better outcomes
- contribute to more equal treatment for women and men
- save money both in the short and long term

Conclusions

There are moral reasons, effectiveness reasons, and financial reasons for gender-sensitive research, policy, and practice, but it is much easier in theory and even in research than in practice. As the Romanow Report makes clear, health and care are about values and about global political/economic pressures. Policy and practices reflect not only old ways of doing and new evidence, they also reflect power and political choices. In Canada we have made some tentative moves toward gender-sensitive policy and practices, but we still have a very long way to go before we can claim gender-sensitive health care.

References

Armstrong, P., H. Armstrong, I. Bourgeault, J. Choinière, E. Mykhalovskiy, and J.P. White. (2000). *"Heal Thyself"*: *Managing Health Care Reform*. Aurora: Garamond.

Armstrong, P., C. Amaratunga, J. Bernier, K. Grant, A. Pederson, and K. Willson. (2002a). *Exposing Privatization*: *Women and Health Care Reform in Canada*. Aurora: Garamond.

Armstrong, P., M. Boscoe, B. Clow, K. Grant, A. Pederson, and K. Willson. (2002b). *Reading Romanow*. Ottawa: Canadian Women's Health Network.

Benoit, C. (1991). *Midwives in Passage*. St. John's: Institute for Social and Economic Research.

Canadian Institute for Health Information (CIHI). (2001). *Canada's Health Care Providers*. Ottawa: Canadian Institute for Health Information

_____. (2003). *Workforce Trends of Registered Nurses in Canada*. Ottawa: Canadian Institute for Health Information.

_____. (2004a). *The Evolving Role of Canada's Family Physicians: 1992–2001*. Ottawa: Canadian Institute for Health Information.

_____. (2004b). *Giving Birth in Canada*: *Providers of Maternity and Infant Care*. Ottawa: Canadian Institute for Health Information.

_____. (2004c). "Number of Visits by Gender and 5 Year Age Groups." Available on-line at www.qstat.cihi.ca/discovered4i/view, 04-11-30.

Chen, M. (2003). "Outsourcing Played a Role in Ourbreaks: CDC Head" *Taipei Times*. Available on-line at www.tapeitimes.com/chnews/2003/06/10/story.

Cohen, M.G. (2003). *Destroying Pay Equity*: *The Effects of Privatizing Health Care in British Columbia*. Report prepared for the Hospital Employees' Union, Vancouver, B.C.

DesMeules, M., D. Stewart, A. Kazanjian, H. McLean, J. Payne, and B. Vissandjée. (2003a). *Women's Health Surveillance Report*. Ottawa: Health Canada and Canadian Institute for Health Information.

DesMeules, M., L. Turner, and R. Cho. (2003b). "Morbidity Experiences and Disability among Canadian Women." In *Women's Health Surveillance Report*, edited by M. DesMeules et al., 1–14. Ottawa: Health Canada and Canadian Institute for Health Information.

Equal Opportunities Commission of Northern Ireland. (1996). *Report on the Formal Investigation into Competitive Tendering in Health and Education Services in Northern Ireland*. Belfast: Equal Opportunities Commission of Northern Ireland.

Guruge, S., G.J. Donner, and L. Morrison. (2000). "The Impact of Canadian Health Care Reform on Recent Women Immigrants and Refugees." In *Care and Consequences*: *The Impact of Health Care Reform*, edited by D.L. Gustafson, 62–88. Halifax: Fernwood.

Hawkins, M., and S. Knox. (2003). "Midwifery Care Continues to Face Challenges. Canadian Midwifery Is Still Defining Itself, One Mother at a Time." *Network Magazine* 6(2/3): 1–3.

Health Canada. (2003). *Exploring Concepts of Gender and Health*. Ottawa: Health Canada.

Hospital Employees' Union. (2005). "Supreme Court of Canada to Hear Charter Challenge to Campbell Liberals' Contract-Breaking Law." News release, April 21.

Institute of Gender and Health. (2003). *Annual Report of Activities 2001-2002*. Ottawa: Institute of Gender and Health.

Laurence, L., and B. Weinhouse. (1997). *Outrageous Practice: How Gender Bias Threatens Women's Health*. New Brunswick: Rutgers University Press.

McAlister, F.A., A.M. O'Connor, G. Wells, S.A. Grover, and A. Laupacis. (2000). "Why Should Hypertension be Treated? The Different Perspectives of Canadian Family Physicians and Patienrs." *Canadian Medical Association Journal* 163(4) (August 22): 403–408.

Messing, K. (1998). *One-Eyed Science: Occupational Health and Women Workers*. Philadelphia: Temple University Press.

Rochon, P.A., et al. (1998). "Reporting of Gender-Related Information in Clinical Trials of Drug Therapy for Myocardial Infarction." *Canadian Medical Association Journal* 159(4): 321–327.

Romanow, R.J. (2002). *Building on Values: The Future of Health Care in Canada*. Saskatoon: Commission on the Future of Health Care in Canada.

Sachdev, S. (2001). "Contracting Culture: From CCT to PPPs" *The Private Provision of Public Services and the Impact on Employment Relations*. London: UNISON.

Sherwin, S. and the Feminist Healthcare Network. (1998). *The Politics of Women's Health*. Philadelphia: Temple University Press.

● ●

Critical Thinking Questions

1. Should we be giving as much attention to men's health issues as we do to women's health issues? Why or why not?

2. What are the limitations of simply treating gender as an "independent variable" in research?

3. In what ways are health and health care issues related to gender similar to issues related to racialized groups in Canada? How are they different?

4. What are the current dimensions of discussions of "appropriate care"? What should such discussions be about?

5. What questions should we ask when we consider evidence that is applied in clinical practices? What might some of the limitations of such evidence be?

Further Readings

Armstrong, P., M. Boscoe, B. Clow, K. Grant, A. Pederson, and K. Willson. (2002). *Reading Romanow*. Ottawa: Canadian Women's Health Network. Available on-line at www.cewh-cesf.ca/healthreform/publications/summary/reading_romanow.html.
The Romanow Report on the Future of Health Care in Canada was the outcome of a Royal Commission that not only conducted extensive research but also held wider-ranging public hearings. It offered recommendations on how to construct a public health care system that is sustainable and that reflects Canadian values. In spite of submissions that called for a gender-sensitive analysis and in spite of federal government policy requiring such analysis, the report was gender-blind. This document provides an example of gender-sensitive analysis in practice.

Grant, K., C. Amaratunga, P. Armstrong, M. Boscoe, A. Pederson, and K. Willson, eds. (2004). *Caring for/Caring about: Women, Home Care and Unpaid Caregiving*. Aurora: Garamond.
Women account for four out of five caregivers. Women also do the overwhelming majority of unpaid care work. This collection of articles offers a conceptual guide to caregiving as well as an assessment of existing research on gender and caregiving. One article focuses specifically on women with disabilities while another focuses on Aboriginal women. Additional articles develop portraits of women who give and receive care in Quebec and Ontario.

Lorber, J. (2000). *Gender and the Social Construction of Illness*. Oxford: Rowman and Littlefield.
The author explores the interaction between gender and medicine, focusing on how both are social constructions that are understood within a context of power and politics.

Messing, K. (1998). *One-Eyed Science*: *Occupational Health and Women Workers*. Philadelphia: Temple University Press.
Internationally recognized as a definitive work on the importance of gender in occupational health, this book provides a comprehensive assessment of theory and research in this critical field.

Van Esterik, P., ed. (2003). *Head, Heart and Hands*: *Partnerships for Women's Health in Canadian Environments*, vol. 1. York University, Toronto: National Networks on Environments and Women's Health (NNEWH).
This volume brings together papers written under the auspices of the National Network for Environments and Women's Health, a federally funded Centre of Excellence for Women's Health. Beginning with conceptual frameworks and methodological approaches, the collection moves on to consider conditions of

work in care, health and locality, and perceptions of risk. The articles cover a wide range of perspectives, issues, methods, and topics, making it an excellent source for those interested in acquiring an understanding of the breadth of women's health issues.

Relevant Web Sites

Canadian Centre for Policy Alternatives
www.policyalternatives.ca
   The Canadian Centre for Policy Alternatives is a research organization that covers multiple topics directly related to health.

Canadian Health Coalition
www.healthcoalition.ca
   The Canadian Health Coalition Web site offers analysis of current critical issues in health care and the social determinants of health. The coalition brings together brings together community, religious, and union organizations dedicated to protecting and promoting public care.

Canadian Institutes of Health Research, Institute of Gender and Health
www.cihr-irsc.gc.ca/
   This institute funds research on gender and health. It also publishes material on integrating gender-sensitive research.

Canadian Women's Health network
www.cwhn.ca/
   The Canadian Women's Health network Web site not only provides access to publications from the Centres of Excellence for Women's Health, but also links directly to sources around the world on a broad range of issues related to women's health.

World Health Organization, Department of Gender, Women, and Health
www.who.int/gender/en/
   The World Health Organization is a particularly good source for comparative information on research from countries around the world.

Glossary

Feminist political economy: An approach that sees political, economic, social, and ideological aspects as not only integrally linked but gendered. It focuses attention on power and inequalities, on ideas and relations that shape and are shaped by people individually and collectively.

Health care services: The entire range of organizations and individuals who provide health care. The term is usually restricted to services that are paid for by government, insurance companies, or individuals. The term thus excludes unpaid care and often excludes what may be called alternative or complementary therapies such as homeopathy.

Policy and practice in health care: Policy usually refers to the formal, explicit approach to health care while practice refers to what people actually do. The first refers to what is supposed to happen while practice refers to what actually happens. Policy and practice influence each other.

Sex and gender: Sex is often used to indicate biological differences between males and females while gender is most frequently used to describe socially constructed differences. However, biological differences are not always easy to determine nor do they always provide clear markers that divide people into two sexes. Moreover, biology is itself influenced by social, economic, and power relations making it frequently difficult to separate the social from the biological or sex from gender. In any case, "sex" cannot capture the complexity of differences related to gender distinctions.

Social context: The conditions under which we live as well as the relations we have with other people. It thus includes power and politics, income and educational opportunities, household members and work colleagues, among other factors.

CHAPTER THIRTEEN

CONSTRUCTING DISABILITY AND ILLNESS

Marcia Rioux and Tamara Daly

Normal is a lack of variation. There is no such thing as normal. Normal is set up by a certain amount of people who have the power to decide, to define norms.
—Gregor Wolbring (2002)

Bodies that depart from the norm—bodies marked by some condition of disability— disrupt the rules. Striking their own "bond with the natural order," they complicate the metaphors of science, infuse static notions of health with deeper, richer meanings, and challenge law and policy-makers who seek to create conditions of justice for all.
—Catherine Frazee, Joan Gilmour, Roxanne Mykitiuk, and Michael Bach (2002)

Learning Objectives

At the conclusion of this chapter, the reader will be able to

- identify the differences between biomedical, functional, environmental, and rights-outcome approaches to disability and illness
- discuss how social structures construct disability
- identify how disability is experienced by women, as people age, and in certain parts of Canada
- discuss critical appraisals of the disability adjusted life years (DALYs) measurement when compared with statistical analyses of people's experiences of disability or illness
- explain the importance of the Charter for ensuring the equality of disabled people

---

Introduction

In this chapter, we consider the theoretical distinctions between two dominant discourses: disability as an individual pathology and as a social pathology. The former includes biomedical and functional accounts of disability. Both of these accounts locate it in an individual's pathology, and tend to conflate it with illness. The social pathology perspective, by contrast, includes environmental and human rights approaches. These approaches begin with the assumption that "Disability is not Measles" (Rioux and Bach 1994). Scholarly work in this tradition locates disability within the context of the broader social system at the level of societies' inability to flexibly adapt to individuals' different needs, whether in terms of physical reconfigurations such as ramps, or workplace policies that prevent people with disabilities from holding full-time employment. Disability is thus equated with social disadvantage. Viewed in this broader context, someone who is disabled may or may not have medical illnesses, but the illness is separate from the social disadvantage that a person experiences as a result of physical or mental impairment.

Second, we investigate the social construction of disability and illness, and the ways in which the two are conflated. It is important at the outset to distinguish between the two, which are rooted in differing assumptions about where the source of disability is located. The World Bank's disability adjusted life years measure is critically discussed.

Third, we turn to consider disability in Canada. Results of the Statistics Canada Participation and Activity Limitation Post Censal Survey are presented. The results show much higher rates of disability in some provinces. Disability increases with age. Pain and discomfort, mobility, and agility were most frequently reported. Overall, women experience higher rates of disability than men. Finally, recent advances in human rights policy and law are briefly discussed.

Section I: Theoretical Models of Disability

Individual Pathology Frameworks of Disability

Biomedical and functional models approach disability as a field of professional knowledge and expertise (Barton and Oliver 1997; Rioux 2001b, 2003). Scholarly research in this tradition works within a positivist, scientific paradigm. It focuses on the prevention of disability resulting from biological and environmental conditions. Both approaches treat disability as pathology focused on individual deficits or incapacities in relation to non-disabled people. These approaches tend to equate disability with anomaly. Disabled people may be viewed as a social burden. The inclusion of people with disabilities tends to be viewed as a private responsibility. Individuals with a disability are compared with a biomedically constructed idea of what is normal.

Biomedical Approach

The biomedical approach emphasizes diagnosis and treatment of dysfunction. This approach focuses research attention on the condition itself. The emphasis is on individual abnormality and the extent of functional limitations.

The professional aim is to decrease the prevalence of the condition in the overall population. This approach highlights medical diagnosis and treatment, including medical or genetic therapeutic interventions. In conjunction with conventional medical models of care and therapy, institutions, other segregated housing, and all-encompassing service provision centres are also used. As many people with disabilities have been characterized as lacking in potential, life in institutions and other forms of segregated housing were limited to providing for basic needs (e.g., food, shelter, and clothing).

In countries with increases to public benefits and institutional facilities, the medical profession has been put into the position of gatekeeper. In this role, access to education and training, financial benefits, mobility aids and devices, and rehabilitation are all scientifically assessed to determine a person's needs based on criteria evaluating the range of disability.

Functional Approach

Like the biomedical approach, this approach views disability as an individual condition or pathology. From a functional perspective, the pathology is best treated with services that enable the individual to become as socially functional as possible. Services, including physiotherapy, occupational therapy, nursing, and health visiting, are more than therapeutic in nature, and include the development of life skills, pre-vocational training, functional assessments, counselling and job training, and skills for independent living. Services' evaluation is measured by the degree to which people who use the services can approximate the lives of "normal" people.

Two other categories of services include behaviour modification or adaptation and developmental programming. In the former, a number of positive or negative reinforcement techniques are used to elicit socially desirable behaviours and prevent undesirable ones. The latter focuses on levels of knowledge and skills that people usually acquire as they mature, identifies where and why someone is not at the "appropriate" level, and claims to intervene to assist individuals to maximize their "developmental" potential.

The primary critique of this model is that it fails to consider the impact of larger social, economic, and political factors that may play a significant role in preventing an individual from progressing or meeting his or her ambitions. This approach also makes several assumptions about a person's best interests that may be different from what a person actually wants, as well as assuming some method of determining what is appropriate development.

Social Pathology Frameworks of Disability

Early analyses of the social construction of sickness and its related behaviours were rooted in Talcott Parsons's (1951) ideas. Other sociologists explored concepts including stigmatization and the way in which rehabilitation professionals socially construct dependence (Goffman 1968; Scott 1969). Throughout the1970s, scholars continued to interrogate the claims of medicine with social science questions, theories, and methods. For instance, Navarro (1976) presented a class analysis of the United States' lack of a national health insurance program, Illich (1977) questioned the legitimacy of medical knowledge and pioneered research into iatrogenic (doctor-caused) disease, and Friedson (1970) examined the power of the medical profession. Starr (1989) introduced the concept of privatization as an application for studying the state's relative power and policy-making ability. He noted that while economists see the market as part of the private sphere, sociologists and political economists see the market as part of the public sphere.

Since these earlier social critiques of medicine, materialist, feminist, legal, health geography, and postmodern critiques have also challenged the hegemony of the biomedical and functional accounts of disability and disentangled its definition from concepts of illness and impairment. This critical social scholarship firmly locates disability within society, not within the individual. Contributions investigate how people with physical and mental impairments are precluded from undertaking social activities as a consequence of the erection of physical and attitudinal barriers by those who are not disabled (Thomas 2002). For instance, Stone (1984) notes that the medical profession's accumulated power, combined with the state's need to restrict access to state-sponsored welfare, constructs disability socially (Barnes 1997).

Within the social pathology framework, we investigate two models of disability: the environmental and rights-outcome approaches (Barton and Oliver 1997; Rioux 2001a, 2003). Both approaches assume that disability is neither inherent to the individual nor independent of the social structure. In other words, these analyses critique the necessary association between disability and individual impairment. The unit of analysis is the social system, meaning that the political, social, and built environments are important factors in constructing disability. Unlike the biomedical and functional models, critical social science frameworks view disability as difference, not deviance. Similar to feminist critiques of the "gendered" body, more scholars are recognizing that the body is "infused with 'able-bodied' notions" (Barnes et al. 1999: 65). The term "disability" is often used to refer to a type of social oppression, much in the way that sexism and racism are used (Thomas 2002).

Environmental Approach

This approach to disability sees personal abilities and limitations resulting from an individual's characteristics interacting with their environment. Disability arises from the failure of ordinary environments to accommodate people's differences.

The manner in which environments are arranged and ordered constructs disability. For instance, a building lacking a wheelchair ramp creates an access to employment barrier for someone reliant on a wheelchair. Impairment can also be the result when workplace policies are insufficiently flexible to allow people who require time during the day to rest in order to continue to function, while making up for work later in the day.

Policy research demonstrates that an individual's physical or mental limitation can be lessened when environments are appropriately adapted to enable participation. For instance, changes to building codes, employing principles of barrier-free design, adapted curricula, and targeted policy and funding commitments have been usefully employed. When modifications and supports are used in homes, school, work, and leisure environments, people with disabilities are able to participate. This approach is grounded in disability discrimination while the rights-outcome approach is grounded in fundamental human rights and freedoms.

Rights-Outcome Approach

The second social pathology approach builds on the environmental approach recognition that supports such as personal services, aids, and devices are required by some people to enable them to gain access to, participate in, and exercise self-determination as equal members of society. However, the rights-outcome approach moves beyond calls for adaptations to environments, reflecting a shift that has taken place over the past 20 years in the paradigm of disability from a medical welfare model to a human rights model.

The rights-outcome approach is premised on the idea that disability has social causes resulting from the way in which individuals relate to how society is organized (ICIDH 1981; Olivier 1990; Rioux and Bach 1994). The end goals of the latter model are non-discrimination and equality for people with disabilities (Rioux 2001a). While the approach is multidisciplinary, the primary lens of analysis is human rights principles. These principles aim to reduce civic inequalities to address social and economic disadvantage for people with disabilities in Canada and across the world. This approach is macro level in orientation. Its focus is on broad, systemic factors that prevent disabled people from fully participating as equals in society. In addition to legal cases that uphold the principles of non-discrimination and equity in Canada, these goals are also currently being negotiated by a United Nations Ad Hoc Committee on a Comprehensive and Integral International Convention on Protection and Promotion of the Rights and Dignity of Persons with Disabilities.

Minow (1990) focuses on the ways in which difference is used in law to create exclusion and disadvantage. She locates difference not in the individual but in the limitations of society to accommodate multiple individuals' needs. In other words, society marginalizes people with disabilities, even though it is possible to incorporate people's different needs. This approach critiques inflexibility in society for creating and constructing disabilities, while recognizing the need for supporting diversity and empowering marginalized individuals.

Table 13.1 summarizes the source of disability according to each of the four main approaches outlined above, and identifies the primary mode of action proponents use to change the conditions for people with disabilities.

Table 13.1

	Individual Pathology		Social Pathology	
	Biomedical Approach	**Functional Approach**	**Environmental Approach**	**Rights-Outcome Approach**
Source of disability	Disability is due to an individual's abnormality and the extent of his or her functional limitations.	Disability is a pathology that is best treated with services that enable the individual to become as socially functional as possible.	Disability arises from the failure of ordinary environments to accommodate people's differences.	Disability has social causes resulting from the way in which individuals relate to how society is organized.
Primary mode of action	Diagnosis and treatment	Service provision (e.g., rehabilitation)	Policy change (e.g., to building codes)	Human rights principles and legal challenges

Section II: Constructing Disability and Illness

This section explores inherent problems with the conflation of the identities of disability and illness. A biomedical reading of the disabled body as ill and impaired focuses on a narrow concept of health. By contrast, the World Health Organization defines health as "a state of complete physical, mental and social well-being and not merely the absence of disease or infirmity" (World Health Organization 1946: 19). This definition broadly locates health not only within each individual but also within social conditions or determinants. It acknowledges that individuals' health relies also on social well-being, which cannot be guaranteed when systemic discrimination and policies of inequity persist.

Health and social policy, grounded in medical assumptions, conflate disability with illness. In other words, a person with a disability is treated as if ill. In reality, people with disabilities experience periods of ill health and health in the same way as do all people. We also investigate critical perspectives on the use of the disability adjusted year life (DALYs) to measure how many years a person or population loses as a result of ill health compared with an idealized and normalized perspective of health equated with freedom from disability.

Disability as Illness

Critical social science scholarship investigates how disability and illness are constructed, and the complex links among sites of care, power relations, the body, and identity (Dyck 1998). The conflation of disability with ill health is grounded in a narrow definition of health based on the presence of disease or infirmity, the use of medical practitioners as gatekeepers to disability benefits, and an inability to acknowledge the multiple ways in which disabilities are often created by societal norms that inflexibly accommodate multiple needs. First, different assumptions underlie how disability is approached (see Section I of this paper) Social pathology perspectives highlight how tying benefits to medical certification conflates disability with illness, and constructs various disabilities as conditions requiring medical intervention. Grounded in the dominance of a biomedical view of disability as individual pathology, access to welfare state disability benefits, including non-medical benefit programs, is contingent upon medical certification of disability by physician gatekeepers (Stone 1984).

Second, making medical practitioners gatekeepers to disability benefits privileges biomedical and functional approaches to disability in the policy, program, and service realm. These approaches do not sufficiently acknowledge that the organization of society can often create disabilities. As well, human rights provisions stipulate that individuals should be treated not just equally, but also without discrimination. The premise of non-discrimination acknowledges that people need to be treated differently in order to access services and have equal rights. The case of *Eldridge v. B.C.* outlined in Section IV is illustrative.

The question of equitable access to benefits is key in a political climate of welfare state restructuring, which has legitimated distinctions between categories of worthy and unworthy poor, and return us to a "poor laws" position escaped briefly with policies of universalism. People with able bodies and minds unwilling to work are defined as unworthy poor. By contrast, people with disabilities, the aged, and infirm are all classed as worthy poor (Rioux and Prince 2002). Worthy poor are accommodated from within the public sphere, whereas policies have marginalized the unworthy poor so their needs must be accommodated within the private sphere. In terms of the funding of social welfare, the role of the state is alternately expansive or restrictive in response to pressures from the internationalized global capital system (Rioux 2002) and the state's priority placed on efficiency and effectiveness (Stein 2001).

At a policy-making level, neo-liberal policies associated with fiscal conservatism, and neo-conservative policies that marry fiscal conservatism with moral conservatism, have dominated the public agenda since just prior to 1980 (Hall 1992). The result is a change in the role of the state, with significant implications for addressing equity policy goals. This neo-liberal discourse emphasizes individual responsibility and private action, debt and deficit reduction over social expenditure, and rights and responsibilities to accommodate citizens who form the majority or constitute the norm. It also emphasizes a shift from universal provision based on shared rights and pooled risk to the provision of services based on individual needs with implications for concepts of citizenship and entitlement. It is also important in a political climate that privileges a role for the state in health care, while withdrawing the state role in social care for both elderly and people with disabilities, as it is being recast as part of private responsibility (Daly 2003).

Illness as Disability

The inverse—the construction of illness as disability—is also true; policies and practices reconstruct illness as disability, particularly in terms of measurement of the health status of countries with instruments such as the DALYs, which are used to measure a country's health status. The World Bank's use of DALYs to measure a country's level of ill health reconstructs illness as disability by turning all illnesses into measures of disability.

DALYs are used both as a measure of health status and as an instrument of health policy. Designed by researchers at the Harvard School of Public Health, disability adjusted life years were introduced by the World Bank in 1993 to measure the global burden of disease (Metts 2001). A basic assumption built into the use of the DALYs is that there is a "reduced value" to a life lived with a disability (Groce et al. 2000) given the foci on burden and loss. Since then, DALYs have come under increasing criticism resulting from the built-in assumptions and policy implications of using these measures.

DALYs were ostensibly designed to measure the years of life lost resulting from disease and ill health. Unlike earlier measures, such as the quality-adjusted life years (QALYs), in which groups of citizens were consulted, the DALYs relied on input and analysis from an internationally representative group of medical professionals. Twenty-two "indicator disabling conditions" were selected and evaluated by professionals from the list of diseases in the World Health Organization's International Classification of Disease (ICD). The participants assigned a severity weight from zero (denoting perfect health) to one (denoting death). Conditions were then grouped into disability classes. Disabilities were calculated by multiplying the age-adjusted severity weights for each condition, by expected duration calculated based on an amalgamation of community-based epidemiological research, information from health facilities, and expert judgments (Metts 2001: 451).

Critical scholarship has pointed out that DALYs make a false assumption that all conditions or disabilities result in ill health of various severities. This treats these conditions as physical disablements instead of situating disability in broader social, political, environmental, and economic factors. In other words, it locates disabilities within the individual and not within the broader conditions and barriers that create a disability. It also makes a second false assumption that the only way to ameliorate disability is to intervene medically (Metts 2001). Others argue that DALYs is a flawed tool for evaluating a country's or population's gross domestic product of health or to set priorities in health policy (Lyttkens 2003). DALYs does not account for health care costs, or other costs resulting from paid and unpaid care supports. DALYs in its current form cannot be used as an aggregate measure of population health because of the way analysts have derived disability weights (Lyttkens 2003). Furthermore, because the method of determining DALYs equates longevity with health, and disability with ill health, a suggested correspondence is made between the two that does not exist in real life. There are also ethical issues in developing policy around the outcomes of a measure of longevity (Lyttkens 2003).

Section III: Measuring Disability in Canada

In this section rather than use the standard measures of disability such as DALYs, we consider the *self-reported* prevalence and impact of disability among different groups based on the results of Statistics Canada's 2001 *Participation and Activity Limitation Survey*. We also consider the status of Canadian legal disability equality rights through analysis of several key legal challenges.

In general, Statistics Canada data show that the rate of disability varies widely across Canada. Disability disproportionately affects older citizens, and women in all age categories, and pain and discomfort, mobility, and agility are the three most often self-reported activity limitations.

Prevalence of Disability in Canada

Altogether, 3.6 million Canadians living in private households reported activity limitations. Among adults aged over 15 years, mobility is most frequently reported (10.5 percent). Pain is the second most frequently reported activity limitation (10.1 percent) (Statistics Canada 2003).

1. Disability Rates Differ Widely across Canada

The percentage of Canada's population that report having a disability is 12.4 percent. The highest percentage of individuals with reported activity limitations live in Nova Scotia (17.1 percent), followed by Saskatchewan (14.5 percent) and PEI (14.3 percent). Reported rates are lowest in Quebec (8.4 percent), followed by Newfoundland (12.3 percent) and Alberta (12.5 percent) (Figure 13.1).

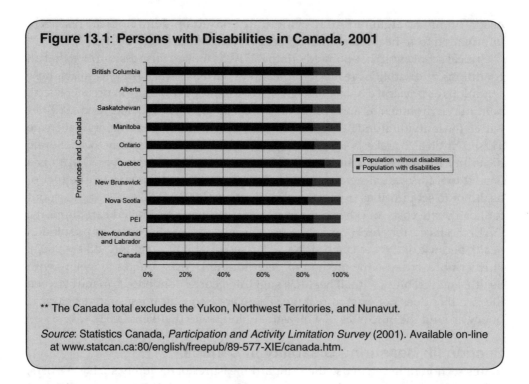

Figure 13.1: Persons with Disabilities in Canada, 2001

** The Canada total excludes the Yukon, Northwest Territories, and Nunavut.

Source: Statistics Canada, *Participation and Activity Limitation Survey* (2001). Available on-line at www.statcan.ca:80/english/freepub/89-577-XIE/canada.htm.

2. Disability Gradually Increases with Age

According to Statistics Canada, the disability rate in Canada gradually increases with age (Statistics Canada 2003). The rate is 3.3 percent among children under 14 years old. Some disabilities are difficult to identify in children under the age of five as they manifest later or result from social barriers. When considering children four years and under, intellectual disability ("developmental delay") is the most often reported.

For adults aged 15 to 64, disability rises to nearly 10 percent and climbs to more than 40 percent among women and men over the age of 65. Among children aged 0 to 14 years, this relationship is reversed with boys more likely to have activity limitations (4 percent) compared with girls (2.5 percent). The disability rate is virtually the same for young men and women between 15 to 24 years of age, but starting at age 25, the prevalence of disability increases for women compared with men. For those aged 65 and over, the rate of disability climbs to 40.5 percent.

3. Disability Affects Women More Frequently Than Men

In general, women (13.3 percent) more frequently report disability than men (11.5 percent) (Statistics Canada 2003). For each age group, except among children under 14, women report higher rates of disability compared with men. As well, for those aged over 15, more women (12.2 percent) than men (8.6 percent) report a mobility-related disability.

Women were less likely than men (32.2 percent compared with 36.4 percent respectively) to report mild degrees of limitation, but the opposite is true when severe levels of activity were reported (28.3 percent compared with 25.1 percent).

Full-time working women also have more days lost, compared with men, due to illness or disability, whether their own or a family member's (Figures 13.2 and 13.3).

4. Pain and Discomfort, Mobility, and Agility Limitations Are Most Prevalent

Activity limitations related to pain or discomfort were reported by 1.5 million people in the working-age population aged 15 to 64 (Statistics Canada 2003). In other words, pain and discomfort affect three-quarters of people reporting activity limitations who are of working age. This translates into nearly 8 percent of all working-age people being in pain or discomfort (Statistics Canada 2003) (Figure 13.4). Pain limited more women (11.4 percent) than men (8.8 percent). Mobility is also an issue for many Canadians. A total of 8.6 percent of men and 12.2 percent of the working-age women reported mobility limitations. Not surprisingly, 11 percent of women and 8.3 percent of men also reported agility limitations.

Of those with disabilities, less than 20 percent (18.2 percent) reported only one disability. Nearly 30 percent reported having three disabilities, while almost as

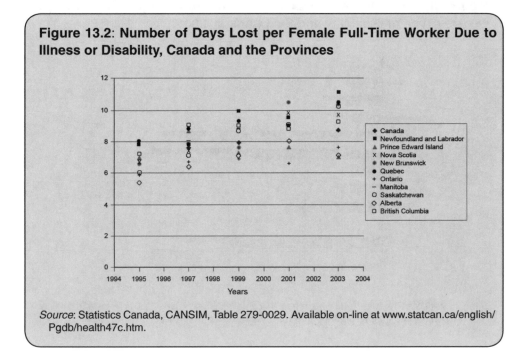

Figure 13.2: Number of Days Lost per Female Full-Time Worker Due to Illness or Disability, Canada and the Provinces

Source: Statistics Canada, CANSIM, Table 279-0029. Available on-line at www.statcan.ca/english/Pgdb/health47c.htm.

Figure 13.3: Number of Days Lost per Male Full-Time Worker Due to Illness or Disability, Canada and the Provinces

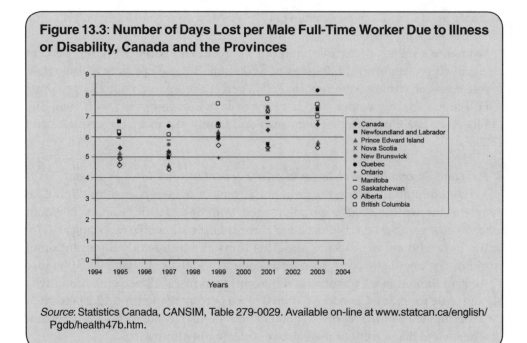

Source: Statistics Canada, CANSIM, Table 279-0029. Available on-line at www.statcan.ca/english/ Pgdb/health47b.htm.

Figure 13.4: Prevalence of Disability Among Adults Aged 15 Years and Over, by Type of Disability and Sex, Canada, 2001

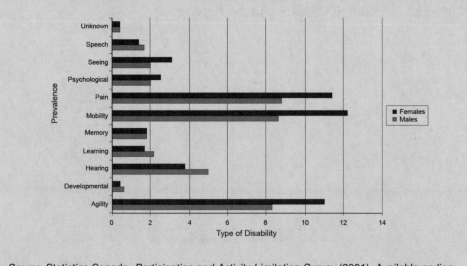

Source: Statistics Canada, *Participation and Activity Limitation Survey* (2001). Available on-line at www.statcan.ca:80/english/freepub/89-577-XIE/adults.htm#prevalence_most-types.

many reported four or five disabilities (27.7 percent). Nearly 10 percent reported six disabilities or more (Statistics Canada 2003).

Figure 13.5 spatially depicts the types of disabilities reported across Canada and for each of the provinces. It shows that some provinces have a higher number of people reporting pain, while for others mobility is the chief condition. Across Canada, 30 percent of people report problems with hearing. Finally, nearly 20 percent identify problems with visual impairment.

Section IV: Disability and Non-discrimination in Accessing Health Services

Principles of non-discrimination, equality, empowerment, freedom, agency, and full participation are enshrined in Section 15 in the Canadian Charter of Rights and Freedoms (1985) for people with "mental and physical disabilities" in Canada (Rioux 2001a). This constitutional provision is applicable at every level of legal authority in Canada (e.g., municipal, provincial, and federal). This section includes both substantive and procedural rights 15(1), and includes the option of affirmative action 15(2). It is based on the entire history of Canada's legislative human rights initiatives. It was included to ensure that disadvantaged groups can participate in society equally and fully. *Andrews v. Law Society* (1989) was the first legal case to address a Section 15 challenge; the court recognized "disadvantage as central to the analysis of discrimination" (Rioux 2001a: 42).

Cases since *Andrews* have continued to ensure that the equality principles are met. The courts rejected an equity model based on equal treatment in favour of a model that recognizes that equality may require different treatment (Rioux 1994, 2001a). The court has taken the position that Section 15 was intended to remedy inequality and disadvantage experienced by people with disabilities. It requires the "spending of public money and the extension of benefits to previously excluded disadvantaged groups" (Lepofsky 1997: 291).

Because there are legislative bans on discrimination, society is obligated to make accommodations to meet the needs of groups that are discriminated against. In terms of non-discriminatory access to health services, *Eldridge v. British Columbia* (1997) involved three deaf applicants who successfully challenged the legislation governing hospital services because sign language interpreter services were not included as an insured service or a requirement for hospitals to provide. First, the court found the province was acting in a discriminatory manner and, more importantly, that the province failed to take action, as opposed to imposing a burden. Second, the court found that failing to make accommodations resulted in discrimination. Third, governments cannot evade responsibility by delegating implementation to private entities (i.e., hospitals). Fourth, the court identified communication as an important part of the delivery of medical services.

While these court decisions are very important milestones, and enable us to move beyond a mindset of accommodation to one of non-discrimination, they have not

Figure 13.5

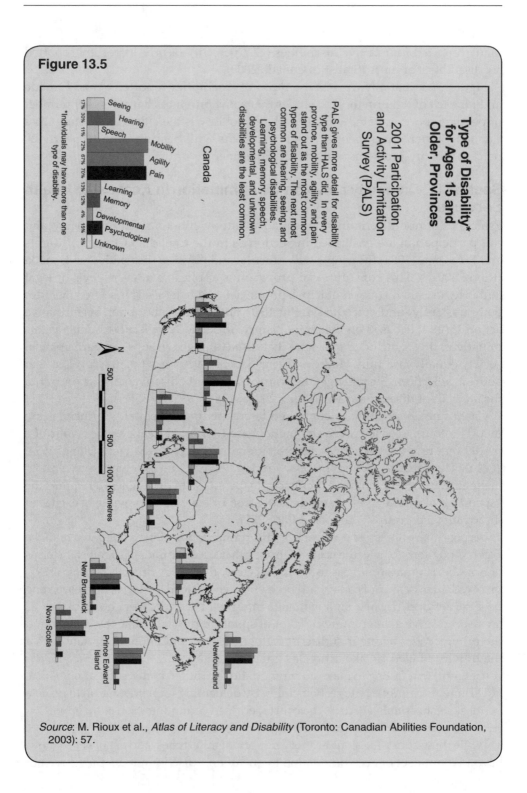

Type of Disability* for Ages 15 and Older, Provinces

2001 Participation and Activity Limitation Survey (PALS)

PALS gives more detail for disability type than HALS did. In every province, mobility, agility, and pain stand out as the most common types of disability. The next most common are hearing, seeing, and psychological disabilities. Learning, memory, speech, developmental, and unknown disabilities are the least common.

Canada

Seeing — 17%
Hearing — 30%
Speech — 11%
Mobility — 72%
Agility — 67%
Pain — 70%
Learning — 13%
Memory — 12%
Developmental — 4%
Psychological — 15%
Unknown — 3%

*Individuals may have more than one type of disability.

Source: M. Rioux et al., *Atlas of Literacy and Disability* (Toronto: Canadian Abilities Foundation, 2003): 57.

eliminated the persistent social and legal exclusion of disabled people. Rioux (2003) argues that both the content of agreements and the ways in which countries meet their commitments to agreements' terms perpetuates the social and legal exclusion of disabled people. In sum, disabled people's human rights are still under threat. Despite these agreements, people with disabilities are still not treated equally, and equality is achieved only when difference is accommodated.

Conclusions

In this chapter, we have explored how disability is often equated with illness, owing to the predominance of biomedical and functional approaches to disability. These approaches tend to focus on the individual origins of disability (e.g., genetics, workplace accident, etc.). By contrast, social science approaches tend to focus on the social origins of disability. These models investigate the ways in which social structures create disability through societies' inability to accommodate difference. In this framework, disability is equated with social disadvantage, and is not simply focused on individual impairment.

We have also explored the prevalence of disability in Canada, and discussed some of the major legal milestones in removing discrimination from Canadians with disabilities. Some of the main ideas include:

- Biomedical and functional accounts of disability equate it with illness. These accounts focus on individuals. Broader critical social science approaches investigate how social structures create disability through societies' inability to accommodate difference.
- Doctors and other medical personnel often serve as gatekeepers to disability benefits, which may unnecessarily perpetuate the conception of disability as illness.
- Social pathology accounts equate disability with social disadvantage, not illness.
- Disability is more often experienced by women, as people age, and in certain parts of Canada.
- The outcome of equality rights for people with disabilities involves more than the removal of physical barriers and adaptation of current structures. It is about achieving a society in which disabled people are free to fully and equally participate.

In 2001, nearly four million Canadians self-reported having at least one disability. Many Canadians reported having more than one. Statistics Canada data show that disability is most frequently experienced by women. It is also more prevalent as people age. As well, there are more people reporting disability depending on where one lives.

Policy making that incorporates a rights-outcome approach is slowly happening through court challenges. Since the Charter, the courts have upheld equality rights for disabled people. These rights encompass more than the removal of physical barriers and the adaptation of current structures. The courts have determined that discrimination is based on imposing a burden and failing to take action to accommodate. This distinction is important because it challenges governments and policy makers to be proactive in eliminating the discrimination that challenges disabled people's ability to fully, equally, and freely participate in society.

Research and education in the humanities, and social and medical sciences must consider human rights issues that identify not only how society constructs barriers, but also the flaw in locating disability solely in the individual. These approaches must separate disability from illness by recognizing that people with disabilities, like other people, have periods of health and ill health. Ameliorating disability is not simply a matter of intervening medically. It is about addressing the physical, social, civic, economic, and cultural rights violations experienced by people with disabilities.

References

Barnes, C. (1997). "A Legacy of Oppression: A History of Disability in Western Culture." In *Disability Studies: Past, Present and Future*, edited by M. Oliver, 3–24. Leeds: The Disability Press.

Barnes, C., G. Mercer, and T. Shakespeare. (1999). *Exploring Disability: A Sociological Introduction.* Cambridge: Blackwell Publishers.

Barton, L., and M. Oliver, eds. (1997). *Disability Studies: Past, Present and Future.* Leeds: The Disability Press.

Daly, T. (2003). "The Grassroots Ceiling: The Impact of State Policy Change on Home Support Nonprofits in Ontario and in Waterloo Region—Wellington-Dufferin (1958–2001)." Department of Health Policy, Management and Evaluation, Faculty of Medicine. Toronto: University of Toronto.

Dyck, I. (1998). "Women with Disabilities and Everyday Geographies." In *Putting Health into Place*, edited by R. Kearns and W. Gesler, 102–119. Syracuse: Syracuse University Press.

Frazee, C., J. Gilmour, R. Mykitiuk, and M. Bach. (2002). "The Legal Regulation and Construction of the Gendered Body and of Disability in Canadian Health Law and Policy." Available on-line at www.yorku.ca/nnewh/netPubs_reports.htm. Retrieved April 3, 2005.

Friedson, E. (1970). *Profession of Medicine.* New York: Dodd, Mead.

Goffman, E. (1968). *Stigma: Notes on the Management of Spoiled Identity.* Harmondsworth: Penguin.

Groce, N.E., M. Chamie, and A. Me. (2000). *Measuring the Quality of Life: Rethinking the World Bank's Disability Adjusted Life Years. Disability World* 3 (June-July). Available on-line at www.disabilityworld.org/June-July2000/Internationl/DALY.html.

Hall, P.A. (1992). "The Movement from Keynesianism to Monetarism: Institutional Analysis and British Economic Policy in the 1970s." In *Structuring Politics: Historical Institutionalism in Comparative Perspective*, edited by S. Steinmo, K. Thalen, and F. Longstreth, 90–113. Cambridge: Cambridge University Press.

ICIDH. (1981). "The Handicap Creation Process." *ICIDH International Network* 4: 1–2.

Illich, I. (1977). *Limits to Medicine: Medical Nemesis: The Expropriation of Health.* Harmondsworth and New York: Penguin.

Lepofsky, D. (1997). "A Report Card on the *Charter's* Guarantee of Equality to Persons with Disabilities after 10 Years—What Progress? What Prospects?" *National Journal of Constitutional Law* 7(3): 263–431.

Lyttkens, C.H. (2003). "Time to Disable DALYs? On the Use of Disability-Adjusted Life Years in Health Policy." *European Journal of Health Economics* 4: 195–202.

Metts, R. (2001). "The Fatal Flaw in the Disability Adjusted Life Year." *Disability and Society* 16(3): 449–452.

Minow, M. (1990). *Making All the Difference: Inclusion, Exclusion and American Law.* Ithaca: Cornell University Press.

Navarro, V. (1976). *Medicine under Capitalism.* New York: Neale Watson.

Olivier, M. (1990). *The Politics of Disablement.* Basingstoke: Macmillan.

Parsons, T. (1951). *The Social System.* Glencoe: The Free Press.

Rioux, M. (1994). "Towards a Concept of Equality of Well-being: Overcoming the Socio-legal Construction of Inequality." *Canadian Journal of Law and Jurisprudence* VII(1): 127–147.

_____. (2001a). "Bending towards Justice." In *Disability, Politics and the Struggle for Change,* edited by L. Barton, 34–48. London: David Fulton Publishers.

_____. (2002). "Social Disability and the Public Good." *Man and Development* (December): 179–198.

_____. (2003). "On Second Thought: Constructing Knowledge, Law, Disability and Inequality." In *The Human Rights of Persons with Intellectual Disabilities,* edited by S. Herr, L. Gostin, and H.H. Koh, 287–317. Oxford: Oxford University Press.

Rioux, M., and M. Bach, eds. (1994). *Disability Is Not Measles.* Toronto: Roeher Institute.

Rioux, M., and M.J. Prince. (2002). "The Canadian Political Landscape of Disability: Policy Perspectives, Social Status, Interest Groups and the Rights Movement." In *Federalism, Democracy and Disability Policy in Canada,* edited by A. Puttee, 11–28. Kingston: McGill-Queen's University Press.

Scott, R.A. (1969). *The Making of Blind Men.* London: Sage.

Starr, P. (1989). "The Meaning of Privatization." In *Privatization and the Welfare State,* edited by S. Kamerman and A. Kahn, 12–48. Princeton: Princeton University Press.

Statistics Canada. (2003). "Disability among Working-Age Adults (aged 15 to 64)." Available on-line at www.statcan.ca/english/freepub/89-577-XIE/workage.htm.

Stein, J.G. (2001). *The Cult of Efficiency.* Etobicoke: Anansi.

Stone, D. (1984). *The Disabled State.* London: MacMillan.

Thomas, C. (2002). "Disability Theory: Key Ideas, Issues and Thinkers." *Disability Studies Today*, edited by M.O. Colin Barnes and Len Barton, 38–57. Cambridge: Blackwell Publishers.

Tindale, J., and E. MacLachlan. (2001). "VON 'Doing Commercial': The Experience of Executive Directors with Related Business Development." In *The Nonprofit Sector and Government in a New Century,* edited by K. Brock and K. Banting, 189–213. Kingston: McGill-Queen's University Press.

Wolbring, G. (2002). "The Tyranny of Normal: Disability, Culture, and Human Engineering." Presentation at the 6th Annual Grassroots Gathering on Genetic Engineering. June 8, 2002, Toronto, Ontario.

World Health Organization. (1946). "Preamble to the Constitution of the World Health Organization as adopted by the International Health Conference," 19–22. New York: World Health Organization.

• •

Critical Thinking Questions

1. In what ways do biomedical and functional accounts of disability equate it with illness?
2. In what ways do social pathology accounts equate disability with social disadvantage and not illness?
3. What issues are associated with doctors and other medical personnel serving as gatekeepers to disability benefits?
4. How do different groups (e.g., gender, age, geographic location) experience disability?
5. In what ways do the outcomes of equality rights for people with disabilities involve more than the removal of physical barriers and adaptation of current structures?

Further Readings

Barnes, C., G. Mercer, and T. Shakespeare. (1999). *Exploring Disability: A Sociological Introduction.* Cambridge: Blackwell Publishers.
This book explores how concepts of disability have changed since the 1970s by addressing both traditional and new theoretical approaches to the field. It also focuses on the social model of disability, and relates scholarship to other areas such as social policy, medical sociology, politics, and cultural studies.

Metts, R. (2001). "The Fatal Flaw in the Disability Adjusted Life Year." *Disability and Society* 16(3): 449–452.
This article argues that the disability adjusted life year, which was developed to measure different countries' health status and to gauge the effectiveness of different health interventions, is flawed. The measure incorrectly assumes that any disabling condition always results in disability regardless of the social and political context.

Minow, M. (1990). *Making All the Difference: Inclusion, Exclusion and American Law.* Ithaca: Cornell University Press.
This book explores how difference in the law is attributed to the individual

as opposed to being located in limitations in the organization of the world. It argues that the concept of difference is used in law to create disadvantage and exclusion.

Rioux, M. (2003). "On Second Thought: Constructing Knowledge, Law, Disability and Inequality." In *The Human Rights of Persons with Intellectual Disabilities*, edited by S. Herr, L. Gostin, and H.H. Koh, 287–317. Oxford: Oxford University Press.
This chapter explores treatments of disability as individual or social pathology. It places disability policy within a human right and social justice framework.

Rioux, M., E. Zubrow, W. Miller, and M. Bunch. (2003). *Atlas of Literacy and Disability.* Toronto: Canadian Abilities Foundation.
This atlas of maps shows, at a glance, the spatial relationships between literacy and disability across Canada. Mapping disability and literacy variables, both on their own and in combination, allowed the researchers to see the issues in inventive ways.

Relevant Web Sites

Disability and Society
www.tandf.co.uk/journals/titles/09687599.asp
  It is an international journal for debate of human rights, discrimination, definitions, policy, and practice.

Disability Peoples' International
www.dpi.org/en/start.htm
  This is a network of national organizations and groups of people with disabilities. It was established to promote disabled people's rights through full participation, equal opportunity, and development.

Disability Studies Quarterly
www.dsq-sds.org/
  It is a multidisciplinary and international journal of interest to social science and humanities scholars and disability rights movement advocates.

Society for Disability Studies
www.uic.edu/orgs/sds/
  Examines scholarly approaches to issues of disability and chronic illness. Members include social science, health, and humanities researchers, and disability rights movement activists. The society is interdisciplinary and promotes the full participation of people in society.

Women with Disabilities in Australia (WWDA)
www.wwda.org.au/
   Founded by women with disabilities in Australia, this group found that their needs and issues were not adequately addressed in the broader disability sector or in the Australian women's sector.

Glossary

Disability adjusted life years (DALYs): Measures the years of life lost resulting from disease and ill health. Measurement is based upon the input and analysis of an internationally representative group of medical professionals. Twenty-two indicators of disabling conditions were selected and evaluated by professionals from the list of diseases in the World Health Organization's International Classification of Disease (ICD).

Disability as individual pathology: Focuses on individual deficits or incapacities in relation to non-disabled people. These approaches tend to equate disability with anomaly.

Disability as social pathology: Locates disability within society's failure to accommodate and not discriminate, not within the individual's attributes and characteristics.

Health: The World Health Organization defines health as "a state of complete physical, mental and social well-being and not merely the absence of disease or infirmity" (World Health Organization 1946).

Hegemony: Dominance or power of one idea, discourse, or group over another.

....

CHAPTER FOURTEEN

PHARMACEUTICAL POLICY

The Dance between Industry, Government, and the Medical Profession

Joel Lexchin

....

Learning Objectives

At the conclusion of this chapter, the reader will be able to
- understand the differences between the corporate and public health viewpoints of pharmaceutical issues in Canada
- be able to discuss the concept of clientele pluralism as it applies to the drug regulatory system in Canada
- explain the differences between the cost of individual drugs and overall drug expenditures in Canada
- understand how the patent system influences drug spending
- understand the interactions between Health Canada and the pharmaceutical industry

---

Introduction

Ever since the late 1990s, spending on prescription medicines has outstripped spending on doctors in Canada and is second only to hospital expenditures. In 2003, the bill for prescription drugs was $15 billion (Patented Medicine Prices Review Board 2004) and costs are rising at 7–8 percent per year, about three times the overall rate of inflation. (See Figure 14.1.) How much Canadians spend and how much value, in terms of improvements in health outcomes, we receive is determined by a series of policy decisions regarding how drugs are approved and monitored once they are on the market, industrial policy, and intellectual property rights. This chapter explores the background to these issues and how decisions about them are made and the interplay between the main actors—the state, the pharmaceutical industry, and the medical profession.

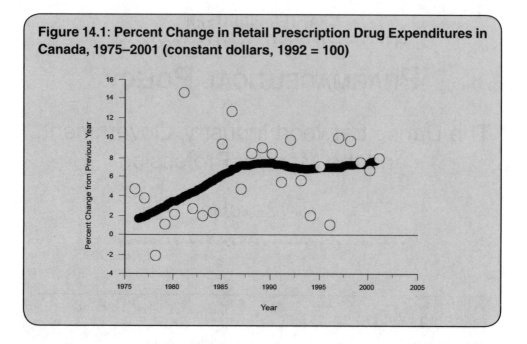

Figure 14.1: Percent Change in Retail Prescription Drug Expenditures in Canada, 1975–2001 (constant dollars, 1992 = 100)

The Drug Regulatory System

The pharmaceutical industry and the Canadian government have long had a close relationship based on clientele pluralism (Atkinson and Coleman 1985). This occurs where the state has a high degree of concentration of power in one agency (the Therapeutic Products Directorate [TPD], a branch of Health Canada), but a low degree of autonomy. With respect to pharmaceuticals, in Canada, government regulation of drug safety, quality, and efficacy is almost solely the responsibility of the TPD. But the state does not possess the wherewithal to undertake the elaborate clinical and pre-clinical trials required to meet the objective of providing safe and effective medications. Nor is the state willing or able to mobilize the resources necessary to undertake these tasks. Therefore, a tacit political decision is made to relinquish some authority to the drug manufacturers, especially with respect to information that forms the basis on which regulatory decisions are made.

On the other hand, the association representing nearly all of the multinational companies operating in Canada, Canada's Researched-Based Pharmaceutical Companies (RxandD), is highly mobilized to assume a role in making and implementing drug policy. It operates an elaborate committee structure, can act on behalf of its members, and can bind member firms to agreements. In clientele pluralism, the state relinquishes some of its authority to private-sector actors, who, in turn, pursue objectives with which officials are in broad agreement (Atkinson and Coleman 1989).

The implications of a clientele pluralist type of relationship take on increasing importance when seen in light of competing visions of what the prime function of a drug-regulatory authority should be. One put forward by the pharmaceutical industry holds that the main function is to facilitate the industry's efforts to develop new products and to approve them as quickly as possible. In this view, medications are commodities and the regulatory authority exists to provide a service to the industry. The second view espoused by consumer groups and public health activists sees the primary purpose as appropriately evaluating products to ensure a high standard of effectiveness and safety. Here medications are seen as an essential element of the health care system and the regulatory authority exists to provide a service to the public.

The Therapeutic Products Directorate: Changing Priorities?

In the Canadian context, the Therapeutic Products Directorate would nominally seem to side with consumer groups. The front page of its bimonthly bulletin contains the following mission statement: "we contribute to the health of Canadians and to the effectiveness of the health-care system by assessing the safety, efficacy and quality of pharmaceuticals ... in a timely manner" (see TPD News at www.hc-sc.gc. ca/hpfb-dgpsa/tpd-dpt).

Over the past decade, financing for the TPD has shifted from coming entirely from government appropriations to now being split about equally between government and user fees from pharmaceutical companies (KPMG Consulting LP 2000). This shift in financing of the regulatory body has raised concerns about whether the TPD's primary commitment is still to public health.

The apparent reorientation of the TPD in favour of business interests is reflected in its business transformation strategy (BTS), which is in the process of being implemented. The BTS was introduced in early 2003 and "builds on the commitments made by the Government of Canada to 'speed up the regulatory process for drug approvals', to move forward with a smart regulations strategy to accelerate reforms in key areas to promote health and sustainability, to contribute to innovation and economic growth, and to reduce the administrative burden on business" (Therapeutic Products Directorate nd: 1).

One of the key phrases in the BTS is "smart regulation." Smart regulation means that Canada should "regulate in a way that enhances the climate for investment and trust in the markets" and "accelerate reforms in key areas to promote health and sustainability, to contribute to innovation and economic growth, and to reduce the administrative burden on business" (Government of Canada 2003). While health is not ignored, the emphasis is clearly on creating a business-friendly environment. The federal External Advisory Committee on Smart Regulation explicitly states that risk management has an essential role in building public trust and business confidence in the Canadian market and regulatory system (External Advisory Committee on Smart Regulation 2004). Once again, the business agenda takes a prominent position.

When applied to drug regulation, risk management would mean weighing potential negative effects against potential advantages. Potential negative effects would be adverse health effects that could occur under reasonably foreseeable conditions (Health Canada 2003a). The shift from the precautionary principle to risk management is subtle but unmistakable. The precautionary principle says that if products cannot be shown to be safe, then they should not be marketed; risk management allows products on the market unless they are shown to be harmful. Realigning regulation to conform to the principles of smart regulation would not totally abandon the concept of precaution, but it seems to imply that there would have to be a threat of serious or irreversible damage before it would come into play.

Timeliness of Drug Approvals

The TPD is devoting significant organizational resources to speed up the drug-approval process. In the budget speech outlining government spending for the 2003 session of the federal Parliament, $190 million was allocated over a five-year period mostly to improving "the timeliness of Health Canada's regulatory processes with respect to human drugs" (Department of Finance Canada 2003). Forty million out of the $190 million was allocated for fiscal 2003–2004. Out of that amount 78 percent ($31.2 million) is going toward "improved regulatory performance," mainly an effort to eliminate the backlog in drug approvals and to ensure timeliness in getting drugs onto the market (Health Canada 2003b). (See Table 14.1.) The TPD justifies spending most of the money on improving the speed at which it approves new drugs largely because this is an area where it has received intense criticism.

Who is criticizing the TPD and why is timeliness so important that it reaches the throne speech? Patient groups are naturally concerned if effective treatments are

Table 14.1: Allocation of $40 million for Improvements in Drug Regulatory System, Fiscal 2003–2004

Program Area	Percent of Money	Dollars ($000,000)
Improved regulatory performance	78	31.2
Enhanced post-marketing safety	6.5	2.6
Optimal drug therapy	6	2.4
Price review capacity	1.25	0.5
Therapeutic access strategy	8.25	3.3

Source: Health Canada, *Improving Canada's Regulatory Process for Therapeutic Products: Building the Action Plan* (Ottawa: Public Policy 7 Forum multi-stakeholder consultation, 2003). Available on-line at www.ppforum.ca/ow/ow_e_05_2003/Presentation%20.

delayed and Canada lags behind other countries in the speed at which it approves drugs given priority status (Rawson 2001). However, fewer than 9 percent of the new active substances marketed in Canada qualify as either breakthrough products or significant therapeutic improvements (Patented Medicine Prices Review Board 2002). (See Figure 14.2.) The loudest and most influential voice calling for faster drug approvals comes from the brand-name industry. In a recently released document, RxandD emphasizes the excessive length of time that it takes to get a drug approved (RxandD 2002). From the point of view of returns on investment, industry's preoccupation with timeliness makes perfect sense, but whether that applies when a public health point of view is adopted is questionable.

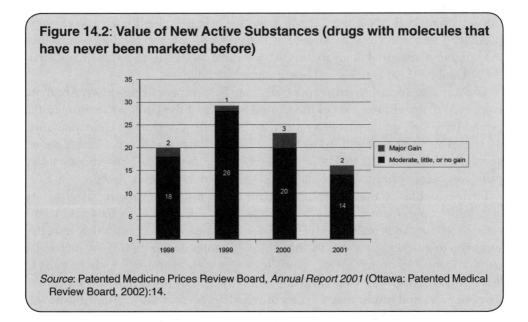

Figure 14.2: Value of New Active Substances (drugs with molecules that have never been marketed before)

Source: Patented Medicine Prices Review Board, *Annual Report 2001* (Ottawa: Patented Medical Review Board, 2002):14.

Timeliness in the approval process may take on even greater importance in the near future. In spring 2004, the private members' Bill C-212 was passed to deal with the user fees that various arms of government collect from industry for delivering services. Strong private-sector interest in this legislation was expressed through the Business Coalition on Cost Recovery, which included the brand-name pharmaceutical companies. The coalition was particularly supportive of aspects of the bill that are meant to ensure that user fees are consistent with the level and value of the services provided (Business Coalition on Cost Recovery 2004). In this regard, Bill C-212 provides for Canadian services to be compared with similar ones offered by Canada's major trading partners. If services are not adequate, government departments stand to forfeit part of the user fees. Setting and measuring timelines for drug approvals is relatively straightforward, but how do you set time standards for how long it should take to act on adverse drug reaction reports? In order to avoid financial penalties, Health Canada may direct even more resources into ensuring that drug-approval times are met at the expense of its other responsibilities.

Drug Safety

In contrast to the $31.2 million given over to faster approvals, only $2.5 million of the $40 million was allocated for the Marketed Health Products Directorate (MHPD), which monitors the safety and performance of drugs already approved. (See Table 14.1.) This discrepancy in the allocation of money came at a time when the MHPD has had to stop trying to assign causality when evaluating adverse drug-reaction reports. Information from each adverse drug-reaction report is entered into a number of fields in the Canada Adverse Drug Reaction Information System (CADRIS) database. Now, because of increased workload and funding constraints, the number of essential fields in the CADRIS database has been reduced, such that the "causality" field is no longer being systematically used.

The move to speed up drug approvals may be compromising safety. Abraham compared drug withdrawals in the United States and the United Kingdom in the period 1971–1992 and reported a ratio of 2.67:1 (24 drugs versus 9). His explanation for the lower number of withdrawals in the United States was that the longer period spent examining the data in the U.S. allowed regulators there to detect serious safety problems before products were marketed (Abraham and Davis 2002).

Further evidence that shorter approval times might adversely affect safety standards comes from a survey of U.S. regulatory officials. User fees paid to the Food and Drug Administration (FDA) by the brand-name pharmaceutical industry were tied to quicker approvals by the FDA, with times dropping for new molecular entities from 27 months in 1993, when user fees were instituted, to 19 months in 2001 (Office of Inspector General 2003). A survey of FDA reviewers by the Office of Inspector General found that 40 percent who had been at the agency at least five years indicated that the review process had worsened during their tenure in terms of allowing for in-depth, science-based reviews (Office of Inspector General 2003).

Pharmaceutical companies place a premium on rapid drug approvals in order to start recouping their investment in their products. Their interest in post-marketing surveillance is decidedly secondary. When companies in the U.S. agreed to supplement the FDA budget with user fees, they stipulated that the fees could be used only to hire new reviewers; none of the money went to post-marketing surveillance.

In Canada, one indication of the interest in drug safety comes from an analysis of the Web site for RxandD. A search of the sight in late 2003 found only a single page dealing with drug safety. The item in question was a news release playing down the significance of a story that had aired on a CBC television show.

Transparency in the Regulatory Process

Another manifestation of the clientele pluralist relationship between the state and the pharmaceutical industry is the agreement between the industry and the TPD that all of the information that companies submit as part of the regulatory approval process is deemed confidential and will not be released without the express consent of the company involved. Health Canada's own Science Advisory Board agrees that "in general, the Health Protection Branch [now the Health Products and Food Branch] has ... taken a very cautious position on what it releases as public information" (Science Advisory Board Committee on the Drug Review Process 2000: 1). As a result, all of the information that the industry submits, including clinical trial data on safety and efficacy, is deemed confidential and can be released only with the permission of the company even with an Access to Information request.

This approach to releasing the clinical information that companies submit reflects a common understanding between officials in Health Canada and the pharmaceutical industry of medical information as a commodity with commercial value that must be protected. Such information can be "loaned" to the government for purposes of review, but the companies do so with the expectation that the review will produce material gains through marketing of their products. This market-based view stands in marked contrast to a view that data on health and safety is something that should be shared directly with the people most affected—those who prescribe and use the products. What we have instead is information filtered through, and protected by, the officials in Health Canada.

There is no good evidence to show that the interests of companies would be harmed by the disclosure of information about safety and effectiveness (McGarity and Shapiro 1980). On the other hand, non-disclosure has serious disadvantages for the TPD, health professionals, and the public. If information submitted to regulatory agencies is never disclosed, then this data will never enter the normal peer review channels and are therefore not subject to scrutiny by independent scientists. Without this type of feedback, TPD reviewers may be more prone to misjudge the accuracy or usefulness of the data submitted, the scientific atmosphere in the agency may be stifled, and the professional growth of its staff severely inhibited (McGarity and Shapiro 1980). Deprived of any independent access to information, health professionals have to accept the TPD's judgment about the safety and effectiveness of products. In the case of well-established drugs, this is probably not much of a concern, but it may be different with new drugs where experience is limited.

Finally, the public may be denied knowledge of the full health effects of products so that they can decide for themselves whether or not to use them. Even if most consumers would never take the time to read health and safety data, consumer-oriented media in consultation with scientific experts could use some of this information to inform the public of the risks and benefits of products (McGarity and Shapiro 1980).

In response to calls for greater transparency, the TPD announced in 2004 that when new drugs and devices are approved, it would publish a document entitled the "Summary Basis of Decision" (SBD). The SBD would outline the scientific and benefit/risk-based reasons for the TPD's decision to grant market authorization for a product (Health Canada 2004). The key part of the SBD of importance to prescribers and consumers is the clinical information on drug effectiveness and safety. Is enough information provided to allow for safe and rational use of new medications or the extended indications for previously approved drugs?

To evaluate the adequacy of information in the SBDs, a colleague and I examined three recent cases in which unpublished data submitted to drug regulators contained important clinical information that was either unavailable or misrepresented within the published literature. The examples we chose were (a) the discovery that a published study on a new arthritis medication (Celebrex®) misrepresented the data by presenting information for only the first six months of a 16-month study; (b) that unpublished studies indicated that newer antidepressants are not any better than placebos; (c) that unpublished studies contained strong clues to the latter finding that hormone-replacement therapy had more harms than benefits for post-menopausal women. We ask whether the same discoveries would have been possible using Health Canada's SBDs. In each of these cases, our conclusion was that it would have been impossible to discover these problems using the SBDs because they did not contain enough detailed information about the studies that had been submitted by the pharmaceutical companies.

Regulation of Promotion

Companies spend significantly more on promotion in Canada than they do on research and development: $2.13 billion per year (see Box 14.1 for calculations) versus $1.19 billion, respectively (Patented Medicine Prices Review Board 2004). This money is not ill spent as surveys show that Canadian doctors rely heavily on promotional sources of information (Angus Reid Group 1991) and large-scale promotion helps to increase early prescribing of new drugs, as shown in Table 14.2. From the perspective of the companies, this process makes good economic sense as it generates large early returns on investment. However, from a public health point of view, prescribing that is driven by promotion should be avoided as there is abundant literature that consistently shows an association between use of promotion and inappropriate prescribing (Lexchin and Mintzes 2002). Furthermore, when drugs reach the market, they have been tested on only a relatively small number of highly selected patients. Consequently, no one has any idea how most people who will be getting the drug will react to it. Prescribing based on promotion, therefore, essentially means that many people are unwittingly participating in an experiment.

Given these negatives associated with promotion, it would seem sensible for governments to keep a tight rein on promotion and to strictly control it. The *Food*

Box 14.1: Calculation of Amount Spent on Promotion

Promotion accounts for about 16 percent of sales. Total prescription drug sales in 2003 were $15 billion. Out of that figure, about $1.7 billion comes from the generic industry, which does little promotion. That leaves sales of $13.3 billion in sales from the brand-name companies. Sixteen percent of $13.3 billion is $2.13 billion.

Table 14.2: Prescribing of Heavily Promoted Drugs

Drug	After Three Months on Market	
	Number of Prescriptions	**Cost ($000,000)**
Xenical (weight loss)	78,200	7.4
Viagra (erectile dysfunction)	65,000 (after one month)	13.3 (after one month)
Celebrex (pain and inflammation)	178,400	20.7

Source: IMS Health Canada, "Xenical Update: New Fat Blocker Is Canada's #1 Anti-obesity Medication" (IMS Health Canada, 2000). Available at www.imshealthcanada.com/htmen/4_2_1_16.htm; IMS Health Canada, "New Arthritis Medication Achieves Fastest Adoption Ever Recorded in Canada." (IMS Health Canada, 2000). Available at www.imshealthcanada.com/htmen/4_2_1_15.htm; IMS Health Canada.

and Drugs Act does give the Canadian government this power, but the government has chosen to turn over its regulatory authority to two bodies: the Pharmaceutical Advertising Advisory Board (PAAB), which controls print advertising, and the pharmaceutical industry, which regulates the behaviour of its sales representatives and how company-sponsored continuing medical education is run.

Voluntary self-regulation seems an attractive option because, lacking government–industry opposition, it is a more flexible and cost-effective option. Government regulators also reason that in a highly competitive industry, individual companies' desire to prevent competitors from gaining an edge can be harnessed to serve the public interest through a regime of voluntary self-regulation run by a trade association (Ayres and Braithwaite 1992). The problem with the foregoing analysis is that industry will always be tempted to exploit the privilege of self-regulation by producing a socially suboptimal level of compliance with regulatory goals. Experience has repeatedly shown this to be the case in the marketing of pharmaceutical products (Kawachi 1992).

In these circumstances few trade associations have made systematic efforts to either monitor the advertising practices of their members or to enforce compliance. The problem is that governments and pharmaceutical manufacturers' associations have different missions and goals. The government's mission is to protect public health by encouraging rational prescribing. The trade associations' mission is primarily to increase sales and profit. From the business perspective, self-regulation is concerned mostly with the control of anti-competitive practices. Therefore, when industrial associations draw up their codes of practice, they deliberately make them vague or do not cover certain features of promotion to allow companies a wide latitude. Self-regulation works well when anti-competitive promotional practices happen to coincide perfectly with government regulators' notions of misleading advertising. Most often, however, the fit is far from perfect because, far from being anti-competitive, many misleading advertising tactics are good for business. Therefore, from the public health perspective, the results of voluntary self-regulation are suboptimal (Lexchin and Kawachi 1996).

Certainly this is the case with the codes promulgated by the PAAB (*Code of Advertising Acceptance* 2002) and RxandD (*Code of Marketing Practices* 2004). Both codes operate under a reactive as opposed to a proactive style of regulation; that is, action is generally taken only upon receipt of complaints, rather than preventing breaches from occurring in the first place. Neither code has effective sanctions where breaches have occurred. PAAB has no authority to levy monetary sanctions, although it can require companies to pull offending advertisements, but by the time a complaint has been made and a ruling taken, the ad may be near to completing its run in any case. The penalty for the third violation of the RxandD code in a single year is a $15,000 fine, which for large drug companies is the equivalent of "lunch money." Neither code has a predefined period after which it needs to be reviewed; there was no major revision to the PAAB code between 1992 and 2004. The PAAB code does not have any specific provision about the type size for safety information and detailed prescribing information does not have to be placed directly after the main body of the ad, but can appear at the back of the journal. The RxandD code does not require sales representatives to provide doctors with specific information about risks, contraindications, and warnings and they do not have to leave a copy of the government-approved official product monograph, which provides detailed information about the drug. According to the RxandD code, companies are required to "support, where possible, the principles and practices of [continuing health education]," but nowhere is it defined what "where possible" means.

A recent example of how Health Canada has abdicated its responsibilities in the area of controlling promotion is the case of direct-to-consumer promotion of prescription drugs. Regulations issued under the *Food and Drugs Act* allow companies to advertise prescription drugs only to the extent that the name, quantity, and price of the product can be displayed (Food and Drugs Act). Policy statements in 1996 and 2000 reinterpreted this regulation to mean that companies were allowed to run "disease awareness" ads as long as the name of a product was not mentioned or firms could name a medication as long as its use was not discussed. The only type of advertising that remained prohibited was one in which a product was named and its use was given (Michols 1996; Rowsell 2000).

Health Canada has been reluctant to enforce even this loose reinterpretation of its own regulations. Ads for Diane-35, an oral contraceptive marketed by Berlex and approved in Canada for use only as a second-line agent for resistant acne, were plastered on bus shelters in Montreal and other cities across Canada with the message "the acne solution for women only." Although the ad did not directly name the drug, the woman featured in the ad was given the name "Diane." The group Women and Health Protection sent a letter to Health Canada complaining about this and other ads in March 2001 following Berlex's launch of a new national billboard, television, and cinema ad campaign for Diane-35. An Access to Information request revealed that 18 months after this letter was sent, there had been no communication between Health Canada and the company. Meanwhile, the Diane-35 ad campaign continued. Print ads continued to run in *Healthy Woman*, a Canadian magazine produced for reading by patients in family physicians and gynecologists' waiting rooms (Barbara Mintzes, personal communication, November 2003).

Intellectual Property Rights and Patent Issues

Intellectual property rights (IPR) and patent issues are key factors in determining how much individual drugs cost and the overall level of expenditure on drugs. Patent life in Canada, for all products, not just pharmaceuticals, lasts for 20 years from the date that the patent is filed. The 20-year period is dictated by the Trade Related Aspects of Intellectual Property Rights (TRIPS) Agreement that Canada is a signatory to as a consequence of its membership in the World Trade Organization (WTO). (See Box 14.2.) The crux of the industry's argument for strong intellectual property rights protection is that it needs a prolonged monopoly time to sell its products in order to recoup the costs entailed in the research and development of new drugs, drugs that may be more expensive than existing ones, but are also more effective and/or more safe.

Box 14.2: Effective Monopoly Time for Patented Drugs

Typically companies take out patents on their drugs once they have synthesized the molecule. At that time it undergoes a variety of testing for things like chemical purity and manufacturing quality. The next step is testing in laboratory animals followed by human testing. Once all of these tests are completed, the company submits files to the Therapeutic Products Directorate to get the drug approved. By the time it has received marketing approval, about 8 to 10 years of patent life have expired.

Table 14.3: Rate of Return on Shareholders' Equity, before Taxes, 1988–1995

Year	Percent Rate of Return	
	Pharmaceutical Industry	All Manufacturing Industries
1988	54.1	21.7
1989	40.1	15.5
1999	26.6	5.8
1991	31.7	0
1992	24.6	2.6
1993	20.8	7.1
1994	21.5	14.4
1995	17.2	18.2
Average	29.6	10.7

Profit Levels

If the industry's message is that it needs a longer period of time to recover its investment, then a natural starting place is to look at how profitable or unprofitable it has been. Profit levels for the pharmaceutical industry have historically been significantly higher than those for other industries. (See Table 14.3.) Even compared to other "high-tech" industries, pharmaceutical companies have fared well; in the mid-1990s the industry had a 16 percent rate of return on capital employed compared to about 14 percent for makers of computer equipment, 10 percent for makers of other types of electronic equipment, and 9 percent for telecommunications carriers (Statistics Canada 1996).

The Cost of Developing New Drugs

The most recent study to look at this question reports that for drugs first tested in humans between 1983 and 1994, the mean cost to bring them to market was U.S. $802 million (DiMasi, Hansen, and Grabowski 2003). It should be noted that these are not costs that need to be recovered solely through Canadian sales. Canada represents about 2 percent of the world pharmaceutical market and therefore a reasonable expectation is that about U.S. $16 million should be recouped in Canada.

Beyond the question of how much Canadians should contribute to R&D costs, there are also fundamental points of dispute around this figure. To begin with, the data used were derived from information self-reported by drug companies and there is no independent way to verify this information. Second, the $802 million amount represents the costs for only one type of drug—new chemical entities (drugs containing ingredients never marketed before)—and excludes drugs that are combinations of previously available medications and reformulations of existing products (e.g., new dosage forms). About 30 percent of R&D expenditures go toward bringing this latter type of drug to market (Frank 2003). Also any drugs developed with funding from non-industry sources—such as government, hospitals, foundations, or medical schools—are excluded. In computing the cost of developing new drugs, it is important to incorporate expenses for products that fail in the development stage. While many drugs are withdrawn because of safety reasons or because of lack of effectiveness, at least 20 percent of drugs in the development stage are terminated for commercial reasons—that is, because they are not deemed profitable enough. As Frank points out, changes in revenue expectations would lead to different decisions about drug terminations and would thus change the average cost figure (Frank 2003).

Recent Rulings by the World Trade Organization (WTO)

Two separate challenges have been launched against Canada in the WTO in recent years. The European Union (E.U.) complained about a provision in the Canadian patent law that allowed generic drug companies to begin testing, manufacturing, and stockpiling drugs for sale before patents expired. When Canada changed from a 17- to a 20-year patent term for drugs approved after October 1, 1989, the change was not made retroactive. The United States charged that a group of about 30 drugs patented before October 1989 should receive an additional three years of patent life. (The complaint by the U.S. did not just cover drugs but patents on all products that were granted before October 1989 and that were still valid.)

Canada lost the case filed by the U.S. (MacKinnon 2000) and the WTO also ruled that generic companies could not stockpile drugs for sale before the patent expired (Scoffield 2000). As a result of these decisions, in mid-2001 Canadian patent laws were amended with the passage of Bill S-17. The extension of the patent term on the 30 drugs is expected to add an estimated $40 million to Canada's prescription drug costs, according to the Canadian Drug Manufacturers Association, the lobbying arm of the generic industry ("Battle to Repeal Automatic Injunctions against Generic Drug Approvals Moves to the Fall" 2001). Prohibiting generic companies from stockpiling drugs until the patent expires will delay the marketing of generic products for weeks.

How Intellectual Property Rights Distort the Pharmaceutical Marketplace

As we saw earlier, the majority of drugs produced through research led by the patent incentive do not represent any significant therapeutic advances. Industry largely engages in R&D of products that are aimed at carving out a share of a lucrative market. The result is drugs that are essentially minor variations of existing medications, for example, additions to the statin group of drugs for lowering cholesterol. Since most drugs offer little or no therapeutic advantage over existing remedies, then it stands to reason that most of the money spent on R&D will go into products that will build market share, not products that will necessarily result in significantly better health outcomes.

Baker and Chatani (2002) itemize an additional five ways that patent protection leads to wasteful rent-seeking behaviour by pharmaceutical companies. The huge costs associated with promotion that were documented earlier are one element of the excess costs.

Gaining a competitive edge on rival firms leads to a restriction in sharing research results and delays in publishing findings because of commercial concerns. Twenty-seven percent of faculty in university life science academic departments who received industry support delayed publication of their results for more than six months compared to 17 percent without such support. Eighty-one percent of life science companies with relationships with academic institutions reported keeping results secret for longer than was necessary to obtain a patent (Blumenthal, Campbell, Anderson, and Louis 1997). Communication is the lifeblood of science, and if it is impeded, so is scientific research. Without knowing what others are doing, scientists may be needlessly repeating work.

There are the direct legal costs associated with filing and protecting patents and the indirect costs that result from successful efforts such as "evergreening," which stall the marketing of generic drugs. When the Canadian Coordinating Office for Health Technology Assessment (CCOHTA) was about to release a report saying that all of the different drugs in the statin group were equivalent, Bristol-Myers Squibb (BMS), the maker of one of these drugs, objected to the release of the report and went to court to block its publication. The case was eventually thrown out, but not before CCOHTA spent 13 percent of its annual budget defending itself (Hemminki, Haley, and Koivusalo 1999).

In the United States the pharmaceutical industry employs over 600 lobbyists and spent U.S. $78.1 million in 2001 partly to ensure that politicians heard its view about IPRs (Public Citizen Congress Watch 2002). Industry in Canada is also into heavy political lobbying. Deputy-Prime Minister John Manley, in his run for the leadership of the Liberal Party in 2002–2003, received tens of thousands of dollars in donations from a group of six pharmaceutical companies, plus RxandD. According to another Liberal parliamentarian, Manley was a key backer of the brand-name pharmaceutical industry's interests in Cabinet discussions and is "part of the Praetorian Guard of status quo on high drug prices"(Clark and McCarthy 2003: A6).

The Cost of Prescription Medications in Canada

The Patented Medicine Prices Review Board (PMPRB) was established in 1987 to protect consumer interests with powers to limit the introductory prices for new patented drugs and prevent prices for existing patented drugs from rising by more than the rate of inflation. Within this context the PMPRB has been a success. Its 2003 report demonstrates that between 1988 to 2000, the rate of inflation for the price of patented medications had risen by just 0.5 percent per year; when Canadian prices are compared to the average of those in seven other countries (France, Germany, Italy, Sweden, Switzerland, the United Kingdom, and the United States) the ratio dropped from 1.23 in 1987 to just 0.95 in 2003 (Patented Medicine Prices Review Board 2004). However, these figures hide a basic failure in the PMPRB's ability to protect consumers from high prices when it comes to the price they pay for a prescription.

The price of a prescription for non-patented medications increased 2.3 percent annually from 1997 to 2001 to a level of $22.94 in 2001. On the other hand, during the same period patented medications went up 6.2 percent annually to a value of $84.36 in 2001 (*Green Shield Report* 2002). Physicians have been substituting these newer, more expensive drugs for older, less costly ones, leading to the rise in the cost of the average prescription as shown by the fact that between 1997 and 2001, sales of patented medications as a proportion of total sales went from 52.3 percent to 65.0 percent (Patented Medicine Prices Review Board 2004).

The prescribing of newer, more expensive drugs in place of older, less expensive, but not necessarily less effective, ones was not something that started in 1987. The practice has been well entrenched for many years. What is different is that prior to 1987 Canada allowed generic drugs to come onto the market typically within five to seven years after the appearance of the originator product through a process known as compulsory licensing. (Compulsory licensing meant that a generic company could obtain permission to market a drug in Canada even while a patent was still in force, even without the consent of the company owning the patent.) The first generic would typically be priced about 25 percent lower than the brand-name product, and when there were three or four generics, then the price differential would be 50 percent (Lexchin 1993). In the absence of compulsory licensing, the originator product typically is in a monopoly situation for about 10–12 years.

The delay in the entry of generics is associated with a continual climb in spending on prescription drugs. Between 1975 and 1987, prescription drugs went from taking up 6.3 percent of the health care dollar to 7.0 percent for an annual increase of 11.5 percent; in comparison the change between 1987 and 2001 was from 7.0 percent to 12.0 percent, a rise of 71 percent per year (Canadian Institute for Health Information 2001). (See Figure 14.3.)

Conclusions

Which pill people eventually put into their mouths is the product of a complex series of decisions that start long before the doctor reaches for his or her prescription pad. This chapter has discussed how these decisions involve economic and political factors at the national and international level and reflect the tensions between private profit and public health. Companies are interested in making as much money as

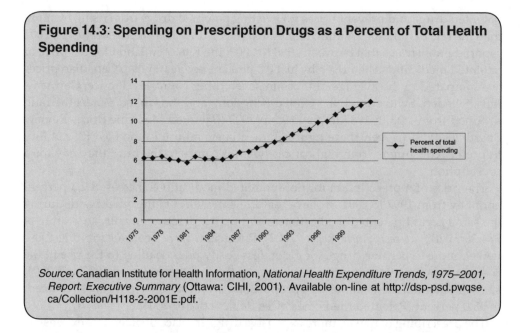

Figure 14.3: Spending on Prescription Drugs as a Percent of Total Health Spending

Source: Canadian Institute for Health Information, *National Health Expenditure Trends, 1975–2001, Report: Executive Summary* (Ottawa: CIHI, 2001). Available on-line at http://dsp-psd.pwqse. ca/Collection/H118-2-2001E.pdf.

possible for their shareholders and develop drugs with the largest markets, but these products usually do not offer any significant advantages over existing therapies. Hundreds of millions of research dollars rest on the decision about which drugs to develop and because such large sums of money are involved, the companies want strong intellectual property rights to protect their investments for the longest time. Once the drug is developed, it still has to get through the regulatory process and then be prescribed by doctors. While government should be looking out for the public's interests in all of these areas, there is increasing concern that government priorities have become reoriented to more closely reflect those of the industry.

A basic understanding of these complex issues is necessary in order to formulate public policy so that Canadian society can decide how to deal with all of the questions regarding prescription drugs and their rapidly escalating costs.

References

Abraham, J., and C. Davis. (2002). *Mapping the Social and Political Dynamics of Drug Safety Withdrawals in the U.K. and the U.S.* London: Economic and Social Research Council.

Angus Reid Group. (1991). *Credibility and the Marketing Mix*. Toronto: Angus Reid Group.

Atkinson, M.M., and W.D. Coleman. (1985). "Corporatism and Industrial Policy." In *Organized Interests and the State*, edited by A. Cawson, 22–44. London: Sage.

_____. (1989). *The State, Business, and Industrial Change in Canada*. Toronto: University of Toronto Press.

Ayres, I., and J. Braithwaite. (1992). *Responsive Regulation: Transcending the Deregulation Debate*. New York: Oxford University Press.

Baker, D., and N. Chatani. (2002). *Promoting Good Ideas on Drugs: Are Patents the Best Way? The Relative Efficiency of Patent and Public Support for Bio-medical Research* (Briefing Paper). Washington: Center for Economic and Policy Research.

"Battle to Repeal Automatic Injunctions against Generic Drug Approvals Moves to the Fall." (2001). *CDMA Viewpoint* 1(6): 1 and 6.

Blumenthal, D., E. Campbell, M. Anderson, and K. Louis. (1997). "Withholding Research Results in Academic Life Science: Evidence from a National Perspective." *Journal of the American Medical Association* 277: 1224–1228.

Business Coalition on Cost Recovery. (2004). *Roy Cullen Congratulated on Passage of C-212.* Toronto: Business Coalition on Cost Recovery.

Canadian Institute for Health Information. (2001). *National Health Expenditure Trends, 1975–2001, Report: Executive Summary.* Ottawa: CIHI.

Clark, C., and S. McCarthy. (2003). "Drug-Company Donations to Manley Spark Controversy." *Globe and Mail* (May 14): A6.

Code of Advertising Acceptance. (2002). Pickering: Pharmaceutical Advertising Advisory Board.

Code of Marketing Practices. (2004). Ottawa: Canada's Research-Based Pharmaceutical Companies.

Department of Finance Canada. (2003). *Building the Canada We Want. Budget 2003: Investing in Canada's Health Care System.* Cat. no. F1-23/2003-4E. Ottawa: Department of Finance.

DiMasi, J., R. Hansen, and H. Grabowski. (2003). "The Price of Innovation: New Estimates of Drug Development Costs." *Journal of Health Economics* 22: 151–185.

External Advisory Committee on Smart Regulation. 2004. "Risk Management." Available on-line at www.pco-bcp.gc.ca/smartreg-regint/en/05/01/ir-01.html.

Food and Drugs Act, C.01.044.

Frank, R. (2003). "New Estimates of Drug Development Costs." *Journal of Health Economics* 22: 325–330.

Government of Canada. (2003). "The Canada We Want: Speech from the Throne to Open the Second Session of the Thirty-Seventh Parliament of Canada." Ottawa: Government of Canada.

Green Shield Report. (2002). Toronto: Green Shield.

Health Canada. (2003a). *Health Protection Legislative Renewal: Detailed Legislative Proposal.* Ottawa: Health Canada.

_____. (2003b). *Improving Canada's Regulatory Process for Therapeutic Products: Building the Action Plan.* Ottawa: Public Policy Forum multi-stakeholder consultation.

_____. (2004). *Issue Analysis Summary: Summary Basis of Decision—Draft 7.* Ottawa: Health Canada.

Hemminki, E., D. Haley, and M. Koivusalo. (1999). "The Courts—a Challenge to Health Technology Assessment." *Science* 285: 203–204.

Kawachi, I. (1992). "Six Case Studies of the Voluntary Regulation of Pharmaceutical Advertising and Promotion." In *For Health or for Profit?*, edited by P. Davis, 269–287. Auckland: Oxford University Press.

KPMG Consulting LP. (2000). *Review of the Therapeutic Products Programme Cost Recovery Initiative,* vol. 1. Ottawa: KPMG Consulting LP.

Lexchin, J. (1993). "The Effect of Generic Competition on the Price of Prescription Drugs in the Province of Ontario." *CMAJ* 148: 35–38.

Lexchin, J., and I. Kawachi. (1996). "Voluntary Codes of Pharmaceutical Marketing: Controlling Promotion or Licensing Deception." In *Contested Ground: Public Purpose and Private Interest in the Regulation of Prescription Drugs*, edited by P. Davis, 221–235. New York: Oxford University Press.

Lexchin, J., and B. Mintzes. (2002). "Direct-to-Consumer Advertising of Prescription Drugs: The Evidence Says No." *Journal of Public Policy and Management* 21(2): 194–201.

MacKinnon, M. (2000). "WTO Rejects Patent Law Appeal." *Globe and Mail* (September 19): B10.

McGarity, T.O., and S.A. Shapiro. (1980). "The Trade Secret Status of Health and Safety Testing Information: Reforming Agency Disclosure Policies." *Harvard Law Review* 93: 837–888.

Michols, D. (1996). *The Distinction between Advertising and Other Activities*. Ottawa: Health Canada, Therapeutics Products Programme.

Office of Inspector General. (2003). *FDA's Review Process for New Drug Applications: A Management Review*. Washington: Department of Health and Human Services.

Patented Medicine Prices Review Board. (2002). *Annual Report 2001*. Ottawa: Patented Medicine Prices Review Board (PMPRB).

_____. (2004). *PMPRB Annual Report 2003*. Ottawa: PMPRB.

Public Citizen Congress Watch. (2002). *The Other Drug War II: Drug Companies Use an Army of 623 Lobbyists to Keep Profits up*. Washington: Public Citizen Congress Watch.

Rawson, N. (2001). "Timeliness of Review and Approval of New Drugs in Canada from 1999 through 2001: Is Progress Being Made?" *Clinical Therapeutics* 25: 1230–1247.

Rowsell, L. (2000). *Advertising Campaigns of Branded and Unbranded Messages*. Ottawa: Health Canada, Therapeutic Products Directorate.

RxandD. (2002). *Improving Health through Innovation: A New Deal for Canadians*. Ottawa: RxandD.

Science Advisory Board Committee on the Drug Review Process. (2000). *Appendix F: Notes on Canadian Law and the Drug Review Process*. Ottawa: Science Advisory Board Committee on the Drug Review Process.

Scoffield, H. (2000). "WTO Upholds Drug Patent Rule." *Globe and Mail* (March 18): B3.

Statistics Canada. (1996). *Financial Performance Indicators for Canadian Business*. Cat. no. 61F0058XPE. Ottawa: Statistics Canada.

Therapeutic Products Directorate. (nd). *Business Transformation Progress Report*. Ottawa: Health Canada.

• •

Critical Thinking Questions

1. How can the contradictions between the profit motive and the public interest be reconciled in the area of research and development?

2. What are the ethical implications when the interests of the public and private corporations are in competition as may be the case when it comes to new drug approvals?

3. Assuming the pharmaceutical promotion will continue to exist, what mechanisms could be used to ensure that it is accurate and unbiased?

4. What can be done to control the increasing expenditure on pharmaceuticals in Canada? How would controls affect economic activity associated with the pharmaceutical industry?

5. Should the pharmaceutical industry be held to higher moral standards than other industries? If so, how could this be accomplished?

Further Readings

Angell, M., MD. (2004). *The Truth about the Drug Companies: How They Deceive Us and What to Do about It.* New York: Random House.
Angell is a former editor of the world's most prestigious medical journal, *The New England Journal of Medicine*, and uses the knowledge that she gained in that position to present a highly critical viewpoint about the pharmaceutical industry.

Commission on the Future of Health Care in Canada (Romanow Commission). (2002). *Building on Values: The Future of Health Care in Canada—Final Report.* Ottawa: Health Canada.
Chapter 9 in this report presents an up-to-date, cogent critique of many of the issues regarding pharmaceutical policy in Canada today along with recommendations for correcting these problems.

Rachlis, M., MD. (2004). *Prescription for Excellence: How Innovation Is Saving Canada's Health Care System.* Toronto: HarperCollins Canada.
Rachlis describes forward-thinking and practical solutions to many of Medicare's most entrenched problems. Although the book deals with the entire health care system, there is an excellent chapter showing how prescription drugs can be made more affordable.

Sanger, M., and S. Sinclair, eds. (2004). *Putting Health First: Canadian Health Care Reform in a Globalized World.* Ottawa: Canadian Centre for Policy Alternatives.
This book draws on material developed for the Romanow Commission to present an in-depth analysis of how trade issues affect Canadian health care, including questions like Pharmacare and drug costs.

Wiktorowicz, M. (2000). "Shifting Priorities at the Health Protection Branch: Challenges to the Regulatory Process." *Canadian Public Administration* 43: 1–22.

Wiktorowicz argues that previous changes in regulatory policy have pushed Canada's regulatory system from one where new agents were considered potentially harmful until proven safe to one where they are considered safe until proven harmful.

Relevant Web Sites

Canada's Research-Based Pharmaceutical Companies
www.canadapharma.org/
Presents the viewpoint of the brand-name pharmaceutical companies on a wide range of issues, including the drug-approval system and patent issues.

Drug Promotion Database
www.drugpromo.info/
An annotated bibliography of more than 2,200 items dealing with the promotion of pharmaceuticals along with four reviews of major issues that are currently being debated in the area of promotion.

Health Care and Intellectual Property
www.cptech.org/ip/health/
Has an extensive listing of articles, letters, and other material on questions like intellectual property rights as they relate to pharmaceuticals in the developed and the developing world.

Therapeutic Products Directorate
www.hc-sc.gc.ca/hpfb-dgpsa/tpd-dpt/index_e.html
Health Canada's Therapeutic Products Directorate is the Canadian federal authority that regulates pharmaceutical drugs and medical devices for human use. This Web site describes the different functions of the TPD and gives policy documents for issues that are currently under discussion.

Women and Health Protection
www.whp-apsf.ca/en/index.html
The group keeps a close watch over the proposed changes in the federal health protection legislation and examines the impact of those changes on women's health. The documents in this Web site make clear recommendations to the government, demanding that Canadian legislation truly provide "health protection."

Glossary

Clientele pluralism: A situation where the state has a high degree of concentration of power in one agency, but a low degree of autonomy, whereas in the private sector an organization has significant resources and the ability to act on behalf of its member firms.

Cost recovery: Companies now pay an annual fee to the Therapeutic Products Programme for each drug that they market and a fee for the evaluation of new drug submissions. This money is used to fund the majority of the operating costs of the TPP.

Generic competition: Generic drugs compete with brand-name products, but are usually priced at least 25 percent lower. They are identical to brand-name products and in Canada are usually produced by Canadian-owned companies.

Patent protection: Once an invention is patented, the individual or company making the discovery is protected from competition for a period of 20 years from the date the patent was filed.

Research and development: The process of discovering a new drug and doing the testing necessary to bring it to market.

· ·

CHAPTER FIFTEEN

PUBLIC HEALTH CONCERNS IN CANADA, THE U.S., THE U.K., AND SWEDEN

Exploring the Gaps between Knowledge and Action in Promoting Population Health

Dennis Raphael and Toba Bryant

· ·

Learning Objectives

At the conclusion of this chapter, the reader will be able to
- identify public health preoccupations in Canada, the U.S., the U.K., and Sweden
- show how these preoccupations both result from—and reinforce—existing models of public health and public policy
- discuss the public health gaps between knowledge and action on the broader determinants of population health
- outline why these gaps exist and their implications for promoting population health
- show how nations can apply advanced thinking about health determinants to public health activities and develop healthy public policy

Introduction

Promoting health comprises three distinct, though potentially related, sets of activities: traditional public health activities; developing healthy public policy; and delivering health care services. Public health and healthy public policy—our focus in this chapter—are concerned with promoting the health of the population while health care services treat individuals who are ill or at risk of being ill. In Canada, these components generally operate independently. With few exceptions, public health agencies carry out one set of activities, policy makers design public policy in their spheres of interest, and health care professionals deliver health services.

The extent to which integration of public health and public policy activities is possible depends upon a variety of factors. The most important is the model of health adhered to within each jurisdiction. If health is seen as a highly individualized issue that reflects biological dispositions and risk behaviours, approaches to public health will focus on managing biomedical and behavioural risk factors (e.g., hypertension, cholesterol levels, weight, tobacco use, and diet).

In contrast, if health is seen as influenced by structural factors (e.g., the organization of society and the distribution of resources), public health will focus on health-supportive public policy such as income, employment, housing, and service provision. Canada has been seen as a leader in broader structural approaches to health. Despite this history, Canada has been surpassed by other nations such as the U.K. and Sweden in applying these concepts to policy development and implementation. Health is a central concern of Canadians, and how the public health community defines it will influence governmental approaches to public policy. This chapter compares approaches to public health and health-supportive policy development in Canada, the U.S., the U.K., and Sweden. We examine the U.S. and the U.K. since policy developments in these nations frequently influence Canada. We look at Sweden as an example of how public health can draw upon the emerging literature on health determinants to influence public policy.

Public Health Preoccupations in Canada and Elsewhere

Public health can be concerned with healthy public policy, health care services, building strong communities, protecting citizens from environmental threats, and promoting healthy behaviours. For decades, Canadian governments and professional associations have stressed the role of "determinants of health and the role of healthy public policy." In practice, however, Canadian public health practice is limited in scope and focused upon protection from environmental threats and modifying individual risk (e.g., safety of water and food supply, infection control, modification of diet, tobacco use, and patterns of physical activity). When working on healthy child development, activities are narrow (e.g., parenting centres, healthy nutrition, etc.), with little effort in influencing family- and child-related public policy.

In the U.S., traditional public health activities include providing health care services to indigent populations. Public health has this responsibility as many Americans lack access to the privately organized health care system. Population health concepts have penetrated into government and health agency documents, yet these same documents emphasize behavioural approaches to health promotion.

There is neglect of public policy as means of influencing the broader determinants of health. Policy options to improve health stress access to health care rather than equitably distributing economic resources.

In contrast, the New Labour government of the U.K. has developed and implemented policies for addressing inequalities in health by addressing broader determinants of health. More recently, however, a spate of policy documents on the need for Britons to modify their health-related behaviours raised concerns that these approaches may detract from action to address health determinants. In Sweden long-standing concern with progressive public policy melds well with increasing knowledge and understandings concerning the broader determinants of health. Public health activities are concerned with strengthening democratic participation, promoting security and well-being of families, and reducing health inequalities. Sweden provides the most developed example of a progressive public health vision that strives to support health through public policy.

In this chapter, we examine governmental statements about health, the structure and activities of public health agencies, and the relationship of public health to other arms of government activity in these four nations. By identifying the principles and concepts that direct public health activities in each nation, we ascertain the extent to which public health preoccupations reflect the emerging theory and research concerning the determinants of population health.

Canada

Canada has been seen as a leader in innovative approaches to public health (Restrepo 1996). Canadians were strong contributors to health-promotion principles of equity and participation and the population health focus on the determinants of health. However, the past decade has seen a retreat from progressive approaches to public health such that Canada has fallen behind other nations in applying its own concepts to promoting health (Canadian Population Health Initiative 2002). Behavioural approaches to health promotion now predominate. Why is this the case?

In Canada, municipalities are responsible for public health. Provincial legislation specifies the mandatory services these local units must provide. Mandatory programs include anti-tobacco, maternal and infant health, dental, school-based programs, infection control, and sanitation, among others. In recent years, provincial governments' increasing emphases on conservative approaches have forced a shift from community-based health promotion to biomedical concerns with disease and infection control and the provision of programs to promote lifestyle changes, such as smoking cessation, increased activity, and dietary changes to reduce obesity (Raphael 2003a).

Canadian Policy Statements on Public Health

The federal government's *A New Vision of Health for Canadians* identified four fields that determined health: human biology, lifestyles, environment, and health care

(Lalonde 1974). Governments and public health officials seized upon the lifestyle aspect—tobacco use, activity level, healthy diet, etc.—to exclude the role played by social conditions. The lifestyle emphasis was balanced by the federal *Achieving Health for All* document, which emphasized structural aspects of society as health determinants (Epp 1986).

The 1990s saw the emphasis upon health promotion—with its explicit concern with community engagement—eclipsed by the field of population health, which focused upon researching how social, economic, and physical environments influence health (Robertson 1998). Health Canada has attempted to maintain the progressive aspects of health promotion in an integrated approach to population health, as shown in Figure 15.1.

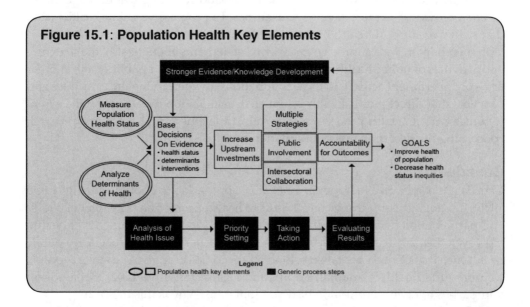

Figure 15.1: Population Health Key Elements

The Canadian Public Health Association (CPHA) has drawn attention to homelessness, employment security, food insecurity, poverty, and other broader determinants of health (Canadian Public Health Association 2001). The CPHA's *Action Statement on Health Promotion* states that since "policies shape how money, power and material resources flow through society and therefore affect the determinants of health …. [A]dvocating for healthy public policies is the single most important strategy for improving health" (Canadian Public Health Association 1996: 3). Similar themes run through federal, provincial, and local public health documents, disease-oriented association mission statements, and Royal Commissions and Senate Committee reports on health. However, translation of these concepts into actions by governments and local public health units—with a few notable exceptions—is rare (Raphael 2003b).

The SARS crisis of 2003, combined with pressure from public health associations, increased concern about public health mandates. In response, the federal government established a National Public Health Agency. The agency consists of the Centres for Healthy Human Development, Chronic Disease Prevention and Control, Infectious Disease Prevention and Control, Emergency Preparedness and Response, and Surveillance Coordination. It is too early to determine whether the agency will concern itself with broader policy issues related to health. To date, the record of Health Canada having its broader vision of health adopted by public health units and other arms of governments has been disappointing (Lavis 2002). Indeed, a widening gap between knowledge and action is apparent.

Healthy Living Initiative

In September 2002, the federal/provincial/territorial Ministers of Health adopted the *Integrated Pan-Canadian Healthy Living Strategy* (Health Canada 2003). It emphasizes the dangers of physical inactivity, unhealthy eating, and tobacco use. The definition of "healthy living" makes no reference to conditions of daily life as determinants of health. Health promotion and population health are reduced to health-related behaviours. The approach contradicts three decades of research and policy statements on health determinants. The *Strategy* argues that broader determinants of health determine individuals' ability to modify health-related behaviours, but says nothing about the direct role the environment plays in determining health or the importance of addressing these health determinants directly.

Chronic Disease Alliance of Canada (CDPAC)

In their "case for change," the CDPAC sees the primary contributors to cardiovascular disease, cancer, respiratory disease, and diabetes as tobacco use, physical inactivity, and poor diets (Chronic Disease Prevention Alliance of Canada 2003). CDPAC fails to mention how material conditions of life directly influence the incidence of chronic disease. No mention is made of research on how the material conditions of life directly influence health or structure health behaviours. Nothing is said on influencing public policy to improve living conditions of those most at risk for chronic disease.

Provincial and Local Public Health Activities

Canadian public health practice is for the most part divorced from modifying the broader determinants of health. Provincial health authorities direct the activities of local health units and, with few exceptions (see Quebec and British Columbia health objectives), provincial focus is on behavioural approaches to health. This is true even when provincial documents detail the importance of broader determinants of health. In Alberta a major report states: "The health of all Albertans should be promoted and improved by taking a global view of all of the factors that determine and affect people's health ... basic public health measures, economic well-being, early childhood development, education, housing, nutrition, employment status, quality of the environment, lifestyle choices and healthy behaviours" (Mazankowski 2001: 41).

Yet, the provincial response to the report was to establish a "wellness program that will encourage Albertans to follow healthier lifestyles, such as increasing their level of physical activity and reducing their use of tobacco" (Government of Alberta 2002: 3). In the other provinces, similar reports that focused on the "obesity epidemic" provide strong direction to local health units (Basrur 2004).

Given these directions, tied to funding, it is not surprising that there is little public health concern with healthy public policy: "Many provinces had no evidence of mandated programs that were explicitly health focused, that addressed broader determinants of health, or used multiple strategies" (Sutcliffe, Deber, and Pasut 1997: 247). Local public health units across Canada are unlikely to have initiatives addressing poverty issues, and among those that do, virtually all deal with the consequences of poverty rather than addressing its causes (Williamson 2001).

Against the Grain: Taking Healthy Public Policy Seriously

Despite public health inaction on broader determinants of health, there are supports for those advancing these issues. Statistics Canada and Health Canada continue to produce documentation of the state of various health determinants. Many non-governmental organizations express concern with issues of income and poverty, housing, child care, food security, employment conditions, and other health determinants (Raphael and Curry-Stevens 2004).

Policy institutes such as the Canadian Centre for Policy Alternatives, the Caledon Institute, and the Canadian Policy Research Networks produce relevant analyses of these issues. The Canadian Population Health Initiative of the federal government provides timely research on the broader determinants of health. Health Canada and its regional offices support investigations and actions upon the broader determinants of health.

The Montreal Health Authority has been a leader in raising and advocating for action on the broader determinants of health (Lessard 1997; Lessard, Roy, Choinière, Lévesque, and Perron 2002). Similar work is being done by scattered health units in Ontario (Waterloo, Peterborough, and Sudbury), Alberta (Chinook Region), and British Columbia (Interior Health Region).

In summary, Canada emphasizes traditional health protection and health-promotion approaches to public health. Health Canada, the CPHA, and various organizations continue to raise issues of healthy public policy and the broader determinants of health. There are only a few isolated instances of public health action to influence healthy public policy.

United States

The U.S. has one of the worst health profiles of modern industrialized nations. It has one of the least developed welfare states. It is the only modern industrialized nation that does not provide health care for citizens as a matter of course. Public health concern with broader determinants of health and healthy public policy is poorly developed. Public health concern is focused on racial and ethnic disparities with little concern about how broader determinants of health cause these disparities. There is a wide gap between knowledge concerning the broader determinants of health and action to address these determinants in the policy sphere.

National Policy Documents and Reports

Healthy People 2010 is the national plan for public health and contains a large number of health objectives (U.S. Department of Health and Human Services 2000). It recognizes developments in theory and findings concerning the broader determinants of health and its model of health is consistent with a broader determinants of health perspective. (See Figure 15.2.) The U.S. assigns a prominent emphasis to issues of access to health care, which is not surprising given that 17 percent or 45 million Americans do not have health insurance coverage.

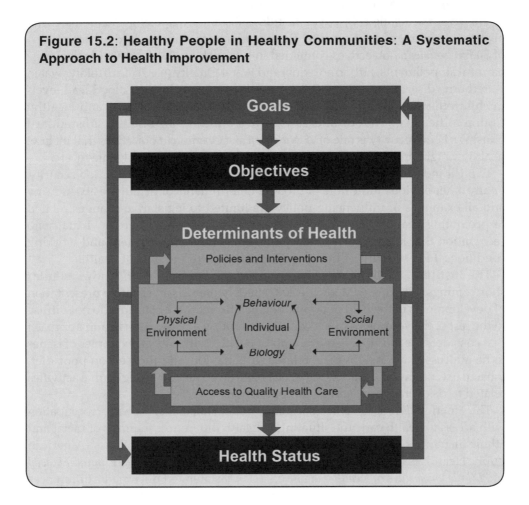

Figure 15.2: Healthy People in Healthy Communities: A Systematic Approach to Health Improvement

Inspection of the document reveals that the role played by broader determinants of health is undeveloped. The *Leading Health Indicators*—that "reflect the major health concerns in the United States at the beginning of the 21st century" (U.S. Department of Health and Human Services 2000: 36)—are low levels of physical activity, excess weight and obesity, tobacco use, substance abuse, irresponsible sexual behaviour, mental health, injury and violence, low environmental quality, immunization, and low access to health care. These are firmly planted in the biomedical and behavioural public health camps.

The *Environmental Quality Leading Indicators*—which could address conditions of daily living of income, food and housing security, early life, employment and working conditions, and social services—are limited to the "proportion of people exposed to air that does not meet the EPA's health-based standards for ozone" and the "proportion of non-smokers exposed to environmental tobacco smoke." There is little explicit recognition of the need to assess the quality of any number of broader determinants of health presented in the health model.

The set of 467 detailed objectives includes substandard housing and food security objectives, but one should consider their prominence. Substandard housing is one of 30 *Environmental* objectives contained in sets such as Outdoor Air Quality (e.g., harmful air pollutants, airborne toxins) and Water Quality (e.g., safe drinking water, waterborne disease outbreaks); Toxics and Waste (e.g., elevated blood lead levels in children, risks posed by hazardous sites); and Healthy Homes and Healthy Communities (e.g., indoor allergens, office building air quality, substandard housing). Food security is one of 18 *Nutrition and Overweight* objectives that include healthy weight and reducing obesity in adults, fruit and vegetable intake, etc.

Explicit indicators for poverty or income rates, unemployment or job security, or any other obvious indicators of broader determinants of health are absent. Any and all examples of influencing policy are limited to legislative changes related to promoting healthy behaviours or access to health care. There is virtually no recognition that factors such as early life, education, employment and working conditions, food security, or housing are primary determinants of health.

The Institute of Medicine's *The Future of the Public's Health* shows similar shortcomings (Institute of Medicine 2002). Its Chapter 2 is an accurate presentation of developments in the field of population health, yet these concepts do not diffuse to the rest of the volume. While it calls for "adopting a population health approach that considers the multiple determinants of health," virtually all examples of issues to be addressed are health care–related or behaviourally focused on poor diet, tobacco use, or physical inactivity. Policy is conceived narrowly: legislative activities related to risk behaviours and health protection.

The American Public Health Association's policy statements show a preoccupation with access to health care, the situating of health differences in terms of racial and ethnic disparities, and behavioural risk factors for disease and illness (American Public Health Association 2004a, 2004b). The *Leave No One Behind: Eliminate Racial and Ethnic Disparities in Health and Life Expectancy* statement documents differences in health status among White, African-American, Hispanics and Latinos, American Indian and Alaskan natives, and Asian-Americans and Pacific Islanders, but highlights recent findings of unequal access to and quality of health care treatment (Institute of Medicine 2003).

A series of fact sheets emphasize health care initiatives. The fact sheet on racial/ ethnic disparities details wide differences in life expectancy, overall health, infant mortality rates, cancer, HIV/AIDS, violence, and diabetes among racial and ethnic minorities. The sheet lists potential reasons for these disparities: unequal (health care) treatment, poverty, insurance, stereotyping (among health care professionals), communication barriers (in health care), frequency of care, and access to care. The fact sheets fail to recognize that conditions of material life influence the incidence of a wide range of diseases, nor do they mention public policy and the importance of influencing the determinants of health.

Broadening the Scope

Some public health agencies concern themselves with broader issues and their influence upon health. The report *America's Health: State Health Rankings* provides data and rankings for states on four sets of indicators that include measures of child poverty, spending on health care and public health, and lack of health insurance (United Health Foundation 2004). Yet, like many other U.S. analyses, the emphasis for action is primarily health care–related with a vague call to address persistent disparities, particularly among racial/ethnic groups.

There are a few innovative public health initiatives that could address broader determinants of health such as the Robert Wood's Johnson Foundation initiative (Turning Point 2004). Our analysis of these initiatives finds that their predominant activity is creating databases and community networks to meet basic public health functions. Only in Minnesota has there been movement to highlight the broader determinants of health and the role they play in health inequalities in the population (Minnesota Department of Health 2001). *A Call to Action: Advancing Health for All through Social and Economic Change* emphasizes public policy action to influence the broader determinants of health (Minnesota Department of Health 2001). However, a new governor has changed the mandate of the health department, threatening this progressive emphasis.

In summary, public health activity in the U.S. that addresses broader determinants of population health is limited. The primary focus is on providing health care access to its citizens and examining racial and ethnic health differences. There is little examination of how the distribution of economic and social resources influences public health, and how public policy can be an appropriate focus of public health action. The harsh public policy environment in the U.S., which includes meagre welfare supports, combines with Americans' generally negative attitudes toward governments to make an activist public health agenda problematic (see Chapter 8 in this volume).

United Kingdom

The U.K. has a long-standing intellectual and academic concern with inequalities in health. In 1980 the Black Report revealed that despite a generation of accessible health care, class-related health inequalities had not only been maintained but in many instances had increased (Black and Smith 1992). The report appeared at the onset of the conservative Thatcher era and its content and recommendations were ignored for two decades. Instead, numerous policies widened income and health inequalities. The election of the New Labour government in 1997 saw the ongoing academic and policy concern with health inequalities translated into a government-wide effort to address health inequalities through the development of public policy. Careful documentation and analysis of these efforts is now available. These reviews illustrate how evidence, combined with the political will to address broader determinants of health, can translate into effective policy development and action.

From the Black Report to the Acheson Inquiry into Health Inequalities

The 1980 Black Report and the 1992 *Health Divide* (Townsend, Davidson, and Whitehead 1992) described how lowest employment-level groups showed a greater likelihood of suffering from a wide range of diseases and dying prematurely from illness or injury at every stage of the life cycle. Among various interpretations available, it was concluded that the material conditions under which people live—availability of income, working conditions, and quality of available food and housing, etc.—were the primary determinants of these findings.

Upon the 1997 change in government, the Labour government commissioned the Acheson Commission into Inequalities in Health. The commission considered a wide range of evidence and concluded that:

> The weight of scientific evidence supports a socioeconomic explanation of health inequalities. This traces the roots of ill health to such determinants as income, education and employment as well as to the material environment and lifestyle. (Acheson 1998: xi)

It offered recommendations across a wide range of health determinants: poverty, income, tax, and benefits; education; employment; housing and environment; mobility, transport, and pollution; nutrition and agriculture policy; mothers, children, and families; young people and adults of working age; older people; ethnicity; gender; and the National Health Service. The most important were: (a) all policies likely to have an impact on health should be evaluated in terms of their impact on health inequalities; (b) high priority should be given to the health of families with children; and (c) further steps should be taken to reduce income inequalities and improve the living standards of poor households.

Government Action Plans

The government responded quickly to these recommendations. Among the major policy initiatives was the document *Reducing Health Inequalities: An Action Report* (Department of Health 1999). The action areas are outlined in Box 15.1.

Box 15.1: Reducing Health Inequalities: The U.K. Agenda for Action

Upon election in 1997, the U.K. Labour government organized a strategy based on nine themes. Specific policies are listed to illustrate its action approach.

- *Raising living standards and tackling low income* by introducing a minimum wage and a range of tax credits and increasing benefit levels
- *Improving education and early years* by introducing policies to improve educational standards, creating "Sure Start," preschool services in disadvantaged areas, free to those on low incomes
- *Increasing employment* by creating a range of welfare-to-work schemes for different priority groups
- *Improving transport and mobility* by setting targets to reduce road traffic accidents, develop safe walking and cycling routes, and standardize concessionary fares for older people
- *Issues for the NHS* include working in partnership with local authorities to tackle the wider determinants of health, reviewing the resource allocation formula to local health care agencies, developing frameworks to standardize care across the country for particular conditions, and broadening the NHS's performance framework to include fair access and improving health
- *Building healthy communities* by investing in a range of regeneration initiatives in disadvantaged areas, including Health Action Zones
- *Improving housing* by changing capital financial rules to promote investment in social housing and introducing special initiatives to tackle homelessness
- *Reducing crime* by investing in a range of community-led crime-prevention schemes and tackling drug misuse
- *Addressing public health issues*—the first-ever Minister for Public Health oversaw a range of initiatives to encourage healthy lifestyles, strengthen the public health workforce, and tackle specific problems such as fluoridation of water supplies

Source: Adapted from M. Benzeval, "England," Box 12.3 in *Reducing Inequalities in Health: European Perspectives*, edited by J. Mackenbach and M. Bakker (London: Routledge, 2002): 207.

There are aspects of the *Agenda for Action* and related documents such as *Opportunity for All—Tackling Poverty and Social Exclusion* (1999), *A New Commitment to Neighbourhood Renewal: National Strategy Action Plan* (2001), and *From Vision to Reality* (2001) that contrast with the public health situation in Canada and the U.S. (Department of Health 2004b). There is recognition that health inequalities are a cause for serious concern not only by health departments but also the entire government.

Goals were set for the elimination of health inequalities. The 2002 Spending Review Public Service Agreement—a kind of business plan—for the Department of Health contained the goal of "by 2010 to reduce inequalities in health outcomes by 10% as measured by infant mortality and life expectancy at birth" (U.K. Government 2002). These initiatives focused on: (a) tackling poverty and low income; (b) improving educational and employment opportunities; (c) rebuilding local communities; and (d) supporting vulnerable individuals and families (Oliver and Nutbeam 2003). To facilitate action, the government set up "cross-cutting spending reviews" focused on health inequalities to be used by a number of departments to inform spending plans for 2003–2006.

Reviews of These Initiatives

A 2003 evaluation concluded that significant progress had been made in tackling health inequalities (Exworthy, Stuart, Blane, and Marmot 2003). Evidence concerning health inequalities had been gathered, health inequalities had been placed on the policy agenda, and a diverse range of activities had been developed. Indicators of outcomes and policy implementation were emerging, though impacts upon health status were not yet apparent. The authors concluded: "Many challenges remain but the prospects for tackling inequalities are good" (Exworthy, Stuart, Blane, and Marmot 2003: 52).

A 2005 evaluation concludes the Labour government has taken seriously the issues of poverty and social exclusion (Hills and Stewart 2005). Evaluations of these initiatives are positive, though effects are modest. Success is apparent in reducing child poverty as a result of the government's tax and benefit reforms. But while overall poverty rates have declined, rates for working-age adults without children had reached all-time high levels by 2002–2003. Their detailed analysis of initiatives, their effects, and issues raised are presented in Table 15.1.

Brewer and Shephard (2004) reached similar conclusions in their analysis of Labour's welfare reform policy of "making work pay" (Brewer and Shephard 2004). In 2004, there are 350,000 fewer children until 16 years in households where no adult has worked since 1997. Child poverty rates have been reduced to levels not seen since the early 1990s.

Against the Grain: Retreating to Individualized Lifestyle Approaches

Potential roadblocks to the continuation of these initiatives need to be considered. Two recent U.K. thrusts have the potential to divert attention from broader policy perspectives on health.

Securing Good Health for the Entire Population

In April 2003, consultant Derek Wanless provided an analysis of how to improve the health of citizens (Wanless 2004). The most striking aspect of the 214-page report is its emphasis upon individual behaviours. The report is sprinkled with references to "wider social costs of particular behaviours," "individuals' poor lifestyles," and "pursuing healthy lifestyles and reducing addictions." Positive changes will be assisted by providing information, marketing healthy lifestyle choices, and by National Health Service staff. Local health authorities, community organizations, and various members of the private sectors will be engaged. The case studies presented are focused on high salt consumption, obesity, falls, and physical activity.

Of concern, the Wanless report reinforces the view that individuals are responsible for their own health "while understating or neglecting entirely the impact of government policies and wider social inequalities on health status" (McDonald and Scott-Samuel 2004). A similar critique is offered by Burstow: "It fails to offer a clear view on the central question of the balance between personal responsibility and state intervention" (Burstow 2004). Some see the report as a tentative step toward healthy public policy (Joffe and Mindell 2004). However, Joffe and Mindell's focus on healthy public policy is limited to reducing behavioural risk factors by supporting individuals through taxation policy, food/agriculture policy, and transportation. The devolution of responsibilities to Scotland and Wales means that the Wanless report does not cover these countries. However, analysis of Scottish and Welsh health documents reveals a similar emphasis upon behavioural, lifestyle-oriented approaches to promoting health. See *Improving Health in Scotland* (Scottish Executive 2004); *The Challenge* and *Health Challenge Wales* (Welsh Assembly Government 2004).

Choosing Health

The government White Paper takes an unambiguous view that individual lifestyle choices are primary determinants of health: "Health is inextricably linked to the way people live their lives and the opportunities available to choose health in the communities where they live (Department of Health 2004a: 9). The 187-page report outlines how concepts of informed choice, personalization of health issues, and organizations working together can reduce the numbers of smokers, reduce obesity and improve diet and nutrition, increase exercise, encourage sensible drinking, and improve sexual and mental health. The health education focus is apparent with sections on marketing health, food labelling, information for the public, information for the media, and working in partnership with local organizations and the private

Table 15.1: Recognition, Targets, Policies, Impacts, and Gaps in Selected U.K. Policy Areas

	Recognition, Targets, and Policies	Impacts	Problems and Gaps
Child poverty	Prominent reduction target; major tax benefit reforms benefiting low-income families with children	Fall in relative child poverty 1996–1997 to 2002–2003 on or close to 2004–2005 target; falls in deprivation and higher child-related spending by parents	Still above E.U. average; long way to be "best in Europe"; adult elements of family benefits are price-linked
Working-age poverty	Policy focus on worklessness, not poverty in itself; policies aimed at employment and income at work	Fell against absolute line, but only slight fall in relative poverty, which has increased for those without children	Despite fall in registered unemployment, many remain without income from work and are dependent on price-linked benefits
Income inequality	Reduction in overall income inequality not an aim; focus on relative poverty for selected groups and on life chances; income inequality monitored at E.U. level	Inequality not changed greatly since 1997; gap between incomes at the very bottom and very top has grown a little, but the gap between those near the bottom and those in the middle or near the top has fallen a little	Incomes and earnings at the very top continue to increase the fastest; some at the bottom are left behind through price-linked benefits or lack of take-up of services

Employment	Clearest initial priority; action through New Deals and "active" policy toward the unemployed	Lowest unemployment for 30 years, but economic inactivity falling only slowly; jobless households are still high	Initial impact of New Deals slowed; high unemployment remains for 16- to 17-year-olds
Education	Blair stated three priorities for government: education, education, and education; targets for school attainment; higher spending since low point of 1999	Positive impacts at primary level, with poorest schools improving fastest; more mixed picture at secondary level	Large social class differences remain; tension between improvements for all and closing gaps
Health inequalities	Unprecedented focus of analysis: Acheson report and follow-up; however, main thrust of policy is on overall health and NHS spending	Too early to judge, but few attributable impacts are yet visible; time trends show little evidence of narrowing gaps	Gap between analysis and implementation
Political participation	Aspects of constitutional reform and parts of Social Exclusion Unit agenda for neighbourhood renewal; participation requirements in nearly all policy areas; targets for volunteering and confidence in institutions	Formal political participation continues to decline; better responsiveness of providers to participation; positive evidence of quality of involvement and better targeting of excluded groups	Many low-income families feel they "have no influence at all"; achievements have not led to excitement about participation and involvement

Source. Adapted from *Policies towards Poverty, Inequality and Exclusion since 1997* (London: U.K. Rowntree Foundation, 2005). Available on-line at www.jrf.org.uk/knowledge/findings/socialpolicy/0015.asp.

sector. The National Health Service will provide health trainers and personal health kits to assist individuals in changing their lifestyle choices.

Scott-Samuel states: "Consistent with the Government's consumerist, market-driven agenda for the public sector, the White Paper enthusiastically espouses health education (supporting individuals in making informed health choices) and more hesitantly, health promotion (supporting healthy choices through healthy public policies)" (Scott-Samuel 2004). The report shows little awareness of Labour's need to address upstream origins of poor health related to material inequalities, excessive deference to the market in trade and services, and promoting egalitarian public policies.

Campbell points out that "while there is mention of health inequalities issues, the measures proposed to address these often assume that they can be tackled through improving access to health services and through changing behaviour and 'choices' on a market/consumer model" (Campbell 2004). Similarly, "nor does the individualistic choice-based analysis of health acknowledge the social and economic determinants of health."

In summary, public health and health policy attention in the U.K. is directed to addressing inequalities in health. Compared to Canada and the U.S., there is a strong public policy concern with addressing the basic determinants of health. It is difficult to avoid the conclusion that "debate on policy to inform health inequalities is alive and well in the UK" (Oliver and Nutbeam 2003: 286).

Sweden

The 2001 Swedish Ministry of Health and Social Affairs document *Towards Public Health on Equal Terms* illustrates government understandings of the nature of health:

> The health of the population is affected by a range of what are known as determinants. These are factors that in part relate to the structure of society and in part to people's lifestyles and habits. The Government's work in the public health field extends to both these types of factors. (Swedish Ministry of Health and Social Affairs 2001: 1)

The 2001 document proposes an explicit role for public health policy in reducing health inequalities between various groups in society. Policy areas identified include employment, education, agriculture, culture, transport, and housing. The January 2003 report emphasizes promoting health and closing the major health gaps in society (Swedish Ministry of Health and Social Affairs 2003). The National Committee for Public Health 2000 report to the government proposed national public health objectives: "To ensure that society: reinforces and enhances social capital; promotes favourable conditions for child development; improves conditions in working life; creates a good physical environment; encourages health promoting lifestyles and habits; and develops good public health infrastructures" (Swedish Ministry of Health and Social Affairs 2001: 2).

The 2002/2003 Public Health plan outlines plans for promoting these objectives. Municipalities and county councils are to draw up and evaluate targets, and report on these activities. National coordination of these is led by the minister for Public Health and Social Services and carried out by the National Institute of Public Health. The institute is drawing up a plan for skills development in public health work for those already working in relevant professions. It is—in co-operation with the Swedish Council for Working Life and Social Research—creating a status report aimed at strengthening research in the field of public health in the long term. Regional centres will be developed with the National Board of Health and Welfare and the Swedish Federation of County Councils and the Swedish Association of Local Authorities to facilitate these activities.

The Swedish National Institute of Public Health objectives that direct these activities focus on the "factors in society or in our living conditions" that influence health (Table 15.2). The first six objectives "relate to what are normally considered to be structural factors, i.e., conditions in society and our surroundings that can be influenced primarily by moulding public opinion and by taking political decisions on different levels." The last five "concern lifestyles which an individual can influence him/herself, but where the social environment normally plays a very important part" (Swedish National Institute for Public Health 2003: 5-6).

Table 15.2: The 11 Target Areas of the New Swedish Public Health Policy

---

The Swedish government has defined 11 target areas for all who work in the field of public health:

- involvement in and influence on society
- economic and social security
- secure and healthy conditions for growing up
- better health in working life
- healthy, safe environments and products
- health and medical care that more actively promotes good health
- effective prevention of the spread of infections
- secure and safe sexuality and good reproductive health
- increased physical activity
- good eating habits and safe foodstuffs
- reduced use of tobacco and alcohol, a drug- and doping-free society and a reduction in the harmful effects of excessive gambling

Source: Swedish National Institute for Public Health, *Sweden's New Public Health Policy* (Stockholm: Swedish National Institute for Public Health, 2003: 6). Available on-line at www.fhi.se/upload/PDF/2004/English/newpublic0401.pdf.

Of particular note is the Swedish health authorities' ability to take the latest work on health determinants and provide it in a form that is understandable to the public. Box 15.2 provides an example of such a presentation.

In summary, it is apparent that a public health approach based on the broader determinants of health is consistent with long-standing Swedish approaches to public policy (see Chapter 8 in this volume). Sweden implemented social welfare policies during the 1920s and the long tradition of establishing and maintaining a strong welfare state makes Swedish public health officials receptive to new developments in health promotion, population health, and the broader determinants of health. The report *Welfare in Sweden: The Balance Sheet for the 1990s* provides a graphic illustration of ongoing and proactive Swedish government concern with societal well-being (Swedish Ministry of Health and Social Affairs 2002). In a sense, public policy has always been focused on the broader determinants of health. New developments from the health sciences only reinforce this approach.

"For many years Sweden has pursued equality-oriented health and social policies, active labour market policies and family-oriented policies that have resulted in higher levels of workplace participation, less income inequality, lower poverty rates and smaller socio-economic inequalities in the distribution of poverty than in most other countries" (Burstrom, Diderichsen, Ostlin, and Ostergren 2002: 281). It should not be surprising that "compared to many other countries, Sweden has low mortality rates, high life expectancy, and favourable health indicators across all socioeconomic groups" (Burstrom, Diderichsen, Ostlin, and Ostergren 2002: 281).

Conclusions

Approaches to public health appear to be driven by dominant political ideologies within jurisdictions. The accumulating evidence concerning the impact upon health and well-being of broader determinants of health is available to policy makers in Canada, the U.S., the U.K., and Sweden. What is striking is the degree of variation in commitment to applying these findings across these nations.

In Canada and the U.S., progressive concepts associated with health promotion and population health are inconsistent with nascent neo-liberal approaches to governance that emphasize individualism, rather than communal approaches, to resource allocation. Concern with newly emerging infections such as SARS and the avian flu virus have reinforced biomedical, epidemiological-oriented approaches focused upon the concrete and observable, rather than the social and conceptual. Canadian and American public health, health policy, and health care communities rarely discuss the reasons for the contradiction between theory and knowledge with practice.

We conclude that leaving the promotion of population health to health professionals — which occurs when government policy makers show little commitment to promoting equity in health outcomes — allows prevailing epidemiological, class, and professional biases to dominate public discourse. As a recent analysis showed, the majority of empirical research in Canada and elsewhere

Box 15.2: Swedish Government Statement on Participation and Influence in Society and Health

The power and possibility of people to influence the world around them is probably of crucial significance for their health. Societies with a low election turnout, where few people feel there is any point in participating in NGO activities or trying to influence development, are also characterized by the occurrence of serious health problems. Increasing people's level of participation in society life is therefore one of the most important national public health objectives.

There is a very clear relationship between the power to influence and health on the individual level. A lack of influence combined with a high workload causes hormone imbalance and increases the risk of heart attack and other diseases. A link has also been established between limited decision-making powers and the incidence of sick leave and it seems in particular as if long-term sick leave is aggravated by a lack of influence. Greater work participation also seems to improve mental health.

It is more difficult to substantiate the positive effects of democracy on health on the societal level. There is a connection between high election turn-out and a high level of trust in authorities and good health, but it is difficult to know how much of this is connected with the degree of influence and how much for example is linked to economic factors. Discrimination, depriving groups of people of their chance to influence, definitely has a negative impact on health and this may explain the much poorer health of a number of immigrant groups. The deteriorated health of the long-term unemployed may be connected to some extent to reduced powers of influence. Less influence probably also leads to less of a chance to "choose" a reasonably healthy lifestyle, which includes physical activity and diet, as well as alcohol and other illicit drugs.

The Public Health Bill emphasizes that efforts to strengthen democracy and defend human rights also reinforce the feeling of affinity in society as a whole and increases trust between people, both of which promote good health. It also stresses the significance of media policy and information and the importance of it reaching all groups in society.

Labour market policy, gender equality, integration, and disability policies are among those fields that are particularly important to allow all citizens the chance to participate in the governing and development of society. Culture, popular movements, youth policy, efforts to strengthen vulnerable metropolitan areas are other examples of activities that strengthen public participation and influence.

Source: Swedish National Institute for Public Health, *Sweden's New Public Health Policy* (Stockholm: Swedish National Institute for Public Health, 2003). Available on-line at www.fhi. se/upload/PDF/2004/English/newpublic0401.pdf.

is focused on individual approaches to health risk. If we allow the dominant perspectives of the professional health communities (i.e., medicine, nursing, nutritionists, health promoters, etc.), reinforced by the beliefs and paradigmatic views of the average health researcher and service worker, to determine the health approach, attention to broader determinants of health will always take a back seat.

Stated another way, "Evidence follows policy, rather than the reverse." That is, governments direct attention to evidence that is consistent with their beliefs about society and health. Despite the accumulating evidence concerning the broader determinants of health—such as the profound, health-threatening effects of poverty—such evidence will not appear on the radar screen of governments whose policy approaches are not consistent with the implications of such evidence (see Chapter 8 in this volume).

In situations, however, where public policy directions are uncertain, the influence of population health perspectives that stress broader determinants of health may be crucial. In the U.K. and Sweden we see that ideological commitments to health equity provide a fertile soil in which policy can be developed from empirical research findings concerning broader determinants of health. The U.S. is an example where the soil is barren. In Canada, the public health community can profoundly influence the public policy environment, and there are many supports for a progressive public health agenda. To date, however, the public health community has not chosen to join in these debates in a serious way. Developments in the U.K. and Sweden show how fruitful such an approach can be.

References

Acheson, D. (1998). *Independent Inquiry into Inequalities in Health*. Stationary Office. Available on-line at www.official-documents.co.uk/document/doh/ih/contents.htm.

ACT Health Promotion. (2004). *History of Health Promotion*. Government of Australia. Retrieved June 3, 2004. Available on-line at www.healthpromotion.act.gov.au/whatis/history/default.htm.

American Public Health Association. (2004a). *Disparities in Health Fact Sheets*. Washington: American Public Health Association.

_____. (2004b). *Leave No One behind: Eliminating Racial and Ethnic Disparities in Health and Life Expectancy*. Washington: American Public Health Association.

Basrur, S. (2004). *Healthy Weights, Healthy Lives*. Toronto: Ontario Ministry of Health.

Black, D., and C. Smith. (1992). "The Black Report." In *Inequalities in Health: The Black Report and the Health Divide*, edited by P. Townsend, N. Davidson, and M. Whitehead, 29–213. New York: Penguin.

Brewer, M., and A. Shephard. (2004). *Has Labour Made Work Pay?* York: Joseph Rowntree Foundation.

Burstow, P. (2004). "Wanless II: Groundhog Day." *PH7 Magazine* 9 (March 22).

Burstrom, B., F. Diderichsen, P. Ostlin, and P.O. Ostergren. (2002). "Sweden." In *Reducing Inequalities in Health: A European Perspective*, edited by J. Mackenbach and M. Bakker, 274–283. London: Routledge.

Campbell, F. (2004). *White Paper on Public Health*. London: Democratic Health Network.

Canadian Population Health Initiative. (2002). *Canadian Population Health Initiative Brief to the Commission on the Future of Health Care in Canada*. CPHI. Retrieved February 20, 2004. Available on-line at http://secure.cihi.ca/cihiweb/en/downloads/cphi_policy_romanowbrief_e.pdf.

Canadian Public Health Association. (1996). *Action Statement for Health Promotion in Canada*. Retrieved July, 2002. Available on-line at www.cpha/cpha.docs/ActionStatement.eng.html.

_____. (2001). *CPHA Policy Statements*. Available on-line at www.cpha.ca/english/policy/pstatem/polstate.htm.

Chronic Disease Prevention Alliance of Canada. (2003). *Who We Are*. Retrieved April 16, 2003. Available on-line at www.chronicdiseaseprevention.ca/content/about_cdpac/mission.asp.

Department of Health. (1999). *Reducing Health Inequalities: An Action Report*. London: Department of Health.

_____. (2004a). *Choosing Health: Making Healthy Choices Easier*. London: Department of Health.

_____. (2004b). *Publications from the Department of Health*. Retrieved January 30, 2005. Available on-line at www.dh.gov.uk/Home/fs/en.

Epp, J. (1986). *Achieving Health for All: A Framework for Health Promotion*. Health and Welfare Canada. Available on-line at www.hc-sc.gc.ca/hppb/hpo/ahfa.htm.

Exworthy, M., M. Stuart, D. Blane, and M. Marmot. (2003). *Tackling Health Inequalities Since the Acheson Inquiry*. Bristol: Policy Press.

Government of Alberta. (2002). *Building a Better Public Health Care System: Alberta Government Response to the Premier's Advisory Council on Health Report*. Edmonton: Government of Alberta.

Health Canada. (2003). *Healthy Living Strategy*. Retrieved April 16, 2003. Available on-line at www.hc-sc.gc.ca/english/media/releases/2003/2003_14.htm.

_____. (2004). *Population Health Approach*. Retrieved January 30, 2005. Available on-line at www.phac-aspc.gc.ca/ph-sp/phdd/approach/approach.html.

Hills, J., and K. Stewart, eds. (2005). *A More Equal Society? New Labour, Poverty, Inequality and Exclusion*. Bristol: Policy Press.

Institute for Medical Education. (2004). *Glossary of Medical Education Terms*. Retrieved January 30, 2005. Available on-line at www.iime.org/glossary.htm#P.

Institute of Medicine. (2002). *The Future of the Public's Health in the 21st Century*. Washington: National Academies Press.

_____. (2003). *Unequal Treatment: Confronting Racial and Ethnic Disparities in Health Care*. Washington: Institute of Medicine.

Joffe, M., and J. Mindell. (2004). "A Tentative Step towards Healthy Public Policy." *Journal of Epidemiology and Community Health* 58(12): 966–968.

Lalonde, M. (1974). *A New Perspective on the Health of Canadians: A Working Document*. Health and Welfare Canada. Available on-line at www.hc-sc.gc.ca/main/hppb/phdd/resource.htm.

Lavis, J. (2002). "Ideas at the Margin or Marginalized Ideas? Nonmedical Determinants of Health in Canada." *Health Affairs* 21(2): 107–112.

Lessard, R. (1997). *Social Inequalities in Health: Annual Report of the Health of the Population.* Direction de la sante publique. Available on-line at www.santepub-mtl.qc.ca.

Lessard, R., D. Roy, R. Choinière, J. Lévesque, and S. Perron. (2002). *Urban Health: A Vital Factor in Montreal's Development.* Direction de la santé publique. Retrieved February 20, 2004. Available on-line at www.santepub-mtl.qc.ca/Publication/autres/annualreport2002.html.

Mazankowski, D. (2001). *A Framework for Reform: Report of the Premier's Advisory Council on Health.* Edmonton: Government of Alberta.

McDonald, R., and A. Scott-Samuel. (2004). "Missed Opportunities? Wanless and the White Paper." *Public Health News* (May 24).

Minnesota Department of Health. (2001). *A Call to Action: Advancing Health for All through Social and Economic Change.* Available on-line at www.health.state.mn.us/divs/chs/hsd/action.pdf.

Nutbeam, D. (1998). *Health Promotion Glossary.* Geneva: World Health Organization.

Oliver, A., and D. Nutbeam. (2003). "Addressing Health Inequalities in the United Kingdom: A Case Study." *Journal of Public Health Medicine* 25: 281–287.

Raphael, D. (2003a). "Addressing the Social Determinants of Health in Canada: Bridging the Gap between Research Findings and Public Policy." *Policy Options* 24(3): 35–40.

_____. (2003b). "Barriers to Addressing the Determinants of Health: Public Health Units and Poverty in Ontario, Canada." *Health Promotion International* 18, 397–405.

Raphael, D., and A. Curry-Stevens. (2004). "Addressing and Surmounting the Political and Social Barriers to Health." In *Social Determinants of Health: Canadian Perspectives,* edited by D. Raphael, 345-359. Toronto: Canadian Scholars' Press.

Restrepo, H.E. (1996). "Introduction." In *Health Promotion: An Anthology,* edited by Pan American Health Organization, ix–xi. Washington: Pan American Health Organization.

Robertson, A. (1998). "Shifting Discourses on Health in Canada: From Health Promotion to Population Health." *Health Promotion International* 13: 155–166.

Scott-Samuel, A. (2004). *New Labour's New Idea—Health Promotion.* Liverpool: Politics of Health Group.

Scott-Samuel, A., M. Birley, and K. Ardern. (2001). *The Merseyside Guidelines for Health Impact Assessment.* Liverpool: International Health Impact Assessment Consortium.

Scottish Executive. (2004). *Improving Health in Scotland: The Challenge.* Edinburgh: Scottish Executive.

Sutcliffe, P., R. Deber, and G. Pasut. (1997). "Public Health in Canada: A Comparative Study." *Canadian Journal of Public Health* 88: 246–249.

Swedish National Institute for Public Health. (2003). *Sweden's New Public Health Policy.* Stockholm: Swedish National Institute for Public Health. Available on-line at www.fhi.se/upload/PDF/2004/English/newpublic0401.pdf.

Swedish Ministry of Health and Social Affairs. (2001). *Towards Public Health on Equal Terms.* Stockholm: Swedish Ministry of Health and Social Affairs.

_____. (2002). *Welfare in Sweden: The Balance Sheet for the 1990s.* Stockholm: Swedish Ministry of Health and Social Affairs.

_____. (2003). *Public Health Objectives.* Stockholm: Swedish Ministry of Health and Social Affairs.

Townsend, P., N. Davidson, and M. Whitehead, eds. (1992). *Inequalities in Health: The Black Report and the Health Divide.* New York: Penguin.

Turning Point. (2004). *States of Change: Stories of Transformation in Public Health*. Seattle: Robert Woods Johnson Foundation.

U.K. Government. (2002). *SR 2002: Public Service Agreements*. London: The Treasury Department.

United Health Foundation. (2004). *America's Health: State Health Rankings*. Minnetonka: United Health Foundation.

U.S. Department of Health and Human Services. (2000). *Healthy People 2010: Understanding and Improving Health*. Washington: U.S. Department of Health and Human Services.

Wanless, D. (2004). *Securing Good Health for the Whole Population*. London: Treasury Office.

Welsh Assembly Government. (2004). *Health Challenge Wales*. Cardiff: Welsh Assembly Government.

Williamson, D. (2001). "The Role of the Health Sector in Addressing Poverty." *Canadian Journal of Public Health* 92: 178–182.

• •

Critical Thinking Questions

1. What are some of the reasons that Canadian public health officials resist integrating findings about the broader determinants of health into their mandates? What would need to change for them to apply these concepts in their practice?

2. What are the reasons for, and the effects of, having racial/ethnic disparities the focus of U.S. public health attention rather than issues of income, social class, and poverty?

3. How might the U.K. initiatives focused on healthy lifestyles complicate action to promote political, economic, and social changes to promote health?

4. What are the lessons that North American policy makers and elected representatives could learn from Swedish approaches to public health?

5. How do public health approaches to the determinants of health shape public understandings of the causes of disease and illness? How could public health agencies educate the public about the sources of health and causes of disease and illness?

Further Readings

Hamilton, N., and T. Bhatti. (1996). *Population Health Promotion: An Integrated Model of Population Health and Health Promotion*. Ottawa: Health Canada. Available on-line at www.phac-aspc.gc.ca/ph-sp/phdd/php/php.htm.

Many health promotion and population health concepts originated in Canada. This paper provides an integrated population health promotion model and explains how it can be applied.

Hills, J., and K. Stewart. (2005). *A More Equal Society? New Labour, Poverty, Inequality and Exclusion*. Bristol: Policy Press.
This volume provides an evaluation of Labour policy toward poverty and social exclusion between 1997 and 2004. It has chapters on employment, inequalities in income, education and health, and political participation. It asks how children, older people, poor neighbourhoods, ethnic minorities, and other vulnerable groups have fared under New Labour.

Institute of Medicine. (2002). *The Future of the Public's Health in the 21st Century*. Washington: National Academies Press.
This text examines the purposes, functions, and roles of American public health agencies and explores practices that can improve public health outcomes.

Mackenbach, J., and M. Bakker, eds. (2002). *Reducing Inequalities in Health*: *A European Perspective*. London: Routledge.
The volume focuses on successful policies and interventions in Europe and provides evaluation studies, issues for research, and draws out policy and research implications for the future.

Swedish National Institute for Public Health. (2003). *Sweden's New Public Health Policy*. Stockholm: Swedish National Institute for Public Health. Available on-line at www.fhi.se/upload/PDF/2004/English/newpublic0401.pdf.
The Swedes require that public health be a priority when public policy decisions are made. This document contains the new health objectives and provides background information about this innovative approach.

Relevant Web Sites

Health Canada Population Health Approach
www.phac-aspc.gc.ca/ph-sp/phdd/approach/index.html
   Health Canada's Web site provides details about the population health approach and Canada's work in this area. It includes links to all the groundbreaking reports for which Canada is known.

Healthy People 2010
www.healthypeople.gov/
   This U.S. government Web site contains details and publications concerned with its national public health objectives.

Professor Raphael's Web site
www.atkinson.yorku.ca/draphael

This Web site contains numerous articles and presentations concerned with public health in Canada and elsewhere.

Swedish Ministry of Health and Social Affairs
www.sweden.gov.se/sb/d/2061/a/16432
   This Swedish government's Web site provides details and publications about the Swedish approach to public health and public policy.

United Kingdom Department of Health
www.dh.gov.uk/Home/fs/en
   The U.K. government Web site provides information on health and social policy, guidance, and all government publications related to public health and public policy toward health.

Glossary

Health impact assessment (HIA): The estimation of the effects of a specified action on the health of a defined population. The actions concerned may range from projects (for instance, a housing development or a leisure centre) to programs (such as an urban regeneration or a public safety program) to policies (like the integrated transport strategy, the introduction of water metering, or the imposition of value-added tax on domestic fuel). HIA builds on the understanding that a community's health is determined not only by its health services, but also by a range of economic, social, psychological, and environmental influences (Scott-Samuel, Birley, and Ardern 2001).

Health promotion: A comprehensive social and political process of enabling people to increase control over the determinants of health and thereby improve their health. It not only embraces actions directed at strengthening the skills and capabilities of individuals, but also action directed toward changing social, environmental, and economic conditions so as to improve health. Participation is essential to sustain health promotion action (Nutbeam 1998).

Healthy public policy (HPP): An explicit concern for health and equity in all areas of policy and accountability for health impact. The aim of HPP is to create a supportive environment to enable people to lead healthy lives. Such a policy makes healthy choices possible or easier for citizens and social and physical environments more health enhancing. In pursuit of HPP, government sectors concerned with agriculture, trade, education, industry, and communications need to take into account health as an essential factor when formulating policy and be accountable for the health consequences of their policy decisions. They should pay as much attention to health as to economics (ACT Health Promotion 2004).

Population health: Focuses on improving the health status of the population rather than individuals. Focusing on the health of populations also requires reducing health inequalities between groups. One assumption of a population health approach is that reductions in health inequities require reductions in material and social inequities (Health Canada 2004).

Public health: The organized efforts of society to protect, promote, and restore people's health. It is the combination of science, skills, and beliefs directed to the maintenance and improvement of the health of all people through collective or social actions. Public health activities change with variations in technology and social values, but the goals remain the same: to reduce the amount of disease, premature death, and disease-produced discomfort and disability in the population. Public health is thus a social institution, a discipline, and a practice (Institute for Medical Education 2004).

CHAPTER SIXTEEN

TOWARD THE FUTURE

Current Themes in Health Research and Practice in Canada

Toba Bryant, Dennis Raphael, and Marcia Rioux

Introduction

Health studies is a complex field that is concerned with a wide range of phenomena. It also has profoundly important—often involving life and death—consequences for individuals, families, communities, and entire nations as exemplified by the title of this volume, *Staying Alive*. These phenomena include the experience and understanding of illness and disability; differential access to both health and health care; the political, economic, and social forces that shape health and health care; and the intersection of social class, gender, and race with all of these issues. Despite the variety of conceptual paradigms and emerging findings available for considering these issues, most of the research and professional health care preoccupations remain strangely narrow, focused on the biology of disease, individual risk factors for these afflictions, and identifying and evaluating the efficacy of medical treatments. Not surprisingly, then, public understanding of key health issues—such as the causes of diseases and the organization of the health care system—are also narrowly focused on access to health care professionals, length of wait for treatment by specialists, and adopting lifestyle approaches to prevent disease.

To help address these narrow preoccupations, this volume has provided the latest conceptual developments and empirical findings concerning the status of health, illness, and health care in Canada. The contributors to Part I provided four important conceptual paradigms—the epidemiological, sociological, political economy, and human rights—that assist in framing health studies questions and providing means of answering these questions. Contributors to Part II provided the latest evidence concerning the role of various social determinants of health in promoting health and explaining health inequalities. Part III focused on the Canadian health care system.

Its history was traced and recent developments in its evolution were outlined. In Part IV, critical issues related to gender, disability, pharmaceuticals, and approaches to promoting public health were carefully explored.

In this final chapter we identify some key themes that run through these contributions. These seven themes are presented in Table 16.1. It is our belief that these issues have been notably neglected by the dominant health sciences paradigms that are customarily applied to the promotion of health, treatment of illness, and analysis and reform of the Canadian health care and public health systems. Many of these concepts have their origins in the social sciences and the related areas of public policy studies and comparative politics.

Table 16.1: Themes Related to Health, Illness, and Health Care in Canada

---

- Defining the field of health studies
- Conflict versus consensus models
- Prevention versus cure
- The public versus private debate
- Constructing illness and disability
- The role of public policy
- The future of the welfare state

Defining the Field of Health Studies

The field of health studies is moving beyond traditional concepts of risk epidemiology and health care treatment evaluation. The complexity of health and health care issues, strides in health care technology, growing understanding and appreciation of the influence of the societal determinants of health, and the increasing gaps in the social and health status of groups in Canada require new innovative approaches to research and practice. The value of these new lines of inquiry is apparent in the contributions in this volume.

Health studies must now consider health, illness, and health care in broader terms than has previously been the case. Health itself is more than the absence of illness and disease, but also the capacity to realize aspirations and access opportunities for human fulfillment. Studies of health are also concerned with how societal structures influence the opportunities for good health for the population as a whole and for specific groups. The contributors to this volume drew upon developments in the disabilities area, gender and women's studies, history of medicine, legal studies, policy studies, political economy, political science, social epidemiology, and sociology to inform their analysis. Virtually all have emphasized the importance of the social determinants of health for understanding health issues. Public policy is also seen as having a key role in influencing health status and the organization of health care. Understanding the policy development and change process would seem essential for those concerned with improving the health of Canadians and improving the health care system through research, advocacy, and policy development.

Conflict versus Consensus Models

The contributors to this book have illustrated the role played by competing political, economic, and social forces in determining health and organizing and delivering health services. These presentations speak to the value of conflict and consensus models for understanding the nature and incidence of health and illness and the organization and delivery of health care. Consensus models such as structural functionalism focus on the interrelationships between social structures and individuals and how societal order is maintained. These approaches are fundamentally driven by an assumption of consensus among different groups in society. The stability of social, economic, and political systems is assumed as is the presence of minimal conflict among various participants and actors in these systems.

Conflict models, however, focus on the tensions inherent in societies and the role played by power. Such tensions lead to fissures in society related to social class, gender, disabilty, and race, and examination of how these fissures influence the experience of health and illness of individuals and groups in society. Conflict models also consider how such tensions influence societal organization—such as the balance between the marketplace and publicly controlled structures—and how these shape the experience of health and health care. And political and economic forces are seen as key contributors to these tensions.

Virtually all contributors drew upon concepts associated with conflict theory. These included the role of political ideology and power relations within society and how these issues proved useful for understanding the sources of social class, gender, and racial differences in health. They also helped elucidate how competing political and economic visions shape public policy, thereby influencing various social determinants of health. Understanding the history and recent evolution of the health care system also seems to benefit from use of these concepts. Armstrong points out (Chapter 12):

> As the Romanow Report makes clear, health and care are about values and about global political/economic pressures. Policy and practices reflect not only old ways of doing and new evidence; they also reflect power and political choices.

Increasing economic globalization, its effects upon public policy, and the competing visions of society that are highlighted in reaction to such globalization lead us to expect that conflict models will continue to be a rich source of insights for understanding the determinants of health and the organization and evolution of health care services. As pointed out by Bourgeault (Chapter 2): "The key approach to take is one that is critical of common and often unquestioned assumptions of how society is and ought to be and in doing so focus on the centrality of power."

Prevention versus Care

There is often conflict between focusing attention on prevention (e.g., the social determinants of health, healthy public policy, and the organization of society, etc.) versus care (e.g., optimizing the quality and accessibility of health care services, etc.). In Canada, government focus and policy making—mirrored by media coverage and public understandings of health—are firmly focused on the health care system. Not surprisingly, public operating funds and research funding are allocated overwhelmingly toward care rather than prevention. Much of this has to do with the immediacy and concrete nature of illness and disease for individuals as opposed to the more abstract concepts associated with the social determinants of health and the development of public policy in support of these determinants. It also reflects the continuing dominance of the medical profession in public discussions of health and the health care system. Media coverage and public understandings reflect these dominant approaches.

In Canada, the ability to raise issues of prevention is complicated by the dominant political economy, which is liberal (or market-oriented), and the growing influence of neo-liberal (even more market-oriented) ideology. Market approaches downplay the collectivity and make it difficult to implement public policy in support of health. The individualism associated with neo-liberalism as a political and economic ideology reinforces biomedical and lifestyle approaches to health and disability advanced by governments, health officials, and service providers.

Even the increased concern with seemingly obvious health issues such as obesity can be misplaced. As Feldberg and Vipond point out (Chapter 9):

> The new diseases, often labelled lifestyle diseases, are actually diseases of circumstance. They reflect living conditions, poverty, and access to housing and income. For historical reasons, Canada has not integrated these social and economic domains into the modern organization or financing of health.

An emphasis upon prevention requires attention to public policies that ensure income security, employment security, housing security, and food security, among others. Since governments consistently neglect these issues, it is not surprising that policy makers—reinforced by the medical profession, media coverage, and public understandings of health and illness—direct their attention to lifestyle approaches to prevention and relatively narrow health care issues such as waiting lists. Despite the evidence provided by most contributors to this volume of the value of looking upstream at the organization of society and the distribution of resources as important determinants of health and health care organizations, raising these issues remains a difficult task. Health-promoting policies discussed by several contributors to this volume will be implemented only when the public comes to a better understand of these issues. As stated by Bezruchka (Chapter 1): "If Canadians want to live as a healthier population, they can take policy steps that are diametrically opposite to the current ones. In a democracy there is this choice. It should be an informed one."

The Public versus Private Debate

The public versus private debate is concerned with issues of ownership and control of both societal resources in general and the health care system in particular. While this issue is usually framed in terms of economic efficiency, it also has strong implications for the health of the population in general and for vulnerable populations such as people with chronic diseases such as HIV/AIDS, people with disabilities, new Canadians, women, and people with low income.

The debate has implications for both the social determinants of health and the quality of health services. More specifically, the move to privatize areas of public activity directly affects the availability of societal resources such as income and housing, the quality and accessibility of health care, and the availability of pharmaceuticals to consumers. Concerning the social determinants of health, nations that have well-developed public services that decommodify resources—that is, that break the link between receiving a benefit and being able to pay for it—have stronger public sectors and better health indicators. Coburn (Chapter 3) argues that acceptance of a neo-liberal—that is, privatized—approach to governance threatens health: "The examples given indicate that the prevailing form of political, economic, and social policy, that of neo-liberalism, has profoundly negative effects on societies generally, and on health and health care specifically."

Bourgeault (Chapter 11) discusses how governments try to control costs by privatizing health care services. Privatization and its concomitant force rationalization emphasize cost containment. Rationalization leads to lowering costs so much that "the least expensive worker performs tasks at the lowest unit cost." While such reforms may seem efficient and necessary to hospital CEOs, these changes ultimately affect the quality of care that is provided, and usually result in poorer-quality care.

As another example of how the privatization of a previously public domain can affect health, Lexchin (Chapter 14) discussed how the regulation of the drug industry in Canada has been weakened by the turning over of these duties to the private sector. Lexchin shows how a political decision to relinquish authority for laboratory testing to the pharmaceutical industry affects the quality and safety of medications available to Canadian consumers. Indeed, Bourgeault (Chapter 11) argued that increased privatization threatens Canadian institutions:

Although some argue that the only conceivable solution to rising costs in health care and other public services is thought to be further market penetration and the adoption of more for-profit practices, Armstrong et al. (2003) argue that the mixing of public and private, for-profit partnerships squeezes out public values and practices. What are left are corporate, for-profit values and methods combined with limited choice.

Constructing Illness and Disability

Disease and disabilities are socially constructed categories that reflect societal values, dominant health paradigms, and societal willingness to adjust to meet the needs of all its members. Marcia Rioux and Tamara Daly (Chapter 13) outlined the different approaches to understanding disability and illness. Biomedical and functional theoretical approaches conflate disability with illness in perceiving disability as individual pathology. In contrast, social pathology approaches such as human rights and political economy situate disability in broader social systems.

Disability and illness can be viewed primarily in terms of disease and variation from an accepted norm. Such a limited view places the power to influence people so defined and related policy firmly in the hands of medical professionals. The concept of DALYs illustrates many of these issues. Use of DALYs imply a "reduced value" to a life lived with a disability. It treats these conditions as physical disablements instead of situating disability in broader social, political, environmental, and economic factors. It also makes a second false assumption that the only way to ameliorate disability is to intervene medically. In contrast, if the limitations of those with disabilities and illness are seen as reflecting society's failures to make accommodations to meet the needs of these individuals, then the area is opened to much broader concepts of societal responsibilities, rules of citizenship, and conforming to ethical principles and values. Rioux and Daly (Chapter 13) comment:

> Social science approaches tend to focus on the social origins of disability. These models investigate the ways in which social structures create disability through societies' inability to accommodate difference. In this framework, disability is equated with social disadvantage, and is not simply focused on individual impairment.

Leaving the field of disabilities to the medical profession has led to perceptions of illness and disability in solely functional terms. The larger point is that we measure health by morbidity and mortality rather than by the conditions that affect them. By doing so, it becomes inevitable that the money (and policy decisions) flow toward investment in medical care because that is what tells us how well we are doing.

This approach has been associated with denial of basic human rights to people with disabilities or other chronic conditions. As noted by Bryant (Chapter 8), Canadian spending on disabilities-related supports and services is among the lowest of any industrialized nation. Disability can be redefined as societies' capacity to adapt to the diverse needs of individual citizens to enable them to participate in civil society. The message that emerges is that of a need to focus on the social origins of disability. There need to be investigations of the ways in which social structures create disability through societies' inability to accommodate difference.

These insights from the disabilities area have profound implications for the treatment of those with chronic illness who then experience some form of disability. The changed state of people that results from chronic illness requires society's attention to continuing their involvement in the activities normally expected of society's members. This opens up discussion to issues of programs, supports, and policies that will make such involvement possible.

The Role of Public Policy

A central aim of this volume is to understand the centrality of public policy in structuring population health and health outcomes. Public policy refers to decisions made by governments and other large organizations on how to address identified problems. Virtually every contributor considered how public policy influences the health and well-being of the population in general and certain groups in particular by shaping the quality of the social determinants of health and the organization and delivery of health care services. The picture that emerges from the analysis of different forms of welfare states and the public policies that each formulate is summarized by Bryant (Chapter 8):

> Public policy decisions made by governments influence the quality of these social determinants of health. These public policy decisions are themselves shaped by political, economic, and social forces within jurisdictions that allow some approaches and exclude others.

Political variables such as union density, left Cabinet share, political ideology, and the electoral system (i.e., proportional representation versus "first-past-the-post" elections) affect the quality of health and social policies that are accepted and implemented. Social democratic nations have the most progressive social and health policies and these reflect a long-standing commitment to social equality and population health and well-being. These welfare states were established prior to the Second World War in contrast to other Western nations such as Canada, the U.S., and the U.K.

Public policy clearly determines the organization and delivery of health care services. All of the debates concerning privatization, competition, and financing of the health care system are essentially debates about public policy, yet health science professionals receive little education and training in public policy analysis. Since social reform and health care system evolution involves having governments and agencies develop and adopt policies, it is essential that the policy process—especially the policy change process—be understood by those researching and advocating for health.

And since public policy in general, and health care policy in particular, is subject to the effects of international forces related to economic globalization and the adoption of international trade agreements, the need for an understanding of the policy process is even more important. Many aspects of our society and its health care systems are increasingly influenced by these developments. Bryant concludes (Chapter 8): "Directing the health sector's gaze to broader political and economic factors may be the most effective means of improving population health and reducing inequalities in health."

The Future of the Welfare State

This volume has outlined several areas for reforming the organization of society, the redistribution of resources in general, and the health care system in particular, to improve the health and well-being of Canadians. These are fundamental issues concerning the nature of the welfare state in Canada. As Coburn argues (Chapter 3), the nature of our economic system varies from nation to nation and affects the welfare state regime that is adopted. And numerous contributors showed how the political economy of a nation determines its willingness to address public policy issues supportive of population health.

The social democratic welfare regimes as described by Coburn (Chapter 3) and Bryant (Chapter 8) are more likely to create the conditions necessary for health than is the case for other welfare regimes. These include equitable distribution of wealth and progressive tax policies that create a large middle class; strong programs that support children, families, and women; and economies that support full employment. They do so through more generous programs and services to their citizens in the form of universal entitlements. In contrast, liberal welfare states such as Canada have means-tested assistance, modest universal transfers, and modest social-insurance plans. While Canadian public policy has been moving toward a neo-liberal model, reversals are possible. New Zealand took a similar neo-liberal course during the 1990s, but has now reversed direction. Ideologies are malleable and national social policies can be changed.

However, Bryant (Chapter 8) points out how recent developments related to economic globalization increase the risk to health:

> Coburn and Teeple describe a state and a process of economic globalization in which the market determines political, social, and economic activity. The rise of neo-liberalism in liberal political economies (e.g., Thatcherism in the United Kingdom, Reaganism in the United States, and Mulroneyism in Canada) has created increased income inequalities and the weakening of social provision.

There are a variety of forces that shape the welfare state. These include the power of left (or progressive) political parties, the strength of labour unions, the presence of proportional representation electoral processes, and attitudes toward the poor and marginalized. The influence of well-organized lobby groups that are striving for increased privatization of public institutions must also be considered. History suggests that public policy in support of health frequently results from social movements that arise from expressed needs of the population. Health researchers and advocates have much to offer by identifying health issues for public discussion and appropriate policy responses.

Conclusions

The current public policy environment in Canada is one of opportunity to effect movement toward public policies supportive of health. There is renewed policy making focused on providing affordable housing and adequate income for the least well off. There is also movement toward a national child care program, and the growing gap between rich and poor has received considerable media coverage. The labour movement has generally maintained its strength—a development different than in the U.S.—and supports a range of progressive public policy initiatives.

Concerning the health care system, the recent Supreme Court of Canada's ruling that banning health insurance for private health care providers is unconstitutional has energized the debate about the organization and delivery of health care services. There are strong forces pushing for increased privatization of health care services. These forces, however, are being opposed by equally strong forces that evoke the spirit of Medicare's founder, Tommy Douglas, in defence of the system. Such active policy environments require that the questions raised in this volume—and their potential solutions—receive the attention from health researchers, policy makers, service providers, and the public that they deserve.

> Medicine, as a social science, as the science of human beings, has the obligation to raise such questions and to attempt their theoretical solutions; the politician, the practical anthropologist, must find the means for their actual solution (Virchow 1848: 217).

Reference

Virchow, R. (1848). "Report on the Typhus Epidemic in Upper Silesia." In *Collected Essays by Rudolph Virchow on Public Health and Epidemiology*, vol. 1, edited by L.J. Rather, 205–319. Canton: Science History Publications.

Contributors' Biographies

Pat Armstrong, PhD, is a professor in sociology and women's studies at York University. She holds a CHSRF/CIHR chair in health services and chairs the National Coordinating Group on Health Care Reform and Women.

Joan Benach, MD, PhD, has a MD degree (Autonomous University of Barcelona), an MPH degree (Barcelona University), and a PhD (Johns Hopkins University). He is also a specialist in preventive medicine and public health and studies in contemporary history (Autonomous University of Barcelona), methodology in social sciences (Barcelona University), and health policy (University of California at Berkeley). His main research fields of interest include topics such as health inequalities, precarious employment, small area geographical analysis, and health policy priorities, where he has published over 100 articles, reports, books, and other publications.

Stephen Bezruchka, MD, was raised in Toronto, received his BSc in mathematics and physics from the University of Toronto and a master's degree in mathematics from Harvard University before completing medical school at Stanford University, and a master's in public health degree from Johns Hopkins University. He is an emergency physician and teaches in the School of Public Health and Community Medicine at the University of Washington. He directs the Population Health Forum.

Carme Borrell, MD, PhD, is head of the Health Information Service, Barcelona Public Health Agency, Catalonia, Spain.

Ivy Lynn Bourgeault, PhD, is an associate professor in health studies and sociology at McMaster University and a Canada research chair in comparative health labour policy.

Toba Bryant, PhD, is a post-doctoral fellow at the Centre for Research on Inner City Health at St. Michael's Hospital in Toronto and an associate of the Centre for Urban and Community Studies at the University of Toronto. She has published numerous book chapters and articles on policy change, housing, and health within a population health perspective, and women's health and quality of life. Dr. Bryant has served as a consultant to Health Canada and the Wellesley Central Health Corporation on urban health issues.

Haejoo Chung, MPH, is a doctoral student at the Johns Hopkins Bloomberg School of Public Health, and conducts research on the political and welfare state determinants of population health, in particular among middle-income countries.

David Coburn, PhD, is a sociologist with interests in the political economy of health and health care. He has carried out research and written on the health professions and on health and income inequalities within and among nations.

Tamara Daly, PhD, is a CHSRF / CIHR post-doctoral award fellow at York's Institute for Health Research. She has a doctorate in health policy from the University of Toronto and a master's degree in political economy from Carleton University. Research interests include health services research, community support services, comparative health policy, and gender and health.

Georgina Feldberg, PhD, is an associate professor of social science at York University, and served as director of the Centre for Health Studies and coordinator of the Health and Society Programme. She writes and teaches on the historical foundations of health care and health policy. The Royal Society of Canada awarded her book *Disease and Class* the Hannah Medal.

Selahadin Ibrahim, MSc, is a statistician with the Institute of Work and Health in Toronto. His research has focused on mental health, social inequalities, and working conditions.

Anton Kunst, PhD, is a social epidemiologist working at Erasmus University. He is the author of numerous studies on social inequalities in health in Europe, and is currently a leading investigator in the Erothyne Project.

Joel Lexchin, MD, graduated from the University of Toronto. He currently teaches health policy at York University and works as an emergency physician in Toronto.

Carles Muntaner, MD, PhD, is a social epidemiologist with the Centre for Addictions and Mental Health, the University of Toronto, and the Institute for Work and Health, all in Toronto. He has conducted public health research and practice in deprived communities in the U.S. (Appalachia, Baltimore), the European Union, Latin America, and western Africa (Mali). At the international level he is involved in the creation of a primary health care system for the poor in Venezuela, affecting 17 million people without access to health care. He conducts research and collaborates with public health investigators and practitioners in Canada, Spain, Sweden, Mali, Mexico, and Chile, and with labour unions in the U.S., Sweden, and Spain.

Ann Pederson, MSc, is the manager of research and policy at the British Columbia Centre of Excellence for Women's Health. She studied public health at the University of Toronto and has worked in the field of health promotion and women's health for 20 years. She participates in a national research group examining the impact of health care reform on women in Canada and is working on studies of what quality health care means to women and how communities are responding to deinstitutionalization in a context of regionalization.

Dennis Raphael, PhD, is an associate professor at the School of Health Policy and Management at York University in Toronto. He is the editor of *Social Determinants of Health: Canadian Perspectives*, published by Canadian Scholars' Press.

Marcia Rioux, PhD (University of California, Berkeley, jurisprudence and social policy) is professor and chair, School of Health Policy and Management, York University, Canada; graduate program director, MA (critical disability studies), and director of the York Institute of Health Research. She has published widely in the area of disability and human rights. Her research interests include health equity, disability and discrimination, education for all, globalization, social welfare, and social justice. Dr. Rioux is internationally known, having taught, researched, and advised on policy issues in numerous countries, including the Americas, Europe, and India. She has been an adviser to federal and provincial commissions, parliamentary committees, international NGOs, and UN agencies. She is currently writing a book on law and disability and is engaged in a number of international research projects.

Robert Vipond, PhD, is professor of political science at the University of Toronto. He has published broadly on Canadian and American politics, especially the history of Canadian federalism.

Mary E. Wiktorowicz, PhD, is an associate professor at the School of Health Policy and Management, Atkinson Faculty of Liberal and Professional Studies, York University. She studies comparative health policy, including mental health sector restructuring, the regulation of pharmaceuticals, and the role of interest groups and social movements in shaping health policy.

INDEX

A

Aboriginal health
Aboriginal women, health of, 175
depression, and Aboriginal women, 167
mortality gap, 175
off-reserve Aboriginal peoples, 175, 176–177
smoking, 163
striking differences in health, 173
systematic reviews of, 174
Aboriginal Peoples Survey, 176–177
absolute poverty, 198
access to health care, 274, 293–298, 317–319
Access to Health Care Services in Canada, 170
Acheson Commission into Inequalities in Health, 356
Achieving Health for All (Govt. of Canada), 350
Action Statement on Health Promotion (CPHA), 350
active labour policy, 215
activities of public health units, 131
age, and disability, 314
age/sex-adjusted mortality rates, 76
age-specific mortality patterns, 150
age-standardized death rates, 147–149
agility limitations, 315–317
agriculture, and health, 26
AIDS, and the right to health, 100–101
allocation, 247
allopathic biomedicine, 224
alternative service delivery, 238
alternative social class measures, 151–152
American Medical Association, 245
American Public Health Association, 354–355

American Sociology Association, Medical Sociology Section, 56
America's Health: State Health Rankings (UHF), 355
Andrews v. Law Society, 317
anti-racism, 47–49, 57
appropriate health care, 293–298
Armstrong, Hugh, 43, 383
Armstrong, Pat, 43, 285, 287–299
Asylums (Goffman), 38–39
Australia, health care system in, 249
Australian Sociological Association, 56
autonomy of medical profession, 246–247
availability of health, 91

B

bacteriologic revolution, 225
Barcelona Health Interview Survey, 142, 143*t*
basic needs, 25–26
Baudrillard, Jean, 49
behavioural gradients, 44
behavioural risk factors, 174
Benach, Joan, 139–154, 383
Bezruchka, Stephen, 11–12, 13–28, 383
Bill C-212, 329
biographical disruption, 39
biomedical approach, 307
biomedical paradigm, 126
biotechnology, 88, 109
The Birth of the Clinic (Foucault), 49, 50
Bitter Medicine, 263
black lung disease, 43, 44–45
Black Report, 43, 356
Blue Cross, 227
Blumer, Herbert, 38
Borrell, Carme, 139–154, 383

387